Dr. Bernstein's
Diabetes Solution

A Complete Guide
to Achieving Normal Blood Sugars

ALSO BY RICHARD K. BERNSTEIN, M.D., F.A.C.E.

Diabetes Type II

*Diabetes: The Glucograf Method for
Normalizing Blood Sugar*

Dr. Bernstein's
Diabetes Solution

A Complete Guide
to Achieving Normal Blood Sugars

Richard K. Bernstein, M.D., F.A.C.E.

Foreword by Frank Vinicor, M.D., M.P.H.
Recipes by Timothy J. Aubert, C.W.C.

LITTLE, BROWN AND COMPANY

Boston   New York   Toronto   London

Theories, no matter how pertinent,

Cannot eradicate the existence of facts.

— *Jean Martin Charcot*

First Edition

Illustrations by Terry Eppridge

The author is grateful for permission to include the following previously copyrighted material:
Figure 1-3. Reproduced from the *Journal of Clinical Investigation*, 1967; 46:1549–1557. By permission of The American Society for Clinical Investigation.
Figure 9-1. Reproduced from *Journal of the American Dietetic Association*, 1995; 45:417–420. Copyright © by The American Dietetic Association. Reprinted by permission of The American Dietetic Association.
Figure 18-1. Reproduced from Humalog PI. Reprinted by permission of Eli Lilly and Company.

Library of Congress Cataloging-in-Publication Data

Bernstein, Richard K.
    Dr. Bernstein's diabetes solution : a complete guide to achieving normal blood sugars / Richard K. Bernstein.
        p.   cm.
    Includes index.
    ISBN 0-316-09344-0
    1. Diabetes — Popular works.   I. Title.
    RC660.4.B464   1997
    616.4'62 — dc21   96-37900

10 9 8 7 6 5 4 3

MV-NY

Published simultaneously in Canada by Little, Brown & Company (Canada) Limited
Printed in the United States of America

CONTENTS

PART TWO
Treatment

Appendices

FOREWORD

by
FRANK VINICOR, M.D., M.P.H.
Director, Division of Diabetes Translation
National Center for Chronic Disease Prevention and Health Promotion
Centers for Disease Control and Prevention
Atlanta, Georgia

We have entered an important and exciting time in diabetes research and treatment. Scientific investigations have now provided us not only with a better understanding of the basic mechanisms of both Type I and Type II diabetes and their associated devastating complications, but also *clear evidence that these complications can be minimized or prevented by normal or near normal blood sugars.*

Studies such as the Diabetes Control and Complications Trial (DCCT) have shown that the severity of diabetic complications can be reduced dramatically. But still there is a substantial gap between the success of the conventional treatment programs being utilized in daily clinical practice and what we know could actually be achieved if only the improved prevention and treatment protocols now available were more widely applied.

This book is an important step in informing the public that we can improve both the quality of care and the quality of life for those afflicted with diabetes, as well as reduce the cost of this disease for our nation. And we can do it now.

Dr. Richard Bernstein has both studied and lived diabetes. As a Type I diabetic and a diabetologist, he has devoted his professional life to helping other people with diabetes secure the opportunities to lead full and rewarding lives. His approaches are innovative, clear, supportive, and successful.

Of the many realities about diabetes care that are now being accepted and acted upon, few are more important than the value of prevention.

Research has shown that by regulation of blood glucose — the corner-stone of Dr. Bernstein's philosophy — we can dramatically decrease the likelihood of serious diabetic complications such as eye, kidney, or nerve problems. Perhaps equally important is the central role of the patient in making judgments about treatment goals, implementation strategies, and necessary daily decisions. The involvement of the person living with diabetes on a moment-to-moment basis is without question the most important issue for health care professionals to accept in diabetes management. Associated with this reality, however, lies our responsibility in the health care profession to provide the individual with the necessary knowledge to make the best decisions under stressful conditions.

There are many ways to involve, inform, and empower people with diabetes, and each of them must be implemented if the individual and societal devastation of diabetes are to be reduced. The challenge to health care providers is formidable. We now have convincing evidence that improved blood sugar control will substantially decrease the likelihood of the development of potential complications of diabetes — blindness, amputations, and kidney failure. Further, this evidence is pertinent to both Type I and Type II diabetes. If in Type II diabetes we cannot normalize blood sugar with diet and appropriate physical activity, a variety of insulins and oral hypoglycemic agents can now be used to bring blood sugar down to normal in an effective and safe manner. There is also convincing evidence that in addition to blood sugar control, if diabetic complications are identified early through screening, preventive treatment interventions can reduce their effects.

The diabetes research agenda remains full, with exciting possibilities in the near future for prevention of Type I and Type II diabetes; islet-cell replacement; genetic approaches to predict and treat diabetes; noninvasive glucose monitoring; better medications; and many other breakthroughs that will soon bring further hope to persons with, or at risk for, diabetes.

Because of the burden of diabetes, especially the cost; because of the advancement in both basic and applied science and knowledge about this disease; because we are learning how to implement preventive treatment strategies to stop the devastation; and because we are finally accepting the central role of the person with diabetes in making daily decisions — we will be entering the next century a mere seventy-five years after the discovery of insulin, with more understanding and hope to ensure better lives for those who at present, and in the future, will be challenged by this vexing condition.

Dr. Bernstein himself is living proof that much can be done that was virtually unheard of in the past. The information and encouragement contained in Dr. Bernstein's book will give readers the knowledge and confidence to really make a difference in the management and control of their own diabetes.

PREFACE

n 1946 I developed diabetes. According to current statistics, I should have been dead years ago, but today I'm in excellent health, routinely work twelve or more hours a day, and have outlived all but a handful of people who developed diabetes when I did.

Twenty-seven years ago, I had already suffered many of the disorders long associated with diabetes, and even my doctor, who was president of the American Diabetes Association, could do nothing to slow their advance. Today the progression of those complications has long been stopped, and some of them have reversed. I'm healthier now than I was then. I still have diabetes. My body still makes no insulin, and I have to have injections every day. How am I different from all those who have died, and all those whose bodies are disintegrating because of chronically high blood sugars? I haven't had any sort of transplant. I haven't had any miracle drug.

Recent research has repeatedly demonstrated what I learned serendipitously more than a quarter-century ago — that the grave long-term consequences of the nation's third leading cause of death can be prevented and even reversed if caught in time. How? By keeping blood sugars normal around the clock.

Despite this knowledge, the procedures for attaining blood sugar normalization are only practiced at a few research centers and by a handful of enlightened physicians.

This book is designed as a tool for patients, to be used under the guidance of their physicians or diabetes educators. It details not only my conquest of diabetes, but covers in a step-by-step fashion virtually everything that must be done to keep blood sugar in the normal range. It builds upon my previous books, *Diabetes Type II* and *Diabetes: The Glucograf Method for Normalizing Blood Sugar.*

This new work attempts to present nearly everything I know about blood sugar normalization, how it can be accomplished and maintained. With it, and with the help of your physician or diabetes educator, I hope that you will learn to take control of your diabetes, whether it's Type I (juvenile-onset), as mine is, or the much more common Type II (maturity-onset) diabetes. To my knowledge, there is no other book in print addressed strictly to blood sugar control for both types of diabetes. This volume updates my earlier books, discussing very new medications, improved techniques, and new tools that were not available when the earlier works were written.

It also contains much material that may be new to many physicians treating diabetes. It is my hope that other doctors and health care professionals will use it, learn from it, and do their best to help their patients take control of this deadly but controllable disease.

This book, though it contains considerable background information on diet and nutrition, is intended primarily as a comprehensive how-to guide to blood sugar control, including detailed instructions on techniques for painless insulin injection and so on. It must, therefore, leave out other related issues, some of which require their own volumes. My office telephone number is listed several times in this book, and we are always happy to hear from readers and patients, so feel free to call if you'd like our latest recommendation for, say, a blood sugar meter or a medication, or would like to pass along a recipe.

If, with your physician's help, you seriously follow the guidelines taught in this book, you should be able to avoid the discomfort of inappropriate blood sugar swings, and perhaps be able to prevent or reverse the development of the grave complications long associated with chronically high blood sugars.

ACKNOWLEDGMENTS

I would like to thank the following people, whose aid and guidance made this book possible:

Frank Vinicor, M.D., M.P.H., past president of the American Diabetes Association, who took time from his overwhelming schedule to write the foreword.

Stephen Stark, novelist, critic, and essayist, whose suggestions about tone, clarity, and structure were of immeasurable value.

Doctors of pharmacology Michael D. Johnson, Stephen M. Setter, and John R. White, Jr., all of Washington State University, who wrote the important appendix "Drugs That May Affect Blood Glucose Levels." Patricia A. Gian, dear friend and director of my medical office, who shared the stresses of this endeavor and gave me invaluable aid and guidance all along the way. Two top-of-the-line professionals, Jennifer Josephy, my editor, and Channa Taub, my literary agent, whose efforts made this undertaking possible. Peggy Leith Anderson, copyeditor nonpareil. Abigail Wilentz, who was always on the spot when help was needed. Amy and Hank Kornfeld and Elise Bahar for their recipes. My beloved teacher and friend, Professor Emeritus Heinz I. Lippmann, M.D., who taught me everything I know about the diabetic foot.

Finally, my love and thanks to my wife, Professor Anne E. Bernstein, M.D., F.A.P.A., who allowed me to steal so much time that really belonged to her.

My First Fifty Years as a Diabetic

There are a number of myths surrounding diet and diabetes, and much of what is still considered sensible nutritional advice for diabetics can over the long run be fatal. I know, because it almost killed me. I developed diabetes in 1946 at the age of twelve, and for more than two decades I was an "ordinary" diabetic, dutifully following doctor's orders and leading the most normal life I could, given the limitations of my disease.

Over the years, the complications from my diabetes became worse and worse, and like many diabetics in similar circumstances, I faced a very early death. I was still alive, but the *quality* of my life wasn't particularly good. I have what is known as Type I, or insulin-dependent, diabetes, which usually begins in childhood (it's also called juvenile-onset diabetes). Type I diabetics must take daily insulin injections just to stay alive.

Back in the 1940s, which were very much still the "dark ages" of diabetes treatment, I had to sterilize my needles and glass syringes by boiling them every day, and use a test tube to test my urine for sugar. Many of the tools the diabetic can take for granted today were scarcely dreamed of back then — there was no such thing as a rapid, finger-stick blood sugar–measuring device, nor disposable insulin syringes. Still, even today, parents of Type I diabetics have to live with the same fear my parents lived with — any morning they could try to wake up their child and discover him dead. For any parent of a Type I diabetic, this is a real and constant possibility.

Because of my chronically elevated blood sugar levels, and the inability to control them, my growth was stunted, as it is for many juvenile-onset diabetics, even to this day.

Back then, the medical community had just learned about the relationship between high blood cholesterol and vascular (blood vessel and heart) disease. It was then widely believed that the cause of high blood cholesterol was consumption of large amounts of fat. Since many diabetics, even children, have high cholesterol levels, physicians were beginning to assume that the vascular complications of diabetes — heart disease, kidney failure, blindness, et cetera — were caused by the fat that diabetics were eating. As a result, I was put on a low-fat, high-carbohydrate diet (45 percent of calories were to be carbohydrates) before such diets were advocated by the American Diabetes Association or the American Heart Association. Because carbohydrate raises blood sugar, I had to compensate with very large doses of insulin, which I injected with a 10 cc "horse" syringe. These injections were slow and painful, and eventually they destroyed all the fatty tissue under the skin of my thighs. In spite of the low-fat diet, my blood cholesterol remained very high. I developed visible signs of this state — fatty growths on my eyelids and gray deposits around the iris of each eye.

During my twenties and thirties, the prime of life for most people, many of my body's systems began to deteriorate. I had excruciatingly painful kidney stones, a stone in a salivary duct, "frozen" shoulders, a progressive deformity of my feet with impaired sensation, and more. I would point these out to my diabetologist, but I was usually told, "Don't worry, it has nothing to do with your diabetes. You're doing fine." But I wasn't doing fine. I now know that most of these problems are commonplace among those whose diabetes is poorly controlled, but then I was forced to accept my condition as "normal."

By this time I was married. I had gone to college and trained as an engineer. I had small children, and even though I was not much more than a kid myself, I felt like an old man. I had lost the hair on the lower parts of my legs, a sign that I had developed peripheral vascular disease — a complication of diabetes that can eventually lead to amputation. During a routine exercise stress test, I was diagnosed with cardiomyopathy, which is a replacement of muscle tissue in the heart with fibrous (scar) tissue — a common cause of heart failure and death among those with Type I diabetes.

Just as the disease had taken its toll on my parents, it also took its toll on my wife and children. Even though I was "doing fine," I suffered a host of other complications. My vision deteriorated; I suffered night blindness, microaneurysms (ballooning of the blood vessels in my eyes), macular edema (swelling of the central portion of my retinas), and early cataracts. Just lying in bed caused pain in my thighs, due to a common but unpronounceable diabetic complication called ilio-tibial band/tensor fascia lata syndrome. Putting on a T-shirt was agonizing because of my frozen shoulders.

I had begun testing my urine for protein and found substantial amounts of it, a sign, I had read, of advanced kidney disease. In those days — the middle and late 1960s — the life expectancy of a Type I diabetic with proteinuria was five years. Back in engineering school, a classmate had told me how his nondiabetic sister had died of kidney disease. Before her death she had ballooned with retained water, and after I discovered my own proteinuria, I began to have nightmares of blowing up like a balloon.

By 1967 I had these and other diabetic complications and clearly appeared chronically ill and prematurely aged. I had three small children, the oldest only six years old, and with good reason was certain I wouldn't live to see them grown.

At my father's suggestion, I started working out daily at a local gym. He thought that if I were to engage in vigorous exercise, I might feel better. Perhaps exercise would help my body help itself. While I did feel slightly less depressed about my condition — at least I felt I was doing something — I couldn't build muscles or get much stronger.

After two years of pumping iron, I remained a 115-pound weakling, no matter how strenuously I worked out. It was at about this time, in 1969, that my wife, a physician, pointed out to me that I had spent much of my life going into, experiencing, or recovering from hypoglycemia, which is a state of excessively low blood sugar. It was usually accompanied by fatigue and headaches. During these episodes, I became confused and unruly and snapped at people. The strain on my family was clearly becoming untenable.

Suddenly, in October of 1969, my life turned around.

I had been the research director of a company that made equipment for hospital laboratories, but recently I had taken a new job as an officer of a housewares corporation. I was still receiving trade journals from my old field, and one day I opened the latest issue of a publication called

Lab World. I came upon an advertisement for a new device to help hospital emergency rooms distinguish between unconscious diabetics and unconscious drunks at night when laboratories were closed. Knowing that an unconscious person was a diabetic and not drunk could easily help hospital personnel save his life. What I stumbled upon was an ad for a blood sugar meter that would give a reading in 1 minute, using a single drop of blood.

Since I'd been experiencing low blood sugars, and since the tests I had been performing on my urine were wholly inadequate (sugar that showed up in the urine was already on its way out of the bloodstream), I figured that if I knew what my blood sugar levels were, perhaps I could catch and correct my hypoglycemic episodes before they made me disoriented and irrational.

I marveled over the instrument. It had a 4-inch galvanometer with a jeweled bearing, weighed 3 pounds, and cost $650, which in those days could have been a month's salary. I tried to order one, but the manufacturer wouldn't sell it to patients — only to doctors and hospitals.

Fortunately, my wife, as I've said, was a physician, so I ordered one in her name. I started to measure my blood sugar about 5 times each day, and soon saw that the levels were on a roller coaster. Engineers are accustomed to solving problems mathematically, but you have to have information to work with. You have to know the mechanics of a problem in order to solve it, and now, for the first time, I was gaining insight into the mechanics and mathematics of my disease. What I learned in my frequent testing was that my own blood sugar levels swung from lows of under 40 mg/dl to highs of over 400 mg/dl about twice daily. A normal blood sugar level is about 85 mg/dl.* Small wonder I was subject to such vast mood swings.

In an effort to balance my blood sugar levels, I began to adjust my insulin regimen, and went from one to two injections a day. I made some experimental modifications to my diet, cutting down on the carbohy-

---

* Although most medical journals and textbooks throughout the world measure blood glucose in mmol/l (millimoles per liter), most physicians, laboratories, and blood glucose meters in the United States measure blood glucose in mg/dl (milligrams per deciliter). Since you will be monitoring your own blood sugar levels with one of these blood glucose meters, blood glucose values in this book will as a rule be given in mg/dl. If you should need to translate from one to the other, 1 mmol/l = 18 mg/dl.

drates to permit me to take less insulin. The very high and low blood sugar levels became less frequent, but few were normal.

Three years after I started measuring my blood sugar levels, my diabetic complications were still progressing, and I was still a 115-pound weakling. My sense of gaining insight into the workings of my diabetes had diminished, and so I ordered a computer search of the scientific literature to see if exercise could prevent diabetic complications. In those days, computer searches were not the simple, almost instant searches they are today. In 1972 you made your request to the local medical library, which mailed it to Washington, D.C., where it was processed. It took about two weeks for my $75 printout to arrive.

There were quite a few entries of interest, and I ordered copies of the original articles. For the most part these were from esoteric journals and dealt with animal experiments. The information I had hoped to find didn't exist. I didn't find a single article pertaining to the prevention of diabetic complications by exercise in humans.

What I did find was that such complications had repeatedly been prevented, *and even reversed,* in animals. Not through exercise, *but by normalizing blood sugars!* To me, this was a total surprise. All of diabetes treatment was heavily focused in other directions, such as low-fat diets, preventing severe hypoglycemia, and preventing a potentially fatal extreme high blood sugar condition called ketoacidosis. Thus it had not occurred to me that keeping blood sugar levels as close to normal as possible for as much of the time as possible would make a difference.

Excited by my discovery, I showed these reports to my physician, who was not impressed. "Animals aren't humans," he said, "and besides, it's impossible to normalize human blood sugars." Since I had been trained as an engineer, not as a physician, I knew nothing of such impossibilities, and since I was desperate, I had no choice but to pretend I was an animal.

I spent the next year checking my blood sugars 5–8 times each day. Every few days, I'd make a small, experimental change in my diet or insulin regimen to see what the effect would be on my blood sugar. If a change brought an improvement, I'd retain it. If it made the blood sugar worse, I'd discard it. I discovered that 1 gram of carbohydrate raised my blood sugar by 5 mg/dl, and ½ unit of the old beef/pork insulin lowered it by 15 mg/dl.

Within a year, I had refined my insulin and diet regimen to the point that I had essentially normal blood sugars around the clock. After years of chronic fatigue and debilitating complications, almost overnight I was no longer continually tired or "washed out." After years of sky-high readings, my serum cholesterol and triglyceride levels had now not only dropped, but were at the low end of the normal ranges.

I started to gain weight, and at last I was able to build muscle as readily as nondiabetics. My insulin requirements dropped by about two-thirds of what they had been a year earlier. With the subsequent development of human insulin, my dosage dropped to one-fifth of the original. The painful, slow-healing lumps the injections of large doses of insulin left under my skin disappeared. The fatty growths on my eyelids vanished. My digestive problems (chronic burning in my chest and belching after meals) and the proteinuria that had so worried me eventually vanished. Today, my results from even the most sensitive kidney function tests are all normal. My deformed feet, the calcified walls of arteries in my legs, and the cystoid macular edema of my eyes are not reversible and still remain.

I had the new sensation of being the boss of my own metabolic state, and began to feel the same sense of accomplishment and reward I had in engineering when I solved a difficult problem. I had taught myself how to make my blood sugar levels whatever I wanted them to be and was no longer on the roller coaster. Things were under *my control.*

Back in 1973, I felt quite exhilarated with my success, and I felt that I was on to something big. Since getting the results of my computer search, I had been a subscriber to all of the English-language diabetes journals, and none of them had mentioned the need for normalizing blood sugars in humans.

In fact, every few months I'd read another article saying that blood sugar normalization wasn't even remotely possible. How was it that I, an engineer, had figured out how to do what was impossible for medical professionals? I was deeply grateful for the fortuitous combination of events that had turned my life, my health, and my family around and put me on the right path. At the very least, I felt, I was obliged to share my newfound knowledge with others. There were no doubt millions of "ordinary" diabetics like me suffering needlessly. I was sure that all physicians treating diabetes would be thrilled to learn how to prevent and possibly reverse the grave complications of this disease.

I hoped that if I could tell the world about the techniques I had stumbled upon, physicians would adopt them for their patients. So I wrote an article detailing my discoveries. I sent a copy to Charles Suther, who was then in charge of marketing diabetes products for Ames Division of Miles Laboratories, the company that made my blood glucose meter. He gave me the only encouragement I received in this new venture, and arranged for one of his company's medical writers to edit the article for me.

I submitted it and its revisions to many medical journals over a period of years — a period during which I was continually improving in health, and continually proving to myself and my family, if to no one else, that my methods were correct. The rejection letters I received are testimony that people tend to ignore the obvious if it conflicts with the orthodoxy of their early training. Typical rejection letters read in part: "Studies are not unanimous in demonstrating a need for 'fine control'" (the *New England Journal of Medicine*), or "How many patients would use the electric device for measurement of glucose, insulin, urine, etc.?" (*Journal of the American Medical Association*). As a matter of fact, since 1980, when these "electric devices" finally were made available to patients, the worldwide market for blood glucose self-monitoring supplies has come to exceed $3 billion annually. Look at the array of blood glucose meters in any pharmacy, and you can get an idea of just how many patients use, and will use, the "electric device."

Trying to cover several routes simultaneously, I joined a few lay diabetes organizations, in the hope of moving up through the ranks, where I could meet physicians and researchers specializing in the disease. This met with mediocre success. I attended conventions, worked on committees, and met many diabetologists. In this country, I met only *three* physicians who were willing to offer their patients the opportunity to put these new methods to the test.

Meanwhile, Charlie Suther was traveling around the country to university research centers with copies of my unpublished article, which by now had been typeset and privately printed at my expense. The rejection by doctors of the concept of blood sugar self-monitoring, even though essential to blood sugar control, was so intense, however, that the management of his company had to turn down the idea of making meters available to patients until many years later. His company and others could clearly have profited from the sale of blood glucose meters and test strips. However, the backlash from the medical establishment prevented it on a number of counts. It was unthinkable that patients be allowed to "doctor" themselves. They knew nothing of medicine — and if they could, how would doctors earn a living? In those days, patients visited their doctors once a month to "get a blood sugar." If they could do it at home for 25 cents (in those days), why pay a physician? But almost no one believed there was any value to normal blood sugars anyway. In some respects, blood glucose self-monitoring remains a serious threat to the incomes of many physicians who specialize in the treatment of the *symptoms* of diabetes and not the disease. Drop into your neighborhood ophthalmologist's office and you will find the waiting room three-quarters filled with diabetics, many of whom are waiting for expensive fluorescein angiography or laser treatment.

With Suther's backing in the form of free supplies, by 1977 I was able to get the first of two university-sponsored studies started in the New York City area. These both succeeded in reversing early complications in diabetic patients. As a result of our successes, the two universities separately sponsored the world's first two symposia on blood glucose self-monitoring. By this time I was being invited to speak at international diabetes conferences, but rarely at meetings in the United States. Curiously, more physicians *outside* the United States seemed interested in controlling blood sugar than did their American colleagues. Some of the earliest converts to blood glucose self-monitoring were from Israel and England.

By 1978, perhaps as a result of Charlie Suther's efforts, a few additional American investigators were trying our regimen or variations of it. Finally, in 1980, manufacturers began to release blood glucose meters for use by patients.

This "progress" was entirely too slow for my liking. I knew that while the medical establishment was dallying there were diabetics dying whose lives could have been saved. I knew also that there were millions of diabetics whose quality of life could be vastly improved, so in 1977, I decided to give up my job and become a physician — I couldn't beat 'em, so I had to join 'em. This way, with an M.D. after my name, my writings might be published, and I could pass on what I had learned about controlling blood sugar.

After a year of premed courses and another year of waiting, I entered the Albert Einstein College of Medicine in 1979. I was forty-five years old. During my first year of medical school I wrote my first book, *Dia-*

betes: The Glucograf Method for Normalizing Blood Sugar, enumerating the full details of my treatment for Type I, or insulin-dependent, diabetes.

In 1983 I finally opened my own medical practice. By that time, I had well outlived the life expectancy of an "ordinary" Type I diabetic. Now, by sharing my simple observations, I was convinced I was in a position to help both Type I and Type II diabetics who still had the best years of their lives ahead of them. I could help others take control of their diabetes as I had mine, and live long, healthy, fruitful lives.

The goal of this new book is to share the techniques and treatments I have taught my patients and used on myself, including the very latest developments. If you or a loved one suffers from diabetes, I hope this book will give you the tools to turn your life around as I did mine.

Dr. Bernstein's
Diabetes Solution

A Complete Guide
to Achieving Normal Blood Sugars

Before and After: Fourteen Patients Share Their Experiences

You're the only person who can be responsible for normalizing your blood sugars. Although your physician may guide you, the ultimate responsibility is in your hands. This task will require significant changes in lifestyle that may involve some sacrifice. The question naturally arises, "Is it really worth the effort?" As you will see in this chapter, others have already answered this question for themselves. Perhaps their experiences will give you the incentive to find out whether you can reap similar benefits.

Thomas G. Watkins is a forty-year-old journalist. His diabetes was diagnosed twenty-three years ago. For the past nine years he's been following one of the treatment protocols described in this book for people who require insulin.

"Following the instructions of several diabetologists over a period of years, I had the illness 'under control.' At least that's what they told me. After all, I was taking two shots a day, and adjusting my insulin doses depending on urine test results, and later on blood sugar measurements. I was also following the common recommendation that carbohydrates fill at least 60 percent of my caloric intake.

"But something was not right; my life was not 'relatively normal' enough. I was avoiding heavy exercise for fear of my blood sugar dropping too low. My meal schedule was inflexible. I still had to eat breakfast, lunch, and dinner even when I wasn't hungry. Aware that recent research seemed to associate high blood sugars with an increased risk of long-term complications, I tried to keep blood sugars normal, but wound up seesawing daily between lows and highs. By the end of 1986, I had ballooned to 189 pounds and was at a loss for how to lose weight. My 'good control' regimen had left me feeling *out* of control. Clearly, something had to be done.

"In that year, I attended a meeting of medical writers at which Dr. Bernstein spoke. It became clear that his credentials were impressive. He himself at that time had lived with the disease for four decades and was nearly free of complications. His approach had been formulated largely through self-experimentation. His knowledge of the medical literature was encyclopedic. Some of his proposals were heretical; he attacked the usual dietary recommendation and challenged dogma surrounding such basics as how insulin ought to be injected. But it seemed like he was doing something right. During his talk, I had to use the bathroom twice; he didn't.

"I decided to spend a day at his office to gather material for an article to be published in the *Medical Tribune*. There, his independence of thought became clear. 'Brittle' diabetes [entailing an endless sequence of wide blood sugar fluctuations] was a misnomer that usually indicated an inadequate treatment plan or poor training, more than any inherent physical deficit, he said. Normal blood sugars round-the-clock were not just an elusive goal, but were frequently achievable, if the diabetic had been taught the proper techniques. Beyond treatment goals, he armed his patients with straightforward methods to attain them. His secret: small doses of medication resulted in small mistakes that were easily correctable.

"By then, my interest had become more personal than journalistic. In early 1987, still wary, I decided to give it a try. The first thing I noticed was that this doctor visit was unlike any previous ones. Most had lasted about 15 minutes. This took 8 hours. Others said I had no complications; Dr. Bernstein found several. Most said my blood sugars were just fine; Dr. Bernstein recommended I make changes to flatten them out and to lower my weight. Those hours were spent detailing the intricacies involved in controlling blood sugar. His whole approach blasted the theory espoused by my first doctor — that I should depend on him to dole out whatever information I needed. Dr. Bernstein made it clear that for diabetics to control their disease they needed to know as much as their doctors did about the disease.

"Two arguments commonly rendered against tight-control regimens are that they increase the incidence of low blood sugar reactions and that they cause subjects to gain weight. I have found the opposite to be true: I shed about 9 pounds within four months after my first visit, and, years later, I have kept them off. And, once the guesswork of how much to inject was replaced by simple calculations, my blood sugar levels became more predictable.

"For the first time since I was diagnosed, I felt truly in control. I no longer am at the mercy of wide mood swings that mirror wide swings in blood sugar. Though I remain dependent on insulin and all the paraphernalia that accompany its use, I feel more independent than ever. I am comfortable traveling to isolated areas of the world, spending an hour scuba diving, or hiking in the wilderness, without fear of being sidetracked by diabetes. Now, if I feel like skipping breakfast, or lunch, or dinner, I do so without hesitation.

"I no longer have delayed stomach-emptying, which can cause very low blood sugars right after a meal followed by high blood sugars many hours later. My cardiac neuropathy, which is associated with an increased risk for early death, has reversed. Though I eat more fat and protein than before, my blood lipids have improved and are now well within normal ranges. My glycosylated hemoglobin measurements, used by life insurance companies to detect diabetics among applicants, would no longer give me away. Most important, I now feel well.

"Many doctors will not embrace Dr. Bernstein's work, for the simple reason that Dr. Bernstein demands a commitment of time, energy, and knowledge not only from patients, but from physicians. Diabetics are the bread and butter of many practices. For decades, the usual treatment scenario has been a blood test, a short interview, a prescription for a one-month supply of needles, a handshake, and a bill. But that is changing. In the past few years, evidence has been amassing in support of Dr. Bernstein's modus operandi. No longer is the old high-carbohydrate diet unquestioned; more and more doctors are espousing a multiple-shot regimen controlled by the patients themselves. Most important, though, tight control is being associated with fewer of the diabetic complications that can ravage every major organ system in the body. Dr. Bernstein's scheme provided me with the tools not only to obtain normal blood sugars, but to regain a feeling of control I had not had since before I was diagnosed."

Frank Purcell is a seventy-six-year-old retiree who, like many of my mar-
ried patients, works closely with his wife to keep his diabetes on track.
Eileen, who goes by the nickname Ike, tells the first part of his story.

IKE: "Frank had been treated for many years for diabetes, and had
been treated orally because he was a Type II. As far as we were aware, he
had a functioning pancreas. The thing was, as a younger man, he'd been
told that he had high blood sugar, but it was ignored. This was going
back to his army days, in 1953 or so. No one suggested medication, no
one called it diabetes, and nothing more was done. They just said he had
high blood sugar. They called it 'chemical' diabetes. It showed up on
blood tests, but not on urinalysis. I guess in those days, having it show
up on a urinalysis was some sort of determinant. He did modify his
diet — he stopped eating so much candy, and he took off weight — he
lost about 30 pounds in those days.

"In about 1983, Frank had a mild heart attack. He began to see a cardiologist, who has been monitoring his health care very carefully since
then. For about two to three years, he took beta blockers and maybe one
or two heart medications. As far as we could tell, his heart problems
were very much in resolution — I mean he'd had a heart attack, he'd
had no surgery, and seemed to be doing okay. But when he started working with the cardiologist, the doctor noted that his blood sugar thing
was ongoing, and he began to feel it was of concern. He prescribed Diabinese, which was the oral medication of choice of the time, I guess, and
he monitored Frank's blood sugar about every four months.

"I might say that I never even *knew* what a normal blood sugar was.
No one *ever* talked about it. I had no idea whether it was 1,000 or 12.
The only thing we were ever told was that it was high or wasn't high.
This went on and on for close to seven or eight years. If he had seen Dr.
Bernstein back then, who knows what could have been different? But
eventually, the cardiologist said he thought Frank ought to see an endocrinologist. He didn't feel he was able to control Frank's blood sugar
well enough himself with medication, and so he felt the condition warranted closer attention.

"We went to see a gentleman who was chief of the diabetes clinic at a
major hospital here in upstate New York, where we live. Now, this is a
very well thought of medical facility. The doctor met with us, and he
kept Frank on the Diabinese, and monitored him every three months or
so. His blood sugars were 253, 240, and he would say, 'Let's try another

pill.' It was always medication. Glyburide, Glucophage — the whole bit. But trying to get his blood sugar down was very difficult. No one ever mentioned diet, really. And rarely was it ever below 200 when we went in. *Rarely.* When I finally found out what the numbers meant, I said to the doctor, 'Don't you think we ought to see a dietitian? I mean, we're eating the same food we always have.' We were on the normal diet that anybody's on. I had friends who are diabetics who watch certain things that they eat, and so I thought it made a certain amount of sense. He said, 'Sure. That's a really good idea.'

"He gave us the name of a young woman, and we saw her three times. She said, 'Eat eleven carbohydrates everyday,' and she gave us the food pyramid — we didn't need *her* for that — and nothing changed, except Frank stopped eating dessert. He would have the occasional bowl of ice cream, or a piece of cake when he felt like it, or a cookie. I always bought the newest foods that came out — low-fat, low-sugar. I was more concerned about fat during that stage, as I recall.

"This went on until God intervened. I mean that. What happened was, Frank had an attack of serious hypoglycemia. No one had warned us that this could happen. No one had told us what hypoglycemia looked like. I thought it was a stroke. He was out of his head. He couldn't answer questions. The only thing that gave me some smidgen of doubt was that he got up and walked to the bathroom and put on his trousers. I called 911. When the medic got here, he hooked him up to some glucose, put him on a gurney and trundled him out of here, and headed for the medical center. In the middle of the ride, Frank woke up and said, 'What the hell am I doing here?' The young man said he certainly seemed to be coming out of his stroke well. By the time we got to the hospital, he was virtually himself. When they decided to do a finger stick, his blood sugar was 26, 26 mg/dl. I didn't have the education in diabetes that I've gotten with Dr. Bernstein, but I knew enough to know that this was not good. Who knows what it was before he got the intravenous?

"Now, we'll never know if he accidentally took his medication twice the night before — it's very possible — but I tell you, however it happened, it was the Lord who was watching over Frank and said, 'Now it's time to do something.' As scary as it was, it was also a blessing.

"I have a doctor friend who's a close colleague of Dick Bernstein's. My friend had had an uncle who'd been very ill with diabetes and its complications, but his life had been prolonged in a much more comfortable fashion by Dick Bernstein. I would talk to my friend about Frank's diabetes, and he'd say to me, 'Nothing's really going to change. You're not going to get his blood sugars down until you see Dick Bernstein.' Even though my friend is a doctor, I brushed off his advice. Frank was seeing a doctor. Why would some private doctor be any more capable than the head of the diabetes clinic at a major medical center? But after this episode with hypoglycemia, Frank went to my friend's office with me, and my friend laid it out for him, told us in grinding detail what we could expect from Dr. Bernstein, what it would be like, and how he hoped we would relate to Dick, because he's rather controversial, and how hard it was going to be — how much of a commitment it was going to take. We went away thinking, 'Let's give it a try.'"

FRANK: "To be honest, when I first met Dr. Bernstein, I felt he was somewhat of a flake. I had worked with doctors in the army, and I was used to a particular kind of guy. Dr. Bernstein — now, he's a horse of another color. Until I came across him, I never met a doctor who was so focused on one thing. He is so completely directed toward this one failing of the human body that I kind of thought that maybe it was a little too intense. But the results have been rather spectacular, and I'm very happy with him. He has specific programs, he has direction, he has goals, and he is not sidetracked by anything other than tending to diabetes. He's given me a regimen. I keep track of my blood sugar, and it's pretty much under control. Instead of blood sugar counts of over 200, I now get them in the range of 85 to 105, which was the goal he set for me. I take insulin in the morning and before midday and evening meals, and before I go to bed. I don't eat ice cream, and I don't do a lot of things I used to do routinely. When I first came to Dr. B., I was looking very pale and wan, and now I'm looking much ruddier and healthier. I'm a little irritated with this constant puncturing of my fingers, but I just do it automatically now, like second nature.

"When I found out I was going to have to inject insulin, I just broke down and cried. It was like the final straw, and I thought, 'My life is over.' Now I hardly think about it. I use Dr. Bernstein's painless injection method and it doesn't bother me at all. It only takes a split second. The needle is so tiny, I almost have no feeling at all. I use the 'love handles' on the sides of my waist. Now, I'm a pretty skinny guy, so there isn't much there, but I can hardly feel it. To do it properly, it took me about two weeks to learn. He made me do it in the office. He showed me — did it to himself — and then he made me do it. Since then, I just do it routinely, all on my own. If I'm out, I do it wherever I am — in a restaurant, in the men's room — I'm not the least bit ashamed and no one seems much to notice."

IKE: "About the insulin, I had the feeling that it was going to be inevitable, and when Frank got the news he just broke into tears and really felt that this was the final insult. He'd had many physical problems, and insulin seemed like a very low blow for him. But he did it, stayed with the program, and within a month to six weeks, we began to feel that we were on top of this, knew what was going on. He can manage his blood sugar when it's a little low, when it's a little high. He knows just what to do. His overall health has improved since the beginning. Dr. Bernstein really gave us an education."

Joan Delaney is a fifty-three-year-old mother and financial editor. Her story is not unusual.

"I must admit that the prospect of following this new regimen for diabetes control seemed daunting at first. My life, I thought, would be dominated by needles, testing, and confusion. However, after a few weeks, the program became a simple part of my day's routine, like putting on makeup.

"Before I became a patient of Dr. Bernstein, I was somewhat resigned to the probability of suffering complications from diabetes. Although I took insulin, I in no way felt I had control of the disease. I had leg pains at night. My hands and feet tingled. I had gained weight, having no understanding of the exchange diet my previous doctor had thrust into my hands. I became chronically depressed and was usually hungry.

"Now that I follow a blood sugar normalizing program I know I am in control of my diabetes, especially when I see that number normal most of the time on the glucose meter. Best of all, I feel good, both physically and emotionally. I am now thin. I eat healthful, satisfying meals and am never hungry. My leg pains have disappeared, as has the tingling in my hands and feet. And now that I am in control of the disease, I no longer find the need to hide from friends the fact that I have diabetes."

About half of all diabetic men are unable to have sexual intercourse, because high blood sugars have impaired the mechanisms involved in attaining erection of the penis. Frequently partial, albeit inadequate, erections are still possible; such "borderline" men may still be able to enjoy adequate erections for intercourse, after extended periods of normal blood sugars. We have seen such improvements in a number of patients — but only in those whose problem was caused mainly by neuropathy (nerve damage), as opposed to blockages of the blood vessels that supply the penis. When we initially saw L.D., he asked us to evaluate his erectile impotence. We found that the blood pressures in his penis and his feet were normal, but that the nerve reflexes in the pelvic region were grossly impaired. L.D.'s comments refer in part to this problem.

"I'm a fifty-nine-year-old male, married, with three children. Approximately four years ago, after being afflicted with Type II diabetes for about ten years, I noticed that I was always tired. In addition, I was quite irritable, short-tempered, and had difficulty maintaining concentration for extended periods of time. Otherwise I was feeling well, with the exception that I was becoming impotent, having difficulty maintaining an erection during sexual intercourse. At the time, I had no knowledge whether these conditions were interrelated.

"After Dr. Bernstein taught me to measure my blood sugars, I discovered that they averaged about 375 mg/dl, which is very high. With my new diet and small doses of insulin, they are now essentially normal all the time.

"I began to feel better than I had in years, both physically and mentally. The problem with impotency has improved. I maintain a daily check of my blood sugars and feel that my overall improvement has also helped me recuperate quickly from a total hip replacement without any complications."

R.J.N., M.D., is board certified in orthopedic surgery. He has been following one of the regimens described in this book for the past three years.

"I am fifty-four years old and have had diabetes since the age of twelve. For thirty-nine years I had been treated with a traditional diet and insulin regimen. I developed severe retinopathy, glaucoma, high blood pressure, and neuropathy that required me to wear a leg brace. Both of my kidneys ceased functioning, and I was placed on kidney dialysis for many months until I received a kidney transplant. The dialysis treatments required me to be in the hospital for about 5 hours per visit, 3 times a week. They were very debilitating and left me totally exhausted.

"Years of widely fluctuating blood sugars affected my mental and physical stability, with great injury to my family life as a result. The resultant disability also forced me to give up my surgical practice, and to suffer almost total loss of income.

"Frequent low blood sugars would cause me to exhibit bizarre behavior, so that people unaware of my diabetes would think I was taking drugs or alcohol. I was hostile, anxious, irritable, or angry, and had extreme mood changes. I would experience severe physical reactions that included fatigue, twitching of limbs, clouding of vision, headaches, and blunted mental activity. I suffered many convulsions from low blood sugars and was placed in hospital intensive care units. When my blood sugars were high, I had no energy and was always sleepy. My vision was blurred and I was usually thirsty and urinating a lot.

"For the past three years, I have been meticulously following the lessons that Dr. Bernstein taught me. I measure my blood sugars a number of times each day and know how to rapidly correct slight variations from my target range. I follow a very low carbohydrate diet, which makes blood sugar control much easier.

"In return for my conscientious attention to controlling blood sugars, I've reaped a number of rewards. My neuropathy is gone, and I no longer require a leg brace. My retinopathy, which was deteriorating, has now actually reversed. I no longer suffer from glaucoma, which had required that I use special eyedrops twice each day for more than ten years. My severe digestive problems have markedly improved. My mental confusion, depression, and fatigue have resolved so that I am now able to work full-time and productively. My blood sugar control has been excellent.

"I now deal with my diabetes in a realistic, organized manner, and as a result I feel stronger, healthier, happier, and more positive about my life."

J.L.F. is seventy-one years old and has three grandchildren. He still works as a financial consultant, and was a naval aviator in World War II. His blood sugars are currently controlled by diet, exercise, and pills called oral hypoglycemic agents. Thanks to the diet described in this book, his cholesterol/HDL ratio, an index of heart disease risk (see page 51), has dropped from a very high risk level of 7.9 to a below-average level of 3.0. His hemoglobin A_{1C} test, which reflects average blood sugar for the prior four *months, has dropped from 10.1 percent (very high) to 5.6 percent (nearly in the nondiabetic range). His R-R interval study (see Chapter 2), an indicator of injury to nerves that control heart rate, has progressed from an initial value of 9 percent variation (very abnormal) to a current value of 33 percent, which is normal for his age.*

"I probably had mild diabetes for most of my adult life without realizing it. It first appeared as lethargy, later as fainting, stumbling, or falling, but as rare occurrences. I also had difficulty attaining full erection of my penis.

"In early 1980, I began to experience dizziness, sweating, arm pains, tendencies to fainting, and the symptoms usually associated with heart problems. An angiogram revealed severe disease of the arteries that supplied my heart. I therefore had surgery to open up these arteries. All was well for the next seven years, and I again enjoyed good health.

"In late 1985, I began to notice a loss of feeling in my toes. My internist diagnosed it as neuropathy probably due to high blood sugar. He did the usual blood test, and my blood sugar was 400. His advice was to watch my diet, especially to avoid sweets. I returned for another checkup in 30 days. My blood sugar was 350. Meanwhile, my neuropathy was increasing, along with the frequency of visits. My blood test results were consistently at the 350 level, my feet were growing more numb, and I was becoming alarmed.

"I felt okay physically, walked at least two miles a day, worked out in the gym once or twice a week, worked a full schedule as a business consultant, and didn't worry a great deal about it. But I did begin to inquire of friends and acquaintances about any knowledge or experience they might have relative to neuropathy or diabetes.

"My first jolt came from a story from one of my friends who had diabetes, foot neuropathy, deep nerve pain in his feet, and a nonhealing ulcer on a toe. He told me that as the neuropathy progressed, amputation of the feet was likely, elaborating by describing the gruesome 'salami surgery' of unchecked diabetes.

"That's when I became emotionally unglued, as they say. One thing about aging and disease, you think a great deal about the utter horror of becoming a cripple, dependent upon others for your mobility. Suddenly foot numbness is no longer a casual matter, more like a head-on crash into reality.

"Then I met a wealthy car dealer at the golf club, with his legs cut off as high as legs go, who explained he hadn't paid too much attention to his diabetes at the time and his doctor couldn't help him. He could never leave his chair, except for relief and sleep, and he had to be lifted for that. Oh, he was cheerful enough. He joked that they would cut him off at the middle of his butt the next time, that is, if he didn't die first. A display of courage to others was a macabre nightmare to me. I got serious about getting someone, somewhere, to tell me what to do about my ever-worsening numbness, which by now had spread to my penis. My condition became an ever-present, gnawing anxiety with me, a creeping presence I couldn't fight against because I simply didn't know how to fight it.

"Then, in early April 1986, my wife and I went to visit Dr. Bernstein. The first visit lasted 7½ hours. Each detail of diagnosis and treatment was discussed. Each symptom of the disease, however minute, was described in great detail, the importance of each balanced with another, with specific remedies for managing them. Take the seemingly insignificant matter of scaly feet, a common, dangerous symptom of diabetes. Dr. B. prescribes mink oil, rubbed into the feet morning and night. Practiced as directed, instead of split skin and running foot sores, you have skin as soft and smooth as velvet. Consider the alternative — feet split, painful, and slow (if at all) to heal — which can change your entire life. Special shoes, debilitating gait, not to mention the horrible possibility of progressive amputation; all things that really can happen if your diabetes is not treated properly.

"What is of highest importance, I believe, is the in-depth explanation of diabetes, its causes, symptoms, and treatment. He gives you the rationale for treatment, so that you have a comprehensive understanding of what is wrong and how it can be corrected.

"First, through frequent finger-stick blood testing, we came to an understanding as to the specifics of how to attack my diabetes. We started with diet. It wasn't just eat this, don't eat that, but eat this for these reasons and eat that for other reasons. Know the reasons and the differences. Knowing the how and why of diet keeps you on the track, and the discipline of that knowledge makes control easy. For without continuous diet observance, you will surely worsen your diabetes. He explains that the effect of uncontrolled diabetes on the heart can be much more deleterious than the other popular demons — cholesterol, fat in the diet, stress, tension, et cetera — demons not to be ignored, obviously, but merely put into proper perspective to the main villain — diabetes.

"Well, the results for me are the numbness of my feet and penis have regressed, and my erections have improved. My feet are now beautifully supple and healthy. The severe belching, flatulence, and heartburn after meals have disappeared. The other ills of diabetes have apparently not greatly affected me, and now that I know that controlling my diabetes is the key to a healthy heart, I expect to reduce greatly any future risk of heart attacks.

"One great result of my ability to normalize my blood sugars has been the stabilizing of my emotional attitude toward the disease. I no longer have a sense of helplessness in the face of it; no longer wonder what to do; no longer feel hopelessly dependent on people who have no answers to my problems. I feel free to exercise, walk vigorously, enjoy good health without worry, enjoy my precious eyesight without fear of diabetic blindness, yes, even have a new confidence in normal sexual activities.

"All of the enjoyments of health that were slowly ebbing away are now within my control, and for that I thank my new knowledge and skills."

LeVerne Watkins is a sixty-eight-year-old grandmother and associate executive director of a social service agency. When we first met, she had been taking insulin for two years, after developing Type II diabetes thirteen years earlier. Her comments relate in part to the effects of large amounts of dietary carbohydrate, covered by large amounts of insulin, while she was following a conventional treatment plan.

"In less than two years, my weight had increased from 125 to 155 pounds; my appetite was always ready for the next snack or the next meal. All my waking hours were focused on eating. I always carried a bag of goodies — unsalted saltine crackers, regular Coca-Cola, and glucose tablets. I always had to eat 'on time.' If I was a half-hour late at mealtime, my hands would begin sweating, I would become very jittery, and if in a social gathering or a conference or meeting at work, I would have to force myself to concentrate on what was taking place. During a meeting that I was chairing, the last thing I remember saying was, 'Oh, I'm so sorry,' before I toppled out of the chair to wake up and find myself in the emergency room of a local hospital.

"During a subway ride which generally took about 25 minutes, the train was delayed for close to 2 hours and — to my utter dismay — I had forgotten my bag of goodies. As I felt myself 'going bananas,' sweating profusely and perhaps acting a little strange, a man sitting across from me recognized my Medic Alert bracelet, grabbed my arm, and screamed, 'She has diabetes!'

"Food, juice, candy bars, cookies, and fruit came from all directions. It was a cold, wintery day, but people fanned and fed me. And I was so grateful and so very embarrassed. I stopped riding the subway, and rescheduled as many meetings and conferences as I could to take place directly after lunch so that I would have more time before the next snack or meal would be necessary.

"I felt that I had no control over my life; I was constantly eating, I outgrew all my clothing, shoes and underwear included. I had been a rather stylish dresser since college days. Now I felt rather frumpy, to say the least. Once, I tried to discuss with my diabetologist how I was feeling about gaining weight and eating all the time. I was told, 'You just don't have any willpower,' and 'If you put your mind to it, you wouldn't eat so much.' I was very, very angry, so much so that I never consulted him again.

"On my own, I tried Weight Watchers, but the diet I had been given by the dietitian to whom the diabetologist had referred me did not mesh with the Weight Watchers diet. So along I limped, trying to accept that I was getting fatter each day, was always hungry, had no willpower, and most of the time was feeling unhappy.

"My husband was my constant support through all this. He would say, 'You look good with a few more pounds. . . . Go buy yourself some new clothes,' especially when I would ask him to zip something that I was trying to squeeze into. He always clipped newspaper and magazine articles about diabetes and would remind me to watch specials on TV. He encouraged me to be active in the local diabetes association, and would accompany me to lectures and various workshops. Then, on Sunday, April 3, 1988 — Easter Sunday — he clipped an article from the *New York Times* entitled 'Diabetic Doctor Offers a New Treatment.' Little did I realize that this thin news article would be a new beginning of my life with diabetes. I must have read it several dozen times before I finally met with Dr. Bernstein. Since that first meeting, I haven't had one single episode of hypoglycemia, which I had formerly experienced very often. Following the regimen of correcting my high and low blood sugars, taking small doses and different kinds of insulin, and eating meals calibrated for specific amounts of carbohydrates and protein, my outlook brightened and I began to feel more energetic and more in charge of myself and my life. I could now hop on the train, ride the subway, drive several hours, and not fear one of those low blood sugar episodes. I started once again to exercise every day. My stamina seemed to increase. I didn't have to push hard to accomplish my daily goals at work and at home. Within a couple of months, I was back to 129 pounds, had gone from size 14 to size 10, and ten months later to size 8 and 120 pounds. Even the swelling and pain in my right knee — arthritis, I was told — subsided. I feel great. My self-esteem and self-worth are whole again. I now take only 8 units of insulin each day, where I had previously been taking 31 units.

"I am also conquering my uneasy and frightening feelings about the long-term consequences of having diabetes. While I once thought that heart disease, kidney failure, blindness, amputations, and many other health problems were what the future probably held for me, I now believe that they are not necessarily outcomes of living with diabetes.

"But my life is not perfect. I still occasionally throw caution to the wind by eating too much and eating foods I know are taboo. Sticking with my diet of no bread, no fruit, no pasta, no milk, seemed easy when it was new, but now it is not easy, and loads of my efforts go into making salads, meat, fish, or poultry interesting and varied. My fantasies are almost always of some forbidden food — a hot fudge sundae with nuts, or my mother's blueberry cobbler topped with homemade ice cream. But when all is told, I feel that I am really lucky. All my efforts have really paid off."

A.D. is a fifty-five-year-old former typesetter whose diabetes was diagnosed fourteen years ago. As with many other people who use our regimen, his test of average blood sugar (hemoglobin A_{1C}) and his tests for cardiac disease risk (cholesterol/HDL ratio) simultaneously dropped from high levels to essentially normal values.

"I watched my mother deteriorate in front of me from the complications of diabetes, finally resulting in an amputation of the leg above the knee, and a sorrowful existence until death claimed her. My oldest brother, who was also diabetic, was plagued with circulatory complications that resulted in the amputation of both feet, with unsightly stumps. Diabetes robbed him of a normal existence.

"When I began to experience the all-too-familiar diabetes symptoms, my future looked bleak and I feared the same fate. I immediately searched for help, but for two years floundered around getting much medical advice but not improving. In fact, I was getting sicker. My doctor had said, 'Watch your weight,' and prescribed a single daily oral hypoglycemic pill for my Type II diabetes. It sounded easy, but it wasn't working. My glucose levels were in the 200 range all too often, and occasionally reached 400. I was constantly exhausted.

"I started Dr. Bernstein's program in 1985. Since then I have recovered my former vitality and zest for life. At my first visit, he switched me to another approach — a fast-acting blood sugar–lowering pill 3 times a day, before meals, along with a slower-acting pill in the morning and at bedtime. My regimen was totally overhauled to eliminate foods that raised blood sugar, and to reduce greatly my consumption of carbohydrates in general. Macaroni and ravioli had been important parts of my diet since birth. I had to give these up. I didn't mind a greater emphasis on protein. I even began to include fresh fish in my diet.

"My initial reaction was that these restrictions were too high a price to pay, and that I would be unable to continue them for long. Also, I was asked to check my blood with a blood sugar meter for a week prior to every visit to Dr. Bernstein. That meant sticking my finger several times a day. I was willing to discipline myself for a short period in order to be able to return to a more active, vigorous life and to put my malaise to rest. At the beach, I was sorely tempted to give up the diet, while watching family and friends eat without restrictions. But since my body was feeling healthier, I continued with the program. After about two months, with many dietary slips on my part, I managed to better discipline myself because I sensed it made me feel better. My glucose level started to descend to 140, 130, and finally to 100 or less on a consistent basis.

"Dr. Bernstein also encouraged me to purchase a pedometer, a device that clipped to my belt and measured the distance that I walked each day. I began to walk daily, holding 3-pound weights and swinging my arms. This was yet another thing to bother with, and I felt it would cut into my free time. But the result was an invigorating high. By this time, I didn't mind pricking my fingers several times each day, as it showed me the way to better blood sugars. Fortunately for me, New Rochelle has many beautiful parks. I chose Glen Island Park because it is near Long Island Sound and nicely kept. This meant getting up earlier in the morning to walk during the week, but that was no problem since I am an early riser. I bought some cast-iron dumbbells for additional exercise. I learned about arm curls, overhead raises, arm circles, and chest pulls. I didn't realize that there were so many different exercises that you could do at home to benefit your health.

"My glucose levels are now consistently within or near the normal range, not at the sorry levels which nearly put me in the hospital. That all-consuming fatigue is gone, and I feel that now I'm in control of my diabetes instead of the reverse. With adherence to the program, I know that I don't have to suffer the same debilitating effects that afflict so many other diabetics."

Harvey Kent is fifty-one. He has known about his diabetes for approximately six years, and we suspect that he probably had it for three to four years prior to his diagnosis. He has a family history of diabetes, and his story is fairly typical.

"I went in for a routine physical. I've always had high risk factors — both my parents had diabetes, my brother had diabetes, and my sister has diabetes. My brother, who was forty-nine, passed away recently from diabetic complications. My sister, who is fifty-nine, is on dialysis. When I found out I had it, I felt I was going down the same slippery slope. I'd been trying to lose weight, but not very successfully. The doctor I was seeing, an endocrinologist, kept upping my medication. Every time I went to see him, I wound up taking more and more, and my blood sugars weren't going anywhere but up.

"I kept having the feeling that as far as treatment went, nothing was happening. I wasn't in bad shape, but then I watched my brother pass away, and I thought, 'I've got to *do* something.'

"I happen to live in Mamaroneck, New York, near Dr. Bernstein, and my wife suggested that I see him for a second opinion. I kept wondering, 'Is there another approach?' That's really how it started. The standard approach was always to tell me to lose weight, to exercise, and to take medication. I was trying to do all those things, but I wasn't having much success at any of them except the taking of medication. As it turned out, Dr. Bernstein still said the same three things, but his approach to each of the categories was *radical,* especially on the diet. The diet has been a major factor — I've lost a lot of weight.

"Once I started getting a sense of what Dr. B. was talking about —

which was really right from the first visit; he's very thorough in his explanations — I kind of figured it out. Just to demonstrate the effects of diet, he told me to stay on my same diet and measure my blood sugars, but I started cutting back on the carbohydrates, so by the time we sat down to negotiate a meal plan, which was maybe the third or fourth session, he just confirmed what I'd already started about a month before.

"Before I met Dr. Bernstein, I'd been under treatment for diabetes by three different doctors. The guy I was seeing before Dr. B. is an endocrinologist/diabetes doctor with a fairly large practice. He never once said to me, 'You know, by controlling your blood sugars, most of these complications are reversible.' When Dr. B. told me that — well, for a diabetic who's stuck with this disease for the rest of his life, that's nice to hear. Nobody ever tells you this. At least I don't remember anyone ever explaining this to me. I've been a member of the ADA [American Diabetes Association] for several years, and *no one* ever said anything like that to me, anywhere. I was lucky. I hadn't developed that many complications — not like my brother and sister — but I knew how fast they could get you.

"With my old doctor, I'd been told to monitor my blood sugars and then come in every three months. What it was supposed to do, I wasn't sure — keep you honest, maybe, but I couldn't figure that out. I was checking my fasting blood sugars in the mornings. They were averaging somewhere about 140 mg/dl. And when I'd go in, the doctor would do blood work, scratch the bottoms of my feet, and check my eyes, then say, 'See me in three months.' The whole thing would take maybe half an hour and then I'd see him again in three months. I wasn't sure what the whole thing was about. The thing is — and I found this out with my sister and my brother — it's a slippery slope. You start out as a Type II and you get this kind of treatment, and you burn out your pancreas, and before long, you're insulin-dependent.

"When I saw Dr. B., he did a very extensive medical exam and uncovered everything there was to uncover. He checked everything. He found that I had an anemia, and so we started doing things to deal with that. I had not had retinopathy or neuropathy. I had some protein in my urine, a potential sign of kidney disease. But he said that could be from my old kidney stone, or it could be from the diabetes. He said we'd wait awhile until my blood sugars were normalized, then test again and find out, because if it was the diabetes, it should clear up.

"The first thing he did was get me off Micronase and onto Glucophage. Micronase is one of those oral hypoglycemic agents that stimulate your pancreas, and he said, 'Why are you doing this? You're burning your pancreas out quick.' He looked at my blood sugars carefully and told me I was low at particular times of the day and told me what I had to do to cover the valleys as well as the peaks. Insulin. I never wanted to take insulin. My father did it, and the idea just brought back horrible memories. My other doctor would say, 'All else is failing, now you have to go on insulin.' What Bernstein says is, 'I want you to take insulin in order to cover your peaks and to keep your pancreas from burning out.' This seems to me a much more sensible approach.

"My wife is very perceptive about the whole thing, and she said what I really needed was a coach, and Bernstein is very much like a coach. Having read up about him and knowing that he was an engineer, you can see the difference in his approach. You can see less of the medical model and more of an engineering model: he's putting you back together, taking your components and manipulating them in order to accomplish something. He's a diabetic himself, he knows the thing inside and out, and so you get the sense that he's much more actively involved. Now I measure my blood sugars 5 times a day, but instead of just jotting them down and saying come back in three months, he adjusts the medication, using it to tweak the peaks and valleys, to get the most optimum response. Now I have excellent control.

"The diet takes some getting used to. Most diabetics, I would surmise, love to eat. Especially if you come from a culture where food is the coin of the realm. People ask me now, 'What do you eat?' I say, 'I have turkey, some salad, and a Diet Coke.' I used to be a big pancake eater. Talk about your carbohydrate! Every Saturday and Sunday morning for years I would make pancakes for my wife. Now I make them for her and for my daughter and don't have any — or occasionally steal just a bite — and I miss it, but I am so much more in control now, and I feel so much better. I've seen so much of my family go down the slippery slope, it seems a small sacrifice for good health.

"Since the time I started seeing Dr. Bernstein, I've lost close to 30 pounds. My blood sugars have dropped by about 35 percent, but my weight loss was not on a weight loss diet, just on Dr. Bernstein's meal plan. I still have a way to go, but for the first time I feel like I'm in control."

J.A.K. is a sixty-seven-year-old business executive who had had Type II di-abetes for twenty-four years, and had been taking insulin for twenty, when he started on our regimen. He writes the following:

"I visited Dr. Bernstein on the recommendation of some good friends, as I had just lost the central vision in my right eye due to sub-retinal bleeding.

"It took hours of instruction, counseling, and explanation to make me clearly understand the relationships between diet, blood sugar control, and physical well-being. I was hoping for the possibility that I might experience an improvement in my already deteriorated physical condition. I have diligently followed up on what I was taught, and the results are obvious:

- I no longer have cramps in my calves and toes.
- The neuropathy in my feet has normalized.
- Various skin conditions have cleared up.
- Tests for autonomic neuropathy (R-R interval study) totally normalized in only two years.
- The difficulty I had with digestion has cleared up completely.
- My weight dropped from 188 to 172 pounds in six months.
- My original cholesterol/HDL ratio of 5.3 put me at increased risk for a heart attack. With a low-carbohydrate diet and improved blood sugars, this value has dropped to 3.2, which puts me at a lower cardiac risk than most nondiabetics of my age.
- My daily insulin dose has dropped from 52 units to 31 units, and I no longer have frequent episodes of severe hypoglycemia.
- My overall physical condition and stamina have improved considerably.

"All these improvements occurred because I learned how to control my blood sugars. As a matter of fact, my glycosylated hemoglobin (a test that correlates with average blood sugar during the prior four months) dropped from 7.1 percent to 4.6 percent, so that I am now in the same range as nondiabetics. I have developed full confidence in my ability to manage my own diabetes. I understand what is happening. I can adjust and compensate my medications as the need arises.

"If I have to miss a meal, for whatever reason, I can adjust accordingly and am not tied to a clock, as I was before I learned these new approaches to blood sugar control.

"I would say that not only has my physical condition improved, but my mental attitude is far better today than it was ten or fifteen years ago. My only regret is that I did not learn how to be in charge of my diabetes years earlier."

Lorraine Candido has had Type I diabetes for more than twenty years and has been my patient for ten. She is in her sixties, and she and her husband, Lou, her "copilot," work together to keep her blood sugars normal. Like a lot of happily married couples, Lorraine and Lou sometimes almost speak as one. When Lorraine comes in for treatment, Lou is with her. When she calls on the phone, Lou is on the other line. They talk about how starting the program changed their lives:

LORRAINE: "I had a lot of complications. Bladder infections, kidney infections — and then my eyes. My feet were numb up to my heels. As a matter of fact, one day I was walking barefoot and I wasn't aware of it but I had a thumbtack in my foot all day long. I had neuropathy of the vagus nerve. I had an ulcer from medication. My mother had had eye problems, and so when I went to an ophthalmologist, he said, 'You have some of your mother's problems. We'll keep an eye on you; come back in a year.' And I thought, 'Uh-oh.' When I saw Dr. Bernstein, he said, 'Oh, I'll make an appointment for you.' Right away I had laser surgery."

LOU: "I firmly believe that if she hadn't gone to Dr. Bernstein, she would've been blind. Her last two visits to the eye doctor she got excellent reports. As a matter of fact, he said he had no idea where the fluid in one eye had gone, but it was all gone."

LORRAINE: "I was elated. He said my left eye had made great progress and I was doing well.

"When I first met Dr. Bernstein, I had no idea what I was getting into. All I knew was that I wasn't feeling well and I was going nowhere. I was kind of scared, didn't know what I was getting into, and didn't know if I wanted to. It was plain and simple. I liked Snickers candy bars. He said, 'No.' I couldn't have anything I liked and wanted, and we kind of butted heads — but then I realized, 'Hey, come on, is there really a candy bar worth dying for?'

"He's a very gentle gentleman. I think he's extremely caring; you're not treated like cattle, you're treated as a person, and he answers all your questions. Between the two of us, at the beginning we had a lot of questions. Really, I don't know if I could live without him.

"We found him — it's kind of embarrassing, but our son used to have a newsstand, and Lou would go help him out on Sundays, and Lou would bring me home the papers to read. Well, in one of those horrible tabloids — you know, when they run out of weird stuff, they run unusual medical stories reprinted from somewhere else — the headline on this was 'Diabetic Heals Himself,' and you know, we didn't think that much about it. But I wasn't feeling well, and so we made some inquiries. Now of course we're in a different state and nobody I knew had ever heard of him, but we called his office. I didn't talk to a nurse or someone, he got on the phone himself and he offered us references. Well, that settled it right there. I mean, how many doctors do you know of who'd offer you references? So Lou said, 'Pack up honey, we're going.'"

Lou: "She had a doctor up here in Springfield, Massachusetts, she was seeing and I was getting pretty concerned about it. Her feet were getting numb, she had kidney problems. I don't have diabetes, but I happened to have the same doctor as my internist, and I said to him, 'Isn't there something you can do for my wife?' He had a son who worked at the Joslin Clinic, which we had heard was very good. 'Can we take her to the Joslin Clinic?' But he said, 'What can he do for her up there that we can't do for her here?' We got sort of scared. They were running her the standard way they treat diabetics — standard but safe. Safe for them, but not much help for Lorraine.

"At Dr. Bernstein's, to start, it was a 10-hour training period — two 5-hour sessions that she had to take at the start."

Lorraine: "It was my husband, me, and the doctor. No waiting room for hours. Now, to be honest, when we walked out of there — it's a 2-hour drive between our house and there — I didn't want to do it. But on the drive back home after the first session, we talked. We talked constantly, and I knew I didn't want to do it, but I also knew I was going to do it. Common sense just dictated it. I wanted to live, and I wanted both feet and both eyes. It was plain and simple. The feeling in my feet has come back almost 100 percent, by the way."

Lou: "We found out about the diet on the first visit, and it took about a month to get her blood sugars into the target range. She had been running 300, 400 mg/dl blood sugars pretty regularly."

Lorraine: "I was kind of reluctant to start with. It was clear that Dr. Bernstein's program wasn't a ride in an amusement park. In some respects, it was a whole new way of living, and we had to change all our grocery lists — but I had a supportive friend here in Lou. When I started on the diet, we pretty much ate the same food. He didn't have to, but he did. He would have a few extras here and there and I wouldn't, but it was *years* before I could go into the supermarket, because it felt like I couldn't have anything there. It was very hard to get used to. I resented being told what to do and how to do it."

Lou: "It's very difficult. You have to understand something. When she started the program she was close to sixty years old, and we were accustomed to living in a particular way."

Lorraine: "We have grandkids — we've been married forty-five years — we have six kids and seven grandkids, and they come over for chocolate chip cookies and ice cream."

Lou: "The program works —"

Lorraine: "Because I'm still here."

Lou: "— but it's difficult to do, because you really have to be dedicated."

Lorraine: "Let's put it this way. There are no hot fudge sundaes here. Ever. Not for Thanksgiving, not for Christmas, birthdays, anniversaries — there are no deviations from the program. The first week, because of the change in diet, I lost 15 pounds. You looked at what you were eating, measured it —"

Lou: "It was a combination of things. The amount of insulin changed a lot. She was taking sometimes 80 to 90 units of insulin on a daily basis, and now she's taking 13½ units. Insulin is the fat-building hormone, so reducing your dosage changes things substantially. And you're changing the amount of carbohydrate you're taking in, and so she lost all this weight."

Lorraine: "Altogether, I lost 85 pounds. I wear junior size clothes. Call me stubborn, but I still resent being told what to eat."

Lou: "Let me put it this way. You live a quality of life and give up what you have to —"

Lorraine: "Like fudge."

Lou: "Or potatoes. The point is, you have to decide somewhere along the line. Are you going to live and enjoy the rest of your life without problems, or are you going to fight the reality of the situation and go down the tubes? It's a choice."

Lorraine: "It's an attitude. I don't like his program, but it works. I'm still here. I miss the goodies I give my grandkids, all the cookies, candy bars, ice cream. And the holidays. Everything's kind of restricted."

Lou: "The irony of this is, my wife, since she lost all the weight, she dresses in very sporty clothes. Now, I'm a race walker. She doesn't exercise, but because of heredity or whatever, she has beautiful, strong legs, and so she wears these spandex tights and such, and people ask her, 'How much do you run?'"

LORRAINE: "He's a champion race walker, very self-disciplined. Not me. I had a conversation with God, and He said, 'Don't sweat.' I'm Lou's cheerleader. I stay home and read books."

LOU: "She walks with me sometimes. But I laugh my ass off."

LORRAINE: "It's fun to go shopping and buy junior sizes with my granddaughters — but I don't let them borrow my clothes. Before I started the program, I never thought about how I looked, how I felt — all I know is, the clothes I was buying were one size fits all."

LOU: "Now look at her."

By the way, Lorraine's cholesterol/HDL ratio has dropped from a high cardiac risk 5.9 to a very low risk 3.3.

It isn't unusual for people with diabetes to make major changes in other aspects of their lives once their blood sugars have been restored to normal after years of poor control. The changes that we see include marriages, pregnancies, and reentry into the workforce. The story of Elaine L. falls into the last category. She also points out the disabling fatigue that she experienced when her blood sugars were high. This problem has led other diabetics, desperate to retain their abilities to function productively, to abuse amphetamines. Elaine is a sixty-year-old mother and artist. Her story is not unusual.

"When I developed diabetes twenty-one years ago, I began a fruitless odyssey to learn all I could about this disease and to have the tools to be able to deal with the psychological and physical roller coaster that I was experiencing.

"The hardest thing to cope with was the total loss of control over my life. I was told that I was a 'brittle' diabetic and that I would just have to endure the very high and very low blood sugars that were totally exhausting me. I feared that my eyes would be damaged. I'm an artist, and this frightened me the most. I knew that this disease was destroying my body every day and that I was helpless.

"We went from doctor to doctor and to major diabetes centers around the country. I never could get a handle on how to become 'controlled.' I was given a gold star for 'good' blood sugar by one doctor; told I 'had imbued the number 150 with mystical significance' by another;

informed that if my blood sugars were high after lunch today, I could correct them before lunch tomorrow. All the while, I was feeling worse and worse. I stopped painting. I was just too tired. I was so scared to read any more of the diabetes magazines, because I kept learning more and more about what was in store for me.

"I'd been diabetic about five years when an uncle in Florida advised me to read Dr. Bernstein's first book. It made a lot of sense, but when I read it, I thought, 'Diabetes has robbed me of so much already, I don't have any more time or effort to give to it — and who wants to be a professional diabetic?' Of course, there was a lot of anger and denial and even attempts to forget about being diabetic. Maybe I could forget about it for a while, but it never forgot about me.

"A seed was now planted, however, in spite of myself. I knew that no matter what happened down the road, I needed to feel that I had tried everything possible, so that I would never have to say, 'I wish I had done more.'

"I was very wary of my first visit to Dr. Bernstein's office. I really thought I would hate having to change my diet yet again. I did not relish the idea of multiple daily injections, testing my blood so often, and keeping records. The fact is that I did hate all of that until I found I was recording better and better blood sugars. The diet wasn't any more restrictive than the American Diabetes Association diet I had been following, and most important, I was feeling better and much less tired. In fact, I began to paint again and soon rented a studio. I now paint full-time, but this time I actually sell my work.

"The regimen that I feared has, in the end, given me the freedom for which I had dreamed."

Although Elaine does not mention it in her story, her cholesterol/HDL ratio dropped from an elevated cardiac risk level of 4.74 to the "cardioprotective" level of 3.4, as her long-term blood sugars approached normal. Furthermore, her weight has dropped from 143 pounds to 134 pounds, and her hemoglobin A_{1C} has dropped from a very high 10.7 percent to a nearly normal 6.0 percent.

Carmine DeLuca is in his early sixties and has had Type II diabetes since about age forty-five. Like many of my patients, he had been in "standard" treatment and found his condition getting progressively worse.

"I was taking pills, tried some diet changes, but after about ten years my diabetes just got worse. Through the years, as a diabetic, I had seen some articles about Dr. Bernstein, and he had appeared several times in the local newspaper. A colleague at work mentioned this Dr. Bernstein to me, the same guy who had been in the paper. She said, 'If you ever want to go to someone, go to this guy.' And I heard from a few other people around the area who said, 'He's excellent.'

"Over the years, I've had trouble with my eyes, my feet, and my hands, but that was before Dr. Bernstein saw me. I had tried to watch my diet, but being Italian, you know, you're always involved with the pasta, the bread, and so forth, and so I really didn't do very well on dieting. Apparently the pill that I was taking was literally burning me out. I was just going to a general doctor, an internist, and what did he know? I used to keep blood sugar about 140 to 160, and then all of a sudden it started hitting the 200 mark, and it was starting to hit it consistently, and then close to 300, and then over 300, and the nerve endings in my feet were gone, and the feeling in my hands. I did have, at age fifty, two cataracts. I don't know if you want to blame it on diabetes, but I guess you can. Finally, when it was so high, I said, 'Well, something has to be done. What have I got to lose?'

"And so when the time came, I thought, let me go to the best. Everybody talks about how excellent he is, so I made an appointment. My blood sugars were very high, in the high 300s, like 375. When I saw Dr. Bernstein, I had no idea what I was getting myself into. I had just heard that he was one of the best, and so I said, 'Lemme do it.' He struck me as very, very knowledgeable. I learned an awful lot — he told me things about diabetes that I just never heard about, even from people with diabetes. He made you feel good, because he literally grew up with it. He was very professional, yet you could sit down and talk to him. He said he was always available, available 24 hours a day, and he has been, no matter what. You go into that, and you feel pretty good.

"I've lost weight since I started seeing him. A few pounds here and there, but the thing is, even though I haven't taken off a lot of weight yet, everybody says, 'Hey, you look great.' But you could see, prior to seeing Dr. Bernstein, that it was tearing me down, people could see I wasn't looking that good.

"Starting the program was tough, but it was carbohydrates that were killing me. He put me on the diet. I never had a problem with cholesterol, but for some reason, every time you turn around, people are talking about high cholesterol this, high cholesterol that, so I thought about it. But I didn't give a damn about carbohydrates; nobody talks about carbohydrates and cholesterol. At least until Dr. Bernstein said, 'You don't eat this, you don't eat that,' and I said, 'These are all carbohydrates.' And so I'm on the diet and, boom, I start losing a little weight.

"The thing was to get used to doing without the carbohydrate, but it's okay, because I like meat, I like salad, I like vegetables. I can eat all the cheese I want — I mean, within reason. My blood sugar has been good, averaging under 100, and I feel like a million.

"I'm strictly on insulin and one pill, and we've reduced the insulin, and as my blood sugar improves, I think we'll reduce it even more. I see him now every two months or so, and for a week prior, I measure my sugars 4 times a day and bring the chart to him. He really analyzes it — you know, 'All right, take this, don't do this. We'll reduce this. Don't eat that.' He's got a system all his own and it's great. It works. It can be a pain in the neck, but hey. He tells me I'm a good patient. I'm here to prove that it's not impossible to change, and the results are there."

Mark Wade, M.D., is one of many physicians with diabetes. He is board certified in pediatric medicine. His lovely wife not long ago gave birth to their third child. His story has a number of parallels with my own.

"Dr. Bernstein's program turned my life around. Prior to meeting Dick Bernstein at age thirty-four, I had spent twenty-two years of my life as what I then considered a well-controlled insulin-dependent, juvenile-onset diabetic. I'd never been hospitalized for ketoacidosis [a serious condition caused by high blood sugar in combination with dehydration] or hypoglycemia [low blood sugar], had what I considered good circulation and nerve function, exercised daily, and ate pretty much whatever I felt like eating.

"However, cuts and lacerations took months or years to heal instead of days, and always left ugly scars. Once or twice each year, I would develop pneumonia that typically lasted four months and had me, without fail, out of school or work for two and a half months per episode. My mood swings went from kind and lovable to short-tempered, hot-headed, and uncaring four to five times daily, congruent with my routine blood sugar swings from high blood sugars (300 to 500) after meals to hypoglycemia (less than 50) before meals. This Dr. Jekyll/Mr. Hyde personality made me very unpredictable and unpleasant to be around, and came close to causing me to lose my wife and the closeness of family and friends. I was forced to eat my meals at exactly the same times each day in order to avoid life-threatening episodes of low blood sugar. Even so, I had to adjust my life around the inevitable periods of hypoglycemia. If I didn't eat, my life was in trouble, and unfortunately so were the people who had to interact with me when I was hypoglycemic. Most of the times those were the ones I loved most.

"My training as a physician, as an intern and resident, averaging 110 hours a week of work, was at times a nightmare, though I did it, trying to balance rounds, clinics, emergency room and ICU schedules, screening patients, long hours of reading, and an unreal demand on physical tolerance, emotional stability, and consistency that almost drove me to the breaking point. My mission was to be an excellent doctor, and I was, with a calm, cool demeanor which I presented externally, but inside I was a mess, and my interactions with my loved ones and close friends were horrible. I was an avid basketball player, jogger, and weight lifter, but despite doing these activities daily, I found my performance and endurance were usually modulated by my blood sugar — and was never really sure whether I would be able to perform for 10 minutes or 2 hours. In addition, despite my high level of exercise, 1 to 1½ hours daily for twelve years, I was never able to develop a muscular or athletic body type, even though I worked hard at it.

"I was never a 'brittle' diabetic. I was always extremely conscientious about testing and exercising and eating and doctor visits, to the point that my friends thought I was neurotic. I was consistently following the conventional guidelines recommended to diabetics, and I thought I was a rather model patient. The problems that I described above, I had been led to believe, were a natural part of life for a diabetic. No one showed me that my life could be better, that I could control my diabetes rather than let my diabetes control me, that with recognition of a few principles that are really just common sense, a few extra finger sticks and a few extra injections and better control of my dietary intake — I could be in charge for real!

"Nine years ago, I met Dick Bernstein. Dr. Bernstein not only gave me the most complete, comprehensive, logical, reasonable, and informative teaching on diabetes that I have ever encountered, but his uniquely expert and comprehensive physical examination and testing illuminated for me the most accurate picture of my overall health and the subtle tolls that the previous management of my diabetes had permitted. Then with a personalized, comprehensive, tightly controlled but reasonable diet, exercise, and a blood sugar–monitoring plan, he put me in control of my diabetes for the first time. Sure, the diet plan, finger sticks, and 5 to 8 insulin injections a day for my program require a high degree of discipline and self-control, but it's doable, it works, and this comparatively small sacrifice brings me the freedom of lifestyle, quality of life, and longevity that nondiabetics take for granted.

"The results have been as follows: I can eat or fast whenever I choose. I plan my day around my activities rather than around my meals, have the ability to be much more flexible in my schedule and participation in activities, and now have the ability to adjust my daily activities easily to accommodate 'emergencies' or sudden changes in schedule — activities and adjustments that nondiabetics take for granted. Best of all, the wild mood swings have been eliminated and I'm sick much less often and less seriously."

PART ONE

Before You Start

1

Diabetes:

THE BASICS

Diabetes is so common in this country that it touches nearly everyone's life — or will. The statistics on diabetes are staggering, and a diagnosis can be frightening: diabetes is the third leading cause of death in the United States. According to the National Institutes of Health (NIH), there are 8 million diagnosed diabetics in America, and equally that many who have not yet been diagnosed. About 700,000 new diabetics will be diagnosed this year, according to NIH statistics; that's *one every 30 seconds.* Each year, tens of thousands of Americans lose their eyesight because of diabetes, the leading cause of blindness for people in the 25–74 age range. Ninety-five percent of diabetics have Type II, or what used to be known as maturity-onset, diabetes. Because 80 percent of Type II diabetics are obese, many inappropriately feel that the disease is their own fault, the result of some failure of character.

Since you are coming to this book, you or a loved one may have been diagnosed recently with diabetes. Perhaps you have long-standing diabetes and are not satisfied with treatment that has left you plagued with complications such as encroaching blindness, foot pain, frozen shoulder, inability to achieve or maintain an erection, or heart or kidney disease.

Although diabetes is still an incurable, chronic disease, it is *very* treatable, and the long-term "complications" are fully preventable. I've had Type I diabetes, also called juvenile-onset or insulin-dependent diabetes mellitus (IDDM), for more than fifty years. This form of diabetes is generally far more serious than Type II, or non-insulin-dependent diabetes mellitus (NIDDM), although both have the potential to be fatal.* Most Type I diabetics who were diagnosed back about the same time I was are now dead from one or more of the serious complications of the disease. Yet, after living with diabetes for more than fifty years, instead of being bedridden or out sick from work, I am more fit than many nondiabetics who are considerably younger than I. I regularly work 12-hour days, travel, sail, and pursue a vigorous exercise routine. If I can take control of my disease, you can take control of yours.

In the next several pages I'll give you a general overview of diabetes, how the body's system for controlling blood sugar (glucose) levels works in the nondiabetic, and how it works — and doesn't work — for diabetics. In subsequent chapters we'll discuss diet, exercise, and medication, and how you can use them to control your diabetes. If talk about diet and exercise sounds like "the same old thing" you've heard again and again, read on, because you'll find that what I've observed is almost exactly the opposite of what you've probably been taught. The tricks you'll learn can help you arrest the diabetic complications you may now be suffering, may reverse many of them, and should prevent the onset of new ones. We'll also talk about new medical treatments and drugs that are now available to help manage blood sugar levels and curtail obesity.

THE BODY IN AND OUT OF BALANCE

Diabetes is the breakdown or partial breakdown of one of the more important of the body's autonomic (self-regulating) mechanisms, and its breakdown throws many other self-regulating systems into imbalance. There is probably not a tissue in the body that escapes the effects of the high blood sugars of diabetes. People with high blood sugars tend to have osteoporosis, or fragile bones; they tend to have tight skin; they

---

* Although until recently many have considered the designations Type I and Type II to be out of date, the current terms, IDDM and NIDDM, are slightly misleading. While it is true that those with Type II can stay alive without injecting insulin, many patients who suffer from so-called NIDDM do inject insulin to preserve their health. I have long thought that the older terms, Type I and Type II, though not precise, are more appropriate. Recently, others in the field of diabetes research have begun to turn away from IDDM and NIDDM as well. Even more precise terms are in the works: "autoimmune diabetes" for Type I, and "insulin-resistant diabetes" for Type II. These are more accurate, but are unlikely to take over for the much-easier-to-say Type I and Type II.

tend to have inflammation and tightness at their joints; they tend to have many other complications that affect every part of their body.

Insulin: What It Is, What It Does

At the center of diabetes is the pancreas, a large gland about the size of your hand, which is located toward the back of the abdominal cavity and is responsible for manufacturing, storing, and releasing the hormone insulin. The pancreas also makes several other hormones, as well as digestive enzymes. Even if you don't know much about diabetes, in all likelihood you've heard of insulin and probably know that we all have to have insulin to survive. What you might not realize is that *only a small percentage of diabetics must have insulin shots.*

Insulin is a hormone produced by the beta cells of the pancreas. Its major function is to regulate the level of glucose in the bloodstream, which it does primarily by facilitating the transport of blood glucose into most of the billions of cells that make up the body. Insulin also stimulates centers in the brain responsible for feeding behavior, and it instructs fat cells to convert glucose and fatty acids in the blood into fat, which the fat cells then store until needed. Insulin is essential for the growth of many tissues and organs. In excess, it can cause excessive growth — as, for example, of body fat and of cells that line blood vessels. Finally, insulin helps to regulate, or counterregulate, the balance of certain other hormones in the body. More about those later.

One of the ways insulin maintains the narrow range of normal levels of sugar in the blood is by regulation of the liver and muscles, directing them to manufacture and store glycogen, a starchy substance the body uses when blood sugar falls too low. If blood sugar does fall too low — as may occur after strenuous exercise or fasting — the alpha cells of the pancreas release glucagon, another hormone involved in the regulation of blood sugar levels. Glucagon signals the muscles and liver to convert their stored glycogen back into glucose (a process called glycogenolysis), which raises blood sugar. When the body's stores of glucose and glycogen have been exhausted, the liver can transform the body's protein stores — muscle mass and vital organs — into sugar.

Insulin and Type I Diabetes

As recently as seventy-five years ago, before the clinical availability of insulin, the diagnosis of Type I diabetes — which involves a severely diminished capacity to produce insulin — was a death sentence. Most people died within a few months of diagnosis. Without insulin, glucose accumulates in the blood to extremely high toxic levels; yet, since it cannot be utilized by the cells, many cell types will starve. The absence of insulin also leads the liver to perform gluconeogenesis, turning the body's protein store — the muscles and vital organs — into even more glucose that the body cannot utilize. Meanwhile, the kidneys, the filters of the blood, try to rid the body of inappropriately high levels of sugar. Frequent urination causes insatiable thirst and dehydration. Eventually, the starving body turns more and more protein to sugar, leaving no organ unaffected. The ancient Greeks described diabetes as a disease that causes the body to melt into sugar water. When tissues cannot utilize glucose, they will metabolize fat for energy, generating by-products called ketones, which are toxic at high levels and cause further water loss as the kidneys try to eliminate them (see ketoacidosis, in Chapter 20, "How to Cope With Dehydrating Illness").

Today Type I diabetes is still a very serious disease, and still eventually fatal if not properly treated with insulin. It can kill you rapidly when your blood glucose level is too low — through impaired judgment or loss of consciousness while driving, for example — or it can kill you slowly, by heart or kidney disease, which are commonly associated with long-term blood sugar elevation. Until I brought my blood sugars under control, I had numerous automobile accidents due to hypoglycemia, and it's only through sheer luck that I'm here to talk about it.

The causes of Type I diabetes have not yet been fully unraveled. Research indicates that it's an autoimmune disorder in which the body's immune system attacks the pancreatic beta cells that produce insulin. Whatever causes Type I diabetes, its deleterious effects can absolutely be prevented. The earlier it's diagnosed, and the earlier blood sugars are normalized, the better off you will be.

At the time they are diagnosed, many Type I diabetics still produce a small amount of insulin, and if they are treated early enough and treated properly, what's left of their insulin-producing capability frequently can be preserved. Type I diabetes typically occurs before the age of forty-five and usually makes itself apparent quite suddenly, with such symptoms as dramatic weight loss and frequent thirst and urination. We now know, however, that as sudden as its appearance may be, its onset is actually quite slow. Routine commercial laboratory studies are available that can detect it earlier, and it may be possible to arrest it in these early stages by aggressive treatment. My own body no longer produces any insulin at all. The high blood sugars I experienced during my first year with diabetes burned out, or exhausted, the ability of my pancreas to produce insulin. I must have insulin shots or I will rapidly die. I firmly believe that if the kind of diet and medical regimen I prescribe for my patients had been available when I was diagnosed, the insulin-producing capability left to me at diagnosis would have been preserved. My requirements for injected insulin would have been lessened, and it would have been much easier for me to keep my blood sugars normal.

Blood Sugar Normalization: Restoring the Balance

According to the American Diabetes Association (ADA), more than 150,000 people die annually from both Type I and Type II diabetes and their long-term complications. Certainly everyone has to die of something, but you needn't die the slow, torturous death of diabetic complications, which often include blindness and amputations. My history and that of my patients supports this. The recently completed Diabetes Control and Complication Trial (DCCT) began as a ten-year study of Type I diabetics to gauge the effects of improved control of blood sugar levels (see the foreword, by Dr. Frank Vinicor). Patients whose blood sugars were nearly "normalized" (my patients' blood sugars are usually closer to normal than were those in the trial) had dramatic reductions of long-term complications. Researchers began the DCCT trying to see if they could, for example, lessen the frequency of diabetic retinopathy by at least 33.5 percent. Instead of a one-third reduction in retinopathy, they found a more than 75 percent reduction in the progression of early retinopathy. They found similarly dramatic results in other diabetic complications and halted the study early in order to make the results available to all. They found a 50 percent reduction of risk for kidney disease, a 60 percent reduction of risk for nerve damage, and a 35 percent reduction of risk for cardiovascular disease.

The patients followed in the DCCT averaged twenty-seven years of age at the beginning of the trial, so reductions could easily have been greater in areas such as cardiovascular disease if they had been older or followed for a longer period of time. The implication is that full normalization of blood sugar could totally prevent these complications. In any case, the results of the DCCT are good reason to begin aggressively to monitor and normalize blood sugar levels. The effort and dollar cost of doing so does not have to be so high as was suggested in the DCCT's findings.

The Insulin-Resistant Diabetic: Type II

Different from Type I diabetes is what is commonly known as Type II. This is by far the more prevalent form of the disease. According to ADA statistics, 90–95 percent of diabetics are Type II. Furthermore, as many as a quarter of Americans between the ages of sixty-five and seventy-four have Type II.

Approximately 80 percent of those with Type II diabetes are overweight and suffer from a particular form of obesity known as truncal, or visceral, obesity. It is quite possible that the 20 percent of the so-called Type II diabetics who do not have visceral obesity actually suffer from a form of Type I diabetes that causes only partial loss of the pancreatic beta cells that produce insulin. If this proves to be the case, then fully all of those who have Type II diabetes may be overweight. (Obesity is usually defined as being at least 20 percent over the ideal body weight for one's height, build, and sex.)

While the cause of Type I diabetes may still be somewhat mysterious, the cause of Type II is less so. As noted earlier, another name for Type II diabetes is insulin-resistant diabetes. Obesity, particularly visceral obesity, and insulin resistance — the inability to fully utilize the glucose-transporting qualities of insulin — are interlinked. For reasons related to genetics (see Chapter 12, "Weight Loss"), a substantial portion of the population has the potential when overweight to become sufficiently insulin-resistant that the increased demands on the pancreas burn out the beta cells that produce insulin. These people enter the vicious circle depicted in Figure 1-1. Note in the figure the crucial role of dietary carbohydrate in the development and progression of this disease. This is discussed in detail in Chapter 12.

Insulin resistance appears to be caused at least in part by inheritance and in part by high levels of fat — in the form of triglycerides — in the branch of the bloodstream that feeds the liver. (Transient insulin resistance can be created in laboratory animals by injecting triglycerides directly into their liver's blood supply.) Insulin resistance by its very nature increases the body's needs for insulin, which therefore causes the pancreas to work harder to produce elevated insulin levels (hyperinsulinemia), which can indirectly cause high blood pressure and damage

Since high blood sugar is the hallmark of diabetes, and the cause of every long-term complication of the disease, it makes sense to discuss where blood sugar comes from and how it is used and not used.

BLOOD SUGARS: THE NONDIABETIC VERSUS THE DIABETIC

Our dietary sources of blood sugar are carbohydrates and proteins. One reason the taste of sugar — a simple form of carbohydrate — delights us is that it fosters production of neurotransmitters in the brain that relieve anxiety and can create a sense of well-being, or even euphoria. This makes carbohydrate quite addictive to certain people whose brains may have inadequate levels of these neurotransmitters, the chemical messengers with which the brain communicates with itself and the rest of the body, or peripheral nervous system. When blood sugar levels are low, the liver can, through a process we will discuss shortly, convert proteins into glucose, but very slowly and inefficiently. The body cannot convert glucose back into protein, nor can it convert fat into sugar. Fat cells, however, with the help of insulin, do transform glucose into fat.

The taste of protein doesn't excite us as much as that of carbohydrate — it would be the very unusual child who'd jump up and down in the grocery store and beg his mother for a steak instead of cookies. Protein gives us a much slower and smaller blood sugar effect, which, as you will see, we diabetics can use to our advantage in normalizing blood sugars.

The Nondiabetic

In the fasting nondiabetic, and even in some Type II diabetics, the pancreas constantly releases a steady, low level of insulin. This baseline, or basal, insulin level prevents the liver from inappropriately converting bodily proteins (muscle, vital organs) into glucose and thereby raising blood sugar, a process known as gluconeogenesis. The nondiabetic ordinarily maintains blood sugar immaculately within a narrow range — usually between 80 and 100 mg/dl (milligrams per deciliter),* with

---

* A deciliter is one-tenth of a liter, or a little over 3 ounces. A milligram is one one-thousandth of a gram, or about one three-thousandth of the weight of a teaspoon of sugar.

most people hovering near 85 mg/dl.* There are times when that range can briefly stretch up or down — as high as 160mg/dl and as low as 65 — but generally, for the nondiabetic, such swings are rare.

You will note that in some literature on diabetes, "normal" may be defined as 60–120 mg/dl, or even as high as 140 mg/dl. This "normal" is entirely relative. No nondiabetic will have blood sugar levels as high as 140 mg/dl except after consuming a lot of carbohydrate. "Normal" in this case has more to do with what is cost-effective for the average physician to treat. Since a postmeal (postprandial) blood sugar under 140 mg/dl is not classified as diabetes, and since the individual who experiences such a value will usually still have adequate insulin production eventually to bring it down to reasonable levels, many physicians would see no reason for treatment. Such an individual will be sent off with the admonition to watch his weight or her sugar intake. Despite the designation "normal," an individual frequently displaying a blood sugar level of 140 mg/dl is a good candidate for full-blown Type II diabetes. I have seen "nondiabetics" with sustained blood sugars averaging 120 mg/dl develop diabetic complications.

Let's take a look at how the average nondiabetic body makes and uses insulin. Suppose that Jane, a nondiabetic, arises in the morning and has a mixed breakfast, that is, one that contains both carbohydrate and protein. On the carbohydrate side, she has toast with jelly and a glass of orange juice; on the protein side, she has a boiled egg. Her basal (i.e., before-meals) insulin secretion has kept her blood sugar level steady during the night, inhibiting gluconeogenesis. Shortly after the sugar in the juice or jelly hits her mouth, or the starchy carbohydrates in the toast reach her saliva, glucose begins to enter her bloodstream. The rise in Jane's blood sugar is a chemical signal to her pancreas to release the granules of insulin it has stored in order to prevent a jump in blood sugar (see Figure 1-2). This rapid release of stored insulin is called phase I insulin response. It quickly corrects the initial blood sugar increase and can prevent further increase from the ingested carbohydrate. As the pancreas runs out of stored insulin, it manufactures more, but it has to do so from scratch. The insulin released now is known as the phase II insulin response, and it's secreted much more slowly. As she eats her

---

* Unless otherwise noted, all values of blood glucose cited in this book refer to levels in capillary blood from finger-stick measurements; venous values are about 5–10 percent higher.

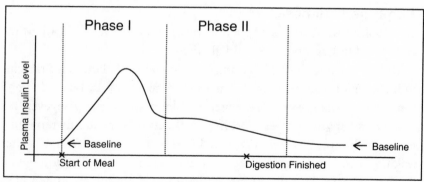

Terry Eppridge

Fig. 1-2. *Phase I and phase II insulin response in normal, nondiabetic person.*

boiled egg, the insulin of phase II can cover the sugar that's slowly produced from the protein of the egg.

Insulin acts in the nondiabetic as the means to admit glucose — fuel — into the cells. It does this by activating the production of glucose "transporters" within the cells. These specialized protein molecules emerge from the nuclei of the cells to grab glucose from the blood and bring it to the interiors of the cells. Once inside the cell, glucose can be utilized to power energy-requiring functions. Without insulin, the cells can absorb only a very small amount of sugar, not enough to sustain the body.

As Jane's blood continues to accumulate sugar, and the beta cells in her pancreas continue to release insulin, some of her blood sugar is transformed to glycogen, a starchy substance stored in the muscles and liver. Once glycogen storage sites in the muscles and liver are filled, excess glucose remaining in the bloodstream is converted to and stored as fat. Later, as lunchtime nears but before Jane eats, if her blood sugar drops too low, the alpha cells of her pancreas will release another pancreatic hormone, glucagon, which will "instruct" her liver and muscles to begin converting glycogen to glucose, to raise blood sugar. When she eats again, her store of glycogen will be replenished.

This pattern of basal, phase I, then phase II insulin secretion is perfect for keeping Jane's blood glucose levels in a healthy range. Her body is nourished, and things work according to design. Her mixed meal is handled beautifully. This is not, however, how things work for either the Type I or Type II diabetic.

The Type I Diabetic

Let's look at what would happen to me, a Type I diabetic, if I had the same breakfast as Jane, our nondiabetic.

Unlike Jane, because of a condition peculiar to diabetics, if I take insulin, I might awaken with normal blood sugar levels, but if I spend some time awake before breakfast, my blood sugar may rise, even if I haven't had anything to eat. Ordinarily, the liver is constantly removing some insulin from the bloodstream, but during the first few hours after waking from a full night's sleep, it clears insulin out of the blood at an accelerated rate. This dip in insulin level is called the dawn phenomenon (see Chapter 6, "Strange Biology"). Because of it, my blood glucose can rise even though I haven't eaten. A nondiabetic just makes more insulin to take care of the increased clearance. Those of us who are severely diabetic have to track the dawn phenomenon carefully by monitoring blood glucose levels, and can learn how to prevent its effect upon blood sugar.

As with Jane, the minute the meal hits my mouth, the enzymes in my saliva begin to break down the sugars in the toast and juice, and almost immediately my blood sugar begins to rise. Even if the toast had no jelly, the enzymes in my saliva and stomach would begin to rapidly transform the toast into glucose upon ingestion.

Since my beta cells have completely ceased functioning, there is no stored insulin to be released by my pancreas, so I have no phase I insulin response. My blood sugar (in the absence of injected insulin) will rise while I digest my meal. None of the glucose will be converted to fat, nor will any be converted to glycogen. Eventually much will be filtered out by the kidneys and passed out through the urine, but not before my body has endured damagingly high blood sugar levels — which won't kill me on the spot but will over the years be an incremental step in the slow, "silent" death from diabetic complications. The natural question is, wouldn't injected insulin "cover" the carbohydrate in such a breakfast? No. This is a common misconception — even by those in the health care profession. Normal phase I insulin is almost instantly in the bloodstream. Rapidly it begins to hustle blood sugar off to where it's needed. Injected insulin, on the other hand, is injected either into fat or muscle (not into a vein) and absorbed slowly. The fastest insulin we have, lispro, starts to work in about 15 minutes, but that isn't fast enough to prevent a damaging upswing in blood sugars if fast-acting carbohydrate, like bread, is consumed.

This is the central problem for Type I diabetics — the carbohydrate and the drastic surge it causes in blood sugar. Because I know my body produces no insulin, I have a shot of insulin before every meal. But I no longer eat meals with fast-acting or large amounts of carbohydrate, because the blood sugar swings they caused were what brought about my complications. Even injection by means of an insulin pump (see discussion at the end of Chapter 18) cannot fine-tune the level of glucose in my blood the way a nondiabetic's body does naturally.

Now, if I ate only the protein portion of the meal, my blood sugar wouldn't have the huge, and potentially toxic, surge that carbohydrates cause. It would rise less rapidly, and a smaller dose of insulin could act rapidly enough to cover the glucose that's slowly derived from the protein. My body would not have to endure wide swings in blood sugar levels. (Dietary fat, by the way, has no effect on blood sugar levels, except that it can slightly slow the digestion of carbohydrate.)

In a sense, you could look at my insulin shot before eating only the protein portion of the meal as mimicking the nondiabetic's phase II response. This is much easier to accomplish than trying to mimic phase I, because of the much lower levels of dietary carbohydrate and injected insulin.

The Type II Diabetic

Let's say Jim, a Type II diabetic, is 6 feet tall and weighs 300 pounds, much of which is centered around his midsection. Remember, at least 80 percent of Type II diabetics are obese. If Jim weighed only 150 pounds, he might well be nondiabetic, but because he's insulin-resistant, Jim's body no longer produces enough excess insulin to keep his blood sugar levels normal.

The obese tend to be insulin-resistant as a group, a condition that's not only hereditary but also directly related to the ratio of visceral fat to lean body mass (muscle). The higher this ratio, the more insulin-resistant a person will be. Whether or not an obese individual is diabetic, his weight, intake of carbohydrates, and insulin resistance all tend to make him produce considerably more insulin than a slender person of similar age and height (see Figure 1-3). Many athletes, because of their low fat mass and high percentage of muscle, tend as a group to require and make low levels of insulin. An obese Type II diabetic like Jim, on the other hand, typically makes *two to three times* as much insulin as the slender nondiabetic. In Jim's case, from many years of having to

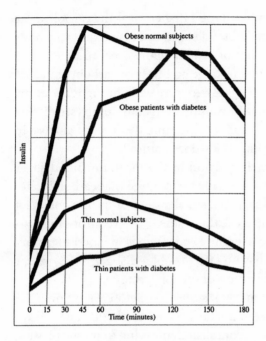

Fig. 1-3. *Serum insulin response of individuals with and without diabetes.*

overcompensate, his pancreas has partially burned out, and despite the huge output of insulin, he no longer can keep his blood sugars within normal ranges. (In my medical practice, a number of patients come to me for treatment of their obesity, not diabetes. However, on examination, most of these very obese "nondiabetics" have slight elevations of their test for average blood sugar.)

Let's take another look at that mixed breakfast and see how it affects a Type II diabetic. Jim has the same toast and jelly and juice and boiled egg that Jane, our nondiabetic, and I had. Jim's blood sugar levels at waking are normal.* Since he has a bigger appetite than either Jane or I, he has two glasses of juice, four pieces of toast, and two eggs. As soon as the toast and juice hit his mouth, his blood sugar level begins to rise. Unlike mine, Jim's pancreas releases insulin, but he has very little or no stored insulin (his pancreas works hard just to keep up his basal insulin level), so he has impaired phase I secretion. His phase II insulin response, however, may be intact. So very slowly, his pancreas will struggle

---

* Waking, or fasting, blood sugars are frequently normal in mild Type II diabetics. After they eat carbohydrate, however, their postprandial blood sugars are usually elevated.

to produce enough insulin to bring his blood sugar down toward the normal range. Eventually it may get there, but not until hours after his meal, and hours after his body has been exposed to high blood sugars. Insulin is not only the major fat-building hormone, it also serves to stimulate the center in the brain responsible for feeding behavior. Thus, in all likelihood, Jim may well grow even more obese, as demonstrated by the cycle illustrated in Figure 1-1.

high-sugar → food cravings

Since he's resistant to insulin, his body has to work that much harder to metabolize the carbohydrate he consumes. Because of insulin's fat-building properties, his body stores away some of his blood sugar as fat and glycogen; but his blood sugar level continues to rise, since his cells are unable to utilize adequate amounts *of insulin* Jim, therefore, still feels hungry. As he eats more, his beta cells work harder to produce more insulin. The excess insulin and the "hungry" cells in his brain prompt him to want yet more food. He has just one more piece of toast with a little more jelly on it, hoping that it will be enough to get him through until lunch. Meanwhile, his blood sugar goes even higher, his beta cells work harder, and perhaps some of them burn out. Even after all this food, he still may feel many of the symptoms of hunger. His blood sugar, however, will probably not go as high as mine would if I took no insulin. In addition, his phase II insulin response could even bring his blood sugar down to normal after many hours without more food.

p. 38 & 87 "insulin resistance"

Postprandial blood sugar levels that I would call unacceptably high — 140 mg/dl, or even 200 mg/dl — may be considered by other doctors to be unworthy of treatment because the patient still produces adequate insulin to bring them periodically down to normal, or "acceptable," ranges. If Jim, our Type II diabetic, had received intensive medical intervention before the beta cells of his pancreas began to burn out, he would have slimmed down, brought his blood sugars into line, and eased the burden on his pancreas. He might even have "cured" his diabetes by slimming down, as I've seen in several patients. But many doctors might decide such "mildly" abnormal blood sugars are only impaired glucose tolerance (IGT), and do little more than "watch" them. Again, it's my belief that aggressive treatment at an early stage can save most patients considerable lost time and personal agony by preventing complications that *will occur* if blood sugar levels are left unchecked. Such intervention can make subsequent treatment of what remains — a mild disease — elegantly simple.

ON THE HORIZON

Researchers are currently trying to perfect a method for cloning, or replicating, insulin-producing pancreatic beta cells in the laboratory. Doing this in a fashion that's comparatively easy and cost effective should not be an insurmountable task, and indeed the preliminary results are quite encouraging. Once cells are replicated, they can be transplanted back into patients to actually cure their diabetes. After such treatment, unless you were to have another autoimmune event that would destroy these new beta cells, you would remain nondiabetic for the rest of your life. If you had another autoimmune attack, you would simply have to transplant more cloned cells. This is the single best opportunity we have for a cure, immeasurably better than all the electronic insulin pumps, and the only one I'd personally have any part of — except I can't.

The catch here for me and other diabetics who no longer have any insulin-producing capacity is that the cells from which new beta cells would be cloned have to be your own, and I have none. Had I gone on insulin, say, a year before I was diagnosed with diabetes, or had my blood sugars been immaculately controlled immediately upon diagnosis, the injected insulin might have taken much of the strain off my remaining beta cells and allowed them to survive.

Many people (including the parents of diabetic children) view having to use insulin as a last straw, a final admission that they are (or their child is) a diabetic and seriously ill. Therefore they will try anything else — including things that will burn out their remaining beta cells — before using insulin. Many people in our culture have the notion that you cannot be well if you are using medication. This is nonsense, but some patients are so convinced that they must do things the "natural" way that I practically have to beg them to use insulin. In reality, nothing could be more natural. Diabetics who still have beta cell function left may well be carrying their own cure around with them — provided they don't burn it out with high blood sugars and the refusal to use insulin.

2

Tests:

A BASELINE MEASURE OF YOUR DISEASE AND RISK PROFILE

The goal in the treatment program laid out in this book is to give you the tools to take control of your disease by normalizing blood sugars. My interest is in treating not just the symptoms of diabetes, but diabetes itself. Essential to treatment is learning to monitor your own blood sugars. But before you begin to monitor and then normalize your blood sugars, you should have a baseline analysis of your disease. How much of your pancreas has "burned out" in part from high blood sugars? Have you already developed some easily measured long-term complications of diabetes? What are your risks for other diabetic complications? Answering these questions will aid you and your doctor in establishing the extent of your disease. Your test results will also serve as valuable baseline data to which you will be able to compare the effects of blood sugar normalization. Once your blood sugars have been normalized, such tests can be repeated from time to time, to show you what you are achieving. Your improvements will give both you and your doctor ongoing incentive for sticking to the program.

The remainder of this chapter describes a number of tests your doctor or his laboratory can perform in order to give you both a picture of your diabetic condition. As some of these tests are costly, any or all may be skipped if you cannot afford them or your insurance or health maintenance organization won't pay for them.

BLOOD AND URINE TESTS

Glycosylated Hemoglobin (HgbA$_{1C}$)

Glucose binds to hemoglobin (the pigment of red blood cells) when new red cells are manufactured. Since the average red cell survives about four months, the percentage of hemoglobin molecules that contain glucose (HgbA$_{1C}$) can provide an estimate of average blood sugar over this time frame. One of the benefits of this test is that it gives your physician an index by which to test the accuracy of your own blood glucose self-monitoring results. If your measurements are strictly normal but your HgbA$_{1C}$ is elevated, then your doctor has a clue that something is awry.

There are, however, a couple of significant drawbacks to this test. First is that the test is only a measure of average blood sugars. Elevated blood sugars may take 24 hours to have any long-term effect on HgbA$_{1C}$, and if blood sugar is elevated for only part of every day and is normalized or too low the rest of the time, your HgbA$_{1C}$ results may appear deceptively low.

The other drawback is that the upper and lower ranges of "normal" values reported by most labs are erroneously high and low, respectively. In other words, the ranges are usually much too wide. Thus, it's up to your physician to decide, based upon his experience, what the proper normal range for his lab should be. Many doctors have their own formulas for estimating average four-month blood sugar levels from HgbA$_{1C}$. A normal value should correspond to blood sugars of about 85–95 mg/dl.

Serum C-Peptide (Fasting)

C-peptide is a protein produced by the beta cells of the pancreas whenever insulin is made. The level of C-peptide in the blood (serum level) is a crude index of the amount of insulin you're producing. The level is usually zero in Type I diabetics, and within or above the "normal range" in mild Type II obese (insulin-resistant) diabetics. If your serum C-peptide is elevated, this would suggest to your physician that your blood sugar may be controllable merely by diet, weight loss, and exercise. If, at the other extreme, your C-peptide is below the limits of measurability, you probably require injected insulin for blood sugar normalization.

Because a physician experienced in treating diabetes can probably make such decisions with only the help of your blood sugar profiles (see Chapter 4), this test, while of interest, is not absolutely necessary.

Complete Blood Count (CBC)

Part of most medical workups, this is a routine diagnostic test that can disclose the presence of ailments other than diabetes. A CBC measures the number of various types of cells found in your blood — white cells, red cells, and platelets. A high level of white blood cells, for example, can disclose the presence of infection, while too few red blood cells can indicate anemia. This test can also detect certain malignancies.

Standard Blood Chemistry Profile

This battery of twelve to twenty-five tests is part of most routine medical examinations. It includes gauges for such important chemical indicators of health as liver enzymes, blood urea nitrogen (BUN), creatinine, alkaline phosphatase, calcium, and others. If you have a history of hypertension, your doctor may want to add red blood cell magnesium to this profile.

Lipid Profile

This is a battery of tests measuring fatty substances (lipids) in the blood that predispose you to arterial and heart disease. A useful profile includes total cholesterol, HDL (high-density lipoprotein), triglycerides, and LDL (low-density lipoprotein). Other lipid measurements, such as "small high-density LDL" and IDL (intermediate-density lipoprotein), may become available in the future.

These tests should be performed after you have fasted for at least 8 hours. The best thing is to have them scheduled in the morning. If you've eaten 2–3 hours before the test, the results will be difficult to interpret.

Maybe you've heard of "good" cholesterol and "bad" cholesterol? Well, this is why a reading for total cholesterol by itself won't necessarily reflect cardiac risk. Most of the cholesterol in our bodies we make ourselves. Some people — because they're obese or have high blood sugars or are genetically predisposed — make more or dispose of less than they should, which can put them at a higher risk for cardiac problems. HDL is a lipid that reduces the risk of heart disease and is the "good" cholesterol. High levels of LDL increase the risk of heart disease, which makes LDL the "bad" cholesterol. So it is the ratio of total cholesterol to HDL (total cholesterol ÷ HDL) that is significant. You could have a high total cholesterol, but because of low LDL and high HDL, you could have a low cardiac risk. Conversely, you could have a low total cholesterol but with a low HDL, which would signify *increased* risk.

The only truly accurate measure of LDL is the direct LDL test. The customary, indirect measure of LDL is estimated mathematically and can result in values that are grossly in error. Direct measurement of LDL, however, may cost more than all the rest of your lipid profile.

Also important to remember is that — as we will discuss in Chapter 9 — fats and cholesterol in the diet do not cause high-risk lipid profiles in most people. On the other hand, diabetics tend to have lipid profiles that reflect increased cardiac risk, if their blood sugars have been elevated for several weeks or months.

Homocysteine

A recently discovered cardiac risk factor (not a lipid) is homocysteine. This is an amino acid that tends to be elevated in poorly controlled diabetes and in individuals with a folic acid or vitamin B-12 deficiency.

Thrombotic Risk Profile

This profile includes levels of fibrinogen, tissue plasminogen activator (tPA), and lipoprotein(a), all of which relate to the increased tendency of blood to clot in people who have had high blood sugars. In my experience, these tests are more potent indicators of impending heart attack than the lipid profile. Because most of these tests are still quite costly, I test only for fibrinogen unless the others are covered by insurance.

Renal Risk Profile

Chronic blood sugar elevation for many years can cause slow deterioration of the kidneys. If caught early, it may be reversible by blood sugar normalization, as it was in my own case. Unless you think frequent hospital visits for dialysis might be a nice way to meet people, it's wise to have periodic tests that reflect early kidney changes. It is also wise to have all these performed together, as the results of each can clarify the interpretation of all.

Several factors can adversely affect the results of these tests, so you should keep them in mind when your doctor schedules the tests. You should avoid strenuous lower-body exercise (which would include motorcycle or horseback riding) in the 48 hours preceding the tests. Additionally, if on the day the tests are to be performed you are menstruating or have a fever, a urinary tract infection, or active kidney stones, you should postpone the tests until these conditions have cleared up.

A basic renal risk profile should include the following:

Urinary kappa light chains. If early diabetic kidney disease is present, this test reports "polyclonal kappa light chains present." This means that small amounts of tiny protein molecules may be entering the urine, due to leaky blood vessels in the kidneys. Because these molecules are so small, they are the first proteins to leak through tiny pores in the blood vessels of the kidneys that may have been affected by disease.

This test requires a small amount of fresh urine. False positive results can be caused by any of the factors listed at the bottom of page 52.

Microalbuminaria. This test can now be performed qualitatively (by dipstick) in your doctor's office, or quantitatively at outside laboratories. It, like the urinary kappa light chain test, can also reflect leaky vessels in the kidneys, but at a later stage since albumin is a slightly larger molecule.

A quantitative measurement requires a 24-hour urine specimen, which means you'll need to collect all the urine you produce in a 24-hour period in a big jug and deliver it to your physician or laboratory. Given the potential embarrassment of carrying a jug full of urine around at work, you might want to schedule your test on a Monday and collect the urine while at home on Sunday.

24-hour urinary protein. This test detects kidney damage at a later stage than the preceding two tests; it also requires a 24-hour urine collection. As with the other tests, false positive results can occur in the presence of one or more of the factors already discussed.

Creatinine clearance. Creatinine is a chemical by-product of muscle metabolism, and is present in your bloodstream all the time. Measuring the clearance of creatinine from the body is a way of estimating the filtering capacity of the kidneys, in comparison with normal kidneys. Test values are usually higher than normal when a person is spilling a lot of sugar in the urine, and eventually lower than normal when the kidneys have been damaged by years of elevated blood sugars. It is not surprising to see a sudden but appropriate drop in creatinine clearance when blood sugars are normalized and urine glucose vanishes.

The creatinine clearance test requires a 24-hour urine collection, and your doctor will draw a small amount of blood. The most common cause of abnormally low values for this test is failure of the patient to collect all the urine produced in a 24-hour period. Therefore, if other kidney tests are normal, tests with low values for creatinine clearance should be repeated for verification.

Serum beta₂ microglobulin. This is a very sensitive test for injury to the tubules of the kidneys, which pass urine filtered from the blood. As with fibrinogen levels, elevated values can also result from inflammation or infection anywhere in the body. Thus an isolated elevation of serum beta₂ microglobulin, without the presence of urinary kappa light chains or microalbumin, is probably due to a viral infection, not to diabetic kidney disease.

24-hour urinary glucose. This test too requires a 24-hour collection of urine, and is of value for proper interpretation of the creatinine clearance.

Note: If, as you've been reading about these tests, you've imagined yourself lugging around multiple jugs of urine, most of us only need one 3-liter jug. This should give you an adequate specimen for your physician to perform creatinine clearance, microalbumin, 24-hour protein, and 24-hour glucose. Nevertheless, it's wise to bring home two empty jugs, just in case your urine output is very high.

OTHER TESTS

R-R Interval Study

The purpose of this study is to test the functioning of the vagus nerve, and it should be part of your initial diabetic physical examination. In the way it's performed, it resembles an ordinary electrocardiogram, but it requires fewer electrical leads.

The vagus nerve is the largest nerve in the body, running from the brain to the lower body. It's the main neural component of the parasympathetic nervous system, or that part of the nervous system that takes

pendix E, I have included the same instructions I give my own patients on how to care for their feet.

Oscillometric Study of Lower Extremities

This inexpensive test utilizes a simple blood pressure cuff connected to a special instrument. It gives an index of the adequacy of circulation to the legs and feet. Since long-standing, poorly controlled diabetes can seriously impair peripheral circulation, this test is fairly important. All diabetics should take special care of their feet, but if you have an abnormal oscillometric study, you have to be extra careful. People who have diminished circulation in the legs usually also have deposits in the coronary arteries that nourish the heart and the arteries necessary for penile erection. Therefore, if this study shows impaired circulation, your doctor may want you to undergo tests that would help diagnose coronary artery disease and narowing of the vasculature that feeds the brain.

WHEN TO PERFORM THESE TESTS

As valuable as they can be to you and your physician, none of the above tests is crucial to our central goal of achieving blood sugar normalization. If you are without medical insurance, or if your insurance won't pay for these tests, and financial considerations are a top priority, all can be deferred. However, if you are experiencing particular problems, such as impairment of vision, you should be tested immediately. Also, examination of your feet, and learning how to care for them properly, is vital and can prevent or forestall serious complications.

The most valuable of these tests for our purposes is the $HgbA_{1C}$, because it alerts your physician to the possibility that your self-monitored blood sugar data may not reflect the average blood sugar for the prior four months. This can occur if your blood sugar measuring technique or supplies are defective. More commonly, some patients, with a scheduled visit to the doctor approaching, will improve their eating habits so that their blood sugar records improve. I have seen several teenagers whose falsified blood sugar data were discovered by this test. I therefore suggest that $HgbA_{1C}$ be measured at regular visits every two to three months. This test costs about $50.

Ideally, the other blood and urine tests should be performed *before* attempting to normalize blood sugar and annually thereafter. If an abnormal value is found, your physician may wish to repeat that test and related tests more often. The exception is the fasting C-peptide test, as there is little value in repeating it except to see if pancreatic function is deteriorating. I certainly like to repeat the thrombotic risk and lipid profiles about two months after blood sugars have been normalized. The improvement that I frequently see tends to encourage patients to continue their efforts at blood sugar normalization. The R-R interval test should be performed every eighteen months.

3

Your Diabetic Tool Kit:

SUPPLIES YOU WILL NEED AND WHERE TO GET THEM

In order to monitor and maintain your blood sugar levels, you're going to need certain tools. This chapter lists and describes them; you'll learn more about them in later chapters. Also included are supplies for foot care and for treating dehydrating illnesses. For most items, approximate costs are listed. Some expenses will be onetime outlays, such as for your blood glucose meter outfit. Others will occur on an ongoing basis.

The tools that all diabetics will need are listed first. Tools that only insulin users will need are listed separately. Some are necessary, and some are optional. You can show your physician the list and he or she can decide which items are appropriate for your needs.

Following the tables of supplies is a brief description of each of them, what they're for, where you can purchase them, whether you'll need a prescription, and where in this book you'll find a complete description of their usage.

If you can't locate some of these supplies in your area, all prescription items and most nonprescription items can be ordered via telephone and credit card, check, or money order from Harrison Chemists at (800) 829-1493. If you have any questions about these products, or which particular brand we're recommending for our patients at any given time, you can call our Diabetes Center at (914) 698-7500.

SUPPLIES FOR ALL DIABETICS

For Measuring and Recording Blood Sugar	**Approximate Cost**
Blood sugar meter outfit	$75
30-gauge lancets (1 box)	$11/box of 200
Blood sugar test strips (at least 1 box of 50)	$35/box
GLUCOGRAF II data sheets	$10.95/pad of 26 double-sided sheets
For Removing Blood from Clothing	
Hydrogen peroxide	$1
For Dehydration	
Nu-Salt Salt Substitute; Morton's Lite Salt; Featherweight Seasoned Salt Substitute; Diamel Salt-It; Adolf's Salt Substitute; etc.	$2
For Severe Vomiting	
Tigan suppositories	$20/box of 10
For Low Blood Sugars *(required only if taking medication that lowers blood sugar)*	
Dextrotabs: 1–3 bottles of 100 tablets. Also, in an emergency, B-D glucose-tablets, Dextrosol, Dextro-Energen, Dex 4, or Sweetarts	$12/bottle of Dextrotabs
Medic Alert identification tags	$35–$700 (gold)
For Urine Testing During Illness	
Ketostix (foil-wrapped) 1 package	$15
For Testing Food	
Clinistix or Diastix, 1 package	$7.50
For Foot Care	
Purified mink oil, vitamin E cream, or Almond Glow Coconut skin lotion	$1–$3/ounce
Bath thermometer	$15

For Menu Planning

The Complete Book of Food Counts, by Corinne T. Netzer	$5.95
Food Values of Portions Commonly Used, by Jane Pennington	$15
Calories and Carbohydrates, by Barbara Kraus	$5
Kosher Calories, by Tziporah Spear	$20

Artificial Sweeteners

Stevia extract	$18.95/2 ounces liquid; $18/1ounce powder
Saccharin tablets	$4.80/1,000 tablets (½ grain)
Equal tablets	$2.95/100 tablets

SUPPLIES FOR INSULIN-USING DIABETICS ONLY

Insulins and Insulin Supplies

Humalog (Lilly), 2 vials	$25/vial
Humulin R (Lilly), 2 vials	$16/vial
Humulin L (Lilly), 2 vials	$16/vial
Humulin U (Lilly), 2 vials	$16/vial
Medicool (to store insulin while traveling in hot climates)	$30
25-unit or 30-unit insulin syringes (get 200 to start)	$20/box of 100

For People Who Won't Learn to Self-Inject Insulin

Autojector push-button injector	$45
Instaject II	$50
Medijector insulin infuser	$600

For Low Blood Sugar Emergencies

Glucose 15	$7.50
Glucagon Emergency Kit	$39
Reglan syrup	$14/4-ounce bottle

FOR ALL DIABETICS

Blood sugar meter outfit. A blood sugar meter outfit should contain a blood sugar meter, a finger-stick device, and a small startup supply of lancets and test strips. The meter does the same job as the one I bought decades ago, although my old one weighed several pounds and some of the new models are smaller than many pocket calculators. They work quite simply: with a sample of blood from a finger stick, the instrument gives you a reading of your blood sugar. (See Chapter 4, "How and When to Measure Blood Sugar.")

If you have difficulty obtaining blood with the puncture device packed with your meter, try the Softclix. This instrument, made by Boeringer Mannheim, has an adjustable puncture-depth control.

Blood sugar meters are available at most pharmacies and chain drugstores. Some are more accurate and reliable than others. Because of the rapid advances in technology, it would be counterproductive to recommend a particular meter. If you want our current recommendation, please call our Diabetes Center.

Disposable 30-gauge lancets. These are used with or without your finger-stick device to puncture your skin for glucose testing. I reuse mine until they become dull.

Blood sugar test strips. When you stick your finger, you'll put the drop of blood on or into one of these. They work with your meter to give your blood sugar readings (see Chapter 4 for complete details).

GLUCOGRAF II data sheets. See Chapter 5, "Recording Blood Sugar Data." These are necessary to record properly the values you get from your self-testing. They are available from Harrison Chemists.

Hydrogen peroxide. Now and then when you're sticking your fingers or injecting through your shirt, as I do, you may get a little blood on your clothing. Hydrogen peroxide is an effective way to eradicate it. You can get small bottles for home, office, car, or travel. Available at any drugstore and at many groceries. (See Chapter 15, page 207.)

For dehydration. If you become dehydrated, these products can help you get rehydrated. Look for potassium chloride on the list of ingredients. These should be available at the supermarket or grocery store. Their use is covered in Chapter 20, "How to Cope with Dehydrating Illness."

For severe vomiting. Vomiting can cause dehydration, which is especially problematic for diabetics. Tigan suppositories are for vomiting and should be used for no more than 1–2 days at a time, unless directed otherwise by your physician. They are available in 100 mg (children and elderly) and 200 mg (adults) dosages. When necessary, use one rectally 4 times daily. (See Chapter 20.) This product requires a prescription.

For low blood sugars. If you experience low blood sugars, Dextrotabs are a good, controlled way of bringing them up by precise increments, while minimizing the risk of overshoot that you might experience with, say, a glass of fruit juice or a soft drink. Each tablet will bring the average adult's blood sugar up about 8 mg/dl. If you run out of Dextrotabs and need an emergency supply of glucose tablets, you can use one of the following: B-D glucose tablets, which will bring up blood sugars approximately 25 mg/dl in most adults; Dextrosol, approximately 15 mg/dl; Dextro-Energen, 15 mg/dl; Dex 4, 20 mg/dl; and Sweetarts, 10 mg/dl. These are available through most drugstores. (See Chapters 13, "Using Exercise," and 19, "How to Prevent and Correct Low Blood Sugars.") As with any other products listed here, contact Harrison Chemists if you cannot locate Dextrotabs locally.

Medic Alert identification tags. These bracelets or necklaces should be worn at all times so that if you happen to become unconscious or confused when you're not with a trained companion, health care professionals will know you're a diabetic and take appropriate action. Available by mail order, using forms that your physician should be able to provide, or phone (800) ID-ALERT.

Ketostix. These dipsticks are for testing your urine for ketones when you are ill. (See Chapter 20.)

Clinistix or Diastix. These are test strips similar to Ketostix, but we use them for testing food (even though they are marketed for testing urine). See Chapter 10, "Diet Guidelines," to learn how you can use them to get an idea if packaged or restaurant foods contain sugar. Available at most pharmacies.

Purified mink oil and other skin lubricants. In Appendix E you will find foot care guidelines, an important part of diabetic self-care. If your feet are dry, you should use an animal or vegetable oil lubricant. Don't use mineral oils or petroleum-based products, as your skin will not absorb them. Available at Harrison Chemists, drugstores, and health food stores.

Bath thermometer. Many diabetics have impaired sensation in their feet. Without knowing it, you can scald and seriously injure your feet if showers or baths are too hot. Don't take foot care lightly. Poor foot care for diabetics can lead to amputation, especially if you have poor circulation. Available at most pharmacies.

Books and publications. There are many books available that can be helpful in trying to figure out your diet plan (see Chapter 11, "Creating a Customized Meal Plan"). They are optional, but here are a few I think are valuable:

- *The Complete Book of Food Counts* (1994), by Corrine T. Netzer, Dell Publishing; available at most bookstores and by mail order from Dell Readers Service, Dept. DCN, Box 5057, Des Plaines, IL 60017
- *Food Values of Portions Commonly Used* (1989), by Jean Pennington, J.B. Lippincott, East Washington Square, Philadelphia, PA 19105
- *Calories and Carbohydrates* (1988), by Barbara Kraus, New American Library; available at most bookstores or from the publisher at 1633 Broadway, New York, NY 10019
- *Kosher Calories* (1985), by Tziporah Spear; available by mail from Mesorah Publications, 4401 Second Avenue, Brooklyn, NY 11223

Artificial sweeteners. As we will discuss in Chapter 10, "Diet Guidelines," the little packets of artificial sweetener you see on restaurant tables are predominantly glucose. Stay away from powdered sweeteners (except stevia extract), and always scan the lists of ingredients for any word ending in *-ose.* Use only the tablet-type or stevia liquid or powder. You can get saccharin or Equal (aspartame) tablets in any drugstore and in many groceries. Stevia is sold at health food stores. If you have a sweet tooth, there is no restriction on how much of these you use. They won't affect your blood sugar.

FOR INSULIN-USING DIABETICS

Insulins. The types of insulins I recommend are Humalog (lispro insulin); Humulin R (regular human insulin); Humulin L (lente human insulin); and Humulin U (ultralente human insulin). I recommend that you keep at least two vials of those insulins selected by your doctor on hand at all times. You must have a prescription, and your physician will select the one(s) appropriate for you. A thorough discussion of their characteristics, use, and administration appears in Chapters 15–18.

Medicool. This is an optional device that will keep insulin cold when you are traveling in hot climates. Insulin need not be kept refrigerated but should not be exposed to high temperatures for prolonged periods.

Insulin syringes. Any 25- or 30-unit insulin syringe. They come in boxes of 100, and you should get at least 200 to start. They are available with a prescription at most pharmacies. Their use is covered in Chapter 15, "Insulin: The Basics of Self-Injection."

"Automatic" insulin injectors. If you are unable or unwilling to learn to self-inject, these may be purchased in a wide variety of configurations. At the low-tech end is Autojector, which performs the entire injection at the push of a button and takes about 20 seconds to prepare with a standard, disposable syringe. Also available is Instaject II, which does the hard part — pushing the needle into the skin — for you; you have to push in the plunger. These are relatively inexpensive. At the high-tech end of the spectrum is the Medijector, which is at least ten times as expensive as either of the low-tech injectors, but utilizes no needles. It sprays the insulin through the skin. Bulky and not convenient to carry around, it must be cleaned and boiled once every two weeks. (See Chapter 15.)

Glutose 15. You will want to show your friends and relatives how to use this glucose syrup if you experience confusion but not unconsciousness from dangerously low blood sugars. Your confusion should lift rapidly as your blood sugar increases toward the normal range. (See Chapter 19, "How to Prevent and Correct Low Blood Sugars.")

Glucagon Emergency Kit. It's important that you have this for the remote possibility that you may become unconscious from dangerously low blood sugars. You will want to train your friends, colleagues, spouse, or other family members in its use. Available at most pharmacies. It's a good idea to attach a bottle of Reglan syrup (below) and a rolled-up handkerchief, by rubber band, to each of your Glucagon Emergency Kits. (See Chapter 19.)

Reglan syrup. Glucagon can cause nausea, and a dose of this syrup when you regain consciousness should keep you from retching.

4

How and When to Measure Blood Sugar

The nondiabetic body is constantly measuring its levels of blood sugar and compensating for values that are either too high or too low. A diabetic's body has lost much or all of this capacity. With a little help from technology, you can take over where your body has left off and do what it once did automatically — normalize your blood sugars.

YOUR BLOOD GLUCOSE PROFILE

No matter how mild your diabetes may be, it is very unlikely that any physician can tell you how to normalize your blood sugars throughout the day without knowing what your blood glucose values are around the clock. Don't believe anyone who tells you otherwise. The only way to know what your around-the-clock levels are is to monitor them yourself.

A table of blood sugar levels, measured at least 4 times daily over several days, is the key element in what is called a blood glucose profile. This profile, described in detail in the next chapter, gives you and your physician or diabetes educator a glimpse of how your medication, lifestyle, and diet converge, and how they affect your blood sugars. Without this information, it's impossible to come up with a treatment plan that will normalize blood sugars. Except in emergencies, I usually won't attempt to treat someone's diabetes until I receive a blood glucose profile that covers at least one week.

Blood glucose data, together with information about meals, medication, exercise, and any other pertinent data that affect blood sugar, is best recorded on a form like the GLUCOGRAF II data sheet, illustrated in Chapter 5.

HOW FREQUENTLY ARE GLUCOSE PROFILES NECESSARY?

If your treatment includes insulin injections before each meal, your diabetes is probably severe enough to render it impossible for your body to automatically correct small deviations from a target blood glucose range. To achieve blood sugar normalization, it therefore may be necessary for you to record blood glucose profiles every day for the rest of your life, so that you can fine-tune any out-of-range values. If you are not treated with insulin, or if you have a very mild form of insulin-treated diabetes, it may only be necessary to prepare blood glucose profiles when needed for readjustment of your diet or medication. Typically, this might be for only *one week* prior to every routine follow-up visit to your physician, or for a few weeks while your treatment plan is being fine-tuned for the first time. After all, your physician or diabetes educator cannot tell if a new regimen is working properly without seeing your blood glucose profiles. I would suggest, however, that you also do a blood glucose profile for 1 day at least every other week, so you will be assured that things are continuing as planned.

SELECTING A BLOOD GLUCOSE MEASURING OUTFIT

The measuring system usually consists of a pocket-sized electronic meter with liquid crystal display. The outfit will include a spring-driven finger-sticking device and a supply of lancets. The meter is designed for use with disposable plastic strips, onto or into which a drop of blood is placed. Some brands of strips change color when exposed to glucose, and the accompanying meter measures color change. Other strips contain electrodes that conduct or generate more or less current, depending upon the amount of glucose in the blood.

About ten different blood glucose metering outfits are presently being marketed in the United States. Only one or two of these have a degree of accuracy acceptable for our purposes. Some systems routinely report blood glucose values that are 40–100 percent in error. This can be very dangerous to the user. How these have secured approval from the Food and Drug Administration (FDA) is a matter of conjecture. Usually the problem involves poor quality control or design of the plastic strips, or inability to calibrate the meter accurately for different batches of strips.

Although your supplier should be in a position to advise you properly on the selection of systems for blood glucose monitoring, this is almost never the case. Even physicians and educators specializing in diabetes rarely conduct the studies necessary to evaluate these products. Reports in medical journals that purport to be evaluating different blood glucose self-measurement systems are frequently financed by one of the manufacturers and often present grossly deceptive conclusions. All this puts you, the consumer, in a difficult position.

Designs advance so rapidly that it's impossible to predict what will be available when you read this book. You can call our Diabetes Center at (914) 698-7500 to find out what system we currently recommend for our patients.

Accuracy is the most important feature to keep in mind when selecting a meter, so do not be seduced by low cost, size, appearance, or special features, such as built-in memory. Buy from a dealer who will refund your money if the system is inaccurate. You can get a rough idea of the precision of the system by performing four blood glucose measurements in succession at the dealer's store. They should be within 5 percent of one another. Ask your physician about the systems he has evaluated. He can secure virtually any system from its manufacturer for study at no cost.

MEASURING YOUR BLOOD SUGARS: IMPORTANT TECHNIQUES

Many instruction booklets give inadequate or erroneous instructions for preparing the finger or putting the drop of blood on the test strip or electrode. If the instructions that follow conflict with what you've been told, believe mine. My techniques aren't based on something I read in medical school or in a medical journal. They're the ones I use on myself every day. I've been measuring my own blood glucose levels for more than twenty-five years and have performed more than 75,000 measurements.

1. If you've handled glucose tablets or any food since last washing your hands, wash them again. Invisible material on your fingers can cause erroneously high readings. Certainly wash your hands if they are soiled. If you are sitting in a car or some other place where you cannot wash your hands, lick the appropriate finger and dry it on a handkerchief or clothing. Don't wipe your fingers with alcohol: this will dry out the skin and can eventually foster the formation of calluses. Neither I nor any of my patients have developed finger infections by not using alcohol.

2. Unless your fingers are already quite warm, it may be necessary to rinse them under warm water. Blood will flow much more readily from a warm hand.

3. Lay out all the supplies you will need at your work area. These usually include a finger-stick device loaded with a lancet, your blood glucose meter, a blood glucose test strip, and a tissue for blotting your finger. If you have no tissue, just suck off the blood. Insert a disposable test strip into your blood sugar meter. (Some test strips are supplied in individual foil packets. The accompanying instruction booklet may tell you not to handle the strips directly but always to hold them in the foil. This assumes that your hands are always dirty, which is absurd, since they must be clean for an accurate result.)

4. Most spring-activated finger-stick devices come with two covers for the end that touches your finger. Usually the light-colored cover is for thin or soft skin, while the darker cover is for thick or callused skin. To get a shallower puncture, use the thicker, light-colored cover; to get a deeper puncture, use the thinner, dark cover. An even deeper puncture may be obtained by strongly pressing your finger against the lancet cover. A very shallow puncture may be obtained by barely touching the fingertip to the cover. The pressure of the finger on the cover determines how deep the puncture will go. It should be deep enough to provide an adequate drop of blood, but not be so deep as to cause bruising or pain. Contrary to common teaching, the best sites for pricking fingers are actually on the back of the hand. Prick your fingers near the

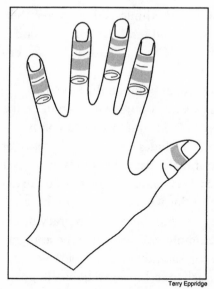 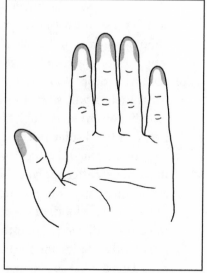

Terry Eppridge

Fig. 4-1. *Sites to prick on the dorsum of your fingers.*   Fig. 4-2. *Sites to prick on the palmar surface of your fingers.*

nails, or between the first and second joints (not over the knuckles), as shown by the shaded areas in Figure 4-1. Pricking these sites should be less likely to cause pain and more likely to produce a drop of blood than will pricking your fingers on the palmar surface of the hand. You will also be free from the calluses that occur after repeated punctures on the palm.* If you find it repugnant to prick the dorsum (back) of your fingers, use the sites on the palmar surface illustrated in Figure 4-2. As you will not be sharing your finger-stick device, you need not discard the disposable plastic lancets with the metal point after every finger stick. It is a good idea to discard them once a week, as they do eventually become dull.

5. Prick any finger. Over a period of time, you should use all the fingers of both hands. There is no reason to prefer one finger over the

---

* My patients and I are much indebted to Mr. Ron Raab of the International Diabetes Institute of Caulfield, Australia, for this not-so-obvious technique. Mr. Raab's attempts to publish this important finding were repeatedly scorned by medical journals and finally came to my attention via personal correspondence. I use Mr. Raab's technique myself and find it far superior to the palmar technique, which I used for years. By the way, this technique was in common use by physicians seventy years ago. Like so many things in medicine, it had to be rediscovered.

others. Squeeze the finger (use a rhythmic action rather than steady pressure) with the opposite hand until the drop of blood is about ⅟₁₆ inch (2 mm) in diameter. If flow is inadequate (see below), perform a deeper finger stick.

6. Touch the drop of blood to the proper point on the test strip.

7. Most meters will start an automatic countdown as soon as the strip has absorbed enough blood. The countdown, in seconds, appears on the display screen and concludes with the appearance of your blood glucose value. If your meter has a timer button, press it immediately after applying blood, *without delay;* do not stop to examine the strip in order to determine whether or not you have applied enough blood. (This comes later.) Since the accuracy of the test usually depends upon the timing, the delay between applying the blood and pressing the button should be no greater than 1 second. This doesn't sound like much time, but you'll be an old pro in short order.

8. Once the timer has started, you may examine the strip to make sure it is adequately covered or filled with blood. If it is not, discard the strip and start again.

9. If you get a little blood on your clothing, rub on a few drops of hydrogen peroxide with a handkerchief. Wait for the foaming to stop. Then blot and repeat the process. Continue until blood has disappeared. This works best while the blood is still wet.

10. If you are measuring someone else's blood sugars, use a fresh lancet each time, and wipe off the end of the finger-stick device with fresh bleach after each use. It is possible to transmit serious infectious diseases from one person to another via finger sticks.

The entire process, from pricking the finger to a final reading, takes as little as 20 seconds, and rarely more than 2 minutes.

PREPARING FOR YOUR FIRST BLOOD SUGAR CONTROL VISIT TO YOUR PHYSICIAN OR DIABETES EDUCATOR

Make sure you have all the supplies you and your physician have checked off in Chapter 3. Put a string on your finger to remind you to ask someone at the doctor's office to watch you measure your blood sugar levels and to correct any errors you may make. (About 80 percent of my new patients are not measuring their blood sugars accurately when I first see them.) Bring along at least one week's worth of your blood glucose profiles. Ideally, these should be written on a GLUCOGRAF II data sheet (see next chapter), which has been designed for quick review by the physician or other health care professional. To compile your profiles, blood sugars should be measured:

- Upon rising in the morning.
- Five hours after every injection of Humalog or "regular" insulin (if you use one of these before meals or to cover elevated blood sugars).
- Two hours after meals and snacks (if you do not take the above insulins before meals).
- At bedtime.
- Before and after exercising, shopping, or running errands.
- Whenever you suspect that your blood glucose may be higher or lower than usual.

5

Recording Blood Sugar Data:

USING THE GLUCOGRAF II DATA SHEET

Your blood sugar levels are affected by a variety of things: what medications you are taking (such as insulin or oral hypoglycemic agents), what exercise you may have performed, whether you're well or ill, what you ate, when you ate it, and many others. All of these — not just your blood sugar levels — need to be recorded and taken into account. Without this detailed information — this blood sugar profile — your physician or diabetes educator cannot assist you in developing an ongoing program for blood sugar normalization. To my knowledge, none of the many forms currently available for this purpose show adequate information in a readily usable format. The GLUCOGRAF II data sheet, like our program, was designed by a diabetic for diabetics.*

GLUCOGRAF II data sheets are printed identically on both sides so that each page provides space for two weeks' worth of data. If your physician wants detailed information about the content of each of your meals, use one side to list meal content and the reverse to list medication, blood sugars, exercise, and the times of your meals. The data sheet is designed

---

* GLUCOGRAF® is a registered trademark owned by Richard K. Bernstein, M.D. The data sheet form is protected by U.S. copyright, and may not be reproduced for sale without permission of the author. Readers of this book who wish to have some practice copies for immediate use may make photocopies of the form, which is reproduced at a reduced size on the next page in order to make it fit into this book. Any photocopying shop can enlarge the page in order to provide you with standard, 8½ x 11 sheets. Pads containing enough pages to cover one year can be ordered by phone from Harrison Chemists (800) 829-1493. 7/21/05 No longer carried

877-987-6882 Trotta

GlucograF II DATA SHEET

NAME

DATA TO REMEMBER

TARGET BG

DOCTOR'S PHONE

USUAL DOSES OF INSULIN OR ORAL AGENT
Upon Arising
Min. before bkfst.
Min. before lunch
Min. before dinner
Min. before snacks
At Bedtime

1 Unit H will Lower Blood Sugar _____ mg/dl

MISCELLANEOUS

BG EFFECTS OF SWEETS (mg/dl)

1 gm CHO ⟶

EXERCISE ADJUSTMENTS

WEIGHT PLAN

ABBREVIATIONS
CHO- Carbohydrate
PRO- Protein
H- Humalog Insulin
R- Regular Insulin
L- Lente Insulin
UL- Ultralente Insulin
B- Breakfast
L- Lunch
S- Supper
SN- Snack
IM- Intramuscular
SC- Subcutaneous

DATE WEEK BEGINS ___/___/___

	SUNDAY			MONDAY			TUESDAY			WEDNESDAY			THURSDAY			FRIDAY			SATURDAY		
	TIME	BLOOD SUGAR	MEDICATION EXERCISE, FOOD, etc.	TIME	BLOOD SUGAR	MEDICATION EXERCISE, FOOD, etc.	TIME	BLOOD SUGAR	MEDICATION EXERCISE, FOOD, etc.	TIME	BLOOD SUGAR	MEDICATION EXERCISE, FOOD, etc.	TIME	BLOOD SUGAR	MEDICATION EXERCISE, FOOD, etc.	TIME	BLOOD SUGAR	MEDICATION EXERCISE, FOOD, etc.	TIME	BLOOD SUGAR	MEDICATION EXERCISE, FOOD, etc.
1 AM THRU 6 AM																					
6 AM THRU 9 AM																					
9 AM THRU 12 NOON																					
12 NOON THRU 3 PM																					
3 PM THRU 6 PM																					
6 PM THRU 9 PM																					
9 PM THRU 1 AM																					

so that you can fold it up and carry it with you. I also recommend carrying a fine-point pen with you as well. It will help when space is tight — which is likely, particularly in the MEDICATION, EXERCISE, FOOD, ETC. column, where much information must be written in a small space.

The rest of this chapter is divided into sections corresponding to column and field headings on the GLUCOGRAF II form, and explains the sorts of things you ought to be recording and the most informative ways for doing so.

DATA FIELDS

Across the top of the data sheet, there are several fields with space for entering important data.

DOCTOR'S PHONE. This field should contain the telephone number at which you can reach your physician when you are asked to phone in blood sugar and other data. If you will be faxing your data sheets, enter your physician's fax number as well.

TARGET BG. This is the blood sugar goal that your physician will assign and that you will try to maintain. Although normal is approximately 85–90 mg/dl, in certain instances your physician may opt for a higher value for a brief period. If you've endured very high blood sugar (BG, for "blood glucose") levels for an extended period of time, your physician will not instantly try to normalize your blood sugars, as you may at first feel uncomfortable (hypoglycemic) in a normal range. If you take insulin, he'll assign a series of intermediate "target ranges" together with instructions for correcting blood sugars to reach this level as you work toward blood sugar normalization. If your initial blood sugars show that you are in the 300–400 mg/dl range, he might set a target of, say, 175 mg/dl for a brief period of time.

USUAL DOSES OF INSULIN OR ORAL AGENT. If you require insulin or an oral hypoglycemic agent* to maintain your target range, you will

---

* Oral hypoglycemic agents are blood sugar–lowering pills. They are discussed in detail in Chapter 14.

have to follow a precise regimen. It will therefore be important to have your medications spelled out so that even if you forget, you can always refer to the doses and times in this field. If your physician asks you to change the dose of one of your blood sugar–lowering medications, put a line through the prior dosage and enter the new dose to the right of the old one, as in the following example:

```
┌──────────────────────────────────────────────────────────┐
│ USUAL DOSES OF INSULIN OR ORAL AGENT                     │
│ Upon Arising ̶2̶U̶L̶  1½ UL _____          │
│ _____Min. before bkfst. _____        │
│ _____Min. before lunch _____         │
│  90  Min. before dinner ̶3̶x̶5̶0̶0̶M̶E̶T̶  2x500 MET ___          │
│ _____Min. before snacks _____        │
│ At Bedtime _____              │
└──────────────────────────────────────────────────────────┘
```

In this fictitious example, the patient had been injecting 2 units of ultralente insulin on arising when this data sheet was started. In addition to insulin, he had been taking three 500 mg tablets of metformin (an oral hypoglycemic agent) 90 minutes before dinner. During the week the sheet covers, his dose of insulin on arising was reduced to 1½ units and his dose of metformin before dinner was reduced to two 500 mg tablets. Retaining the old doses in this field can give your physician an important at-a-glance history of the changes that were made.

1 UNIT H WILL LOWER BLOOD SUGAR. This field is for use only by people who take insulin. Humalog lispro insulin (H) is a fast-acting insulin that we use for the rapid lowering of elevated blood sugars. It is the fastest-acting insulin we have. In Chapter 18, we'll discuss guidelines for calibrating the effect that 1 unit of Humalog insulin will have upon you. Meanwhile, enter on the form the amount of blood sugar reduction that your physician suggests will be achieved by injecting 1 unit.

MISCELLANEOUS. This field is for any other pertinent guidelines or instructions you may have difficulty recalling. Some people enter the times they should check their blood sugars. Thus you might write:

✓ BG on arising,
2 hr post meals,
bedtime

BG EFFECTS OF SWEETS. If you use insulin or oral hypoglycemic agents, you will be taught how to use glucose tablets to raise your blood sugar rapidly. In Chapter 19, we'll discuss how you will calibrate the effect that 1 tablet has on your blood sugar. Thus, if 1 Dextrotab raises your blood sugar 8 mg/dl, you would write:

1 DT → ↑8

Alternately, if your brand of glucose tablet is Wacky Wafers (which might raise your blood sugar 10 mg/dl), you could write:

1 WW → ↑10

You will also learn to calibrate the effect 1 gram of carbohydrate has on your blood sugar. If 1 gram will raise your blood sugar 5 mg/dl, you would write:

1 gm CHO → ↑5

EXERCISE ADJUSTMENTS. This field is also used only if you use insulin or oral hypoglycemic agents. It reminds you what to eat for various forms of exercise to prevent your blood sugar from dropping too low. Thus, if you were planning to spend the afternoon at a shopping mall (which can be treacherous, because this often requires considerably more walking than we realize), you may be advised to eat half a slice of bread at the start of every hour to keep your blood sugar from falling too low. Thus, you might write:

Shopping Mall — ½ brd/hr

WEIGHT PLAN. If a portion of your treatment plan involves a diet regimen that you and your physician have negotiated (for weight loss or gain), you would enter the guidelines for it in this field. Thus, to remind yourself that your goal is to lose 1 pound weekly and that your weight should be checked every Sunday, you might write:

↓1 lb/wk, ✓ Sun

ABBREVIATIONS. Space constraints make it necessary to use abbreviations. You may be tempted to use your own, but in order to avoid confusion, I recommend using the short list of standardized abbreviations provided in the top right-hand corner of the data sheet. Using these abbreviations will help both you and your physician to know immediately the details of "events" that affect your blood sugar.

DAY-BY-DAY RECORD OF EVENTS

As you can see, each day is broken up horizontally into three columns — TIME; BLOOD SUGAR; and MEDICATION, EXERCISE, FOOD, ETC. Vertically, each column is broken up into 3-hour blocks, except the 9 PM THRU 1 AM and 1 AM THRU 6 AM blocks. During each day, you will experience various "events" involving your blood sugar. An event may be a meal, a dose of medication, exercise, or even a blood sugar measurement itself. These should be recorded in the corresponding time block. You needn't record a dose of medication that does not affect your blood sugar levels, such as blood pressure medication.

TIME. In this column, write the exact time of the event. If you measure your blood sugar at 1:30 P.M. on Tuesday, write 1:30 in the 12 NOON THRU 3 PM block of the time column for Tuesday.

BLOOD SUGAR. In this column, write all blood sugar readings. If for some reason you do not have your blood sugar meter with you (a minor crime) and you experience symptoms suggestive of low blood sugar (see Chapter 19), write "low" in this column in the appropriate time block and proceed with the instructions for correcting low blood sugar in Chapters 18 and 19.

MEDICATION, EXERCISE, FOOD, ETC. This column is a catchall where you should record all events other than blood sugar readings. Following are a few examples of events and how you would record them in abbreviated form in the proper block:

Injected 5 units of ultralente insulin	5 UL
Ate breakfast	B
Consumed more protein at dinner than prescribed	DIN — ↑PRO

Took 3 Dextrotabs (glucose tablets)	3 DT
Took two 500 mg Glucophage (metformin) pills	2 × 500 MET
Walked 2 miles	Walk 2 mi
Went shopping for 3 hours	Shop 3 hr
Injected 1½ units Humalog insulin, intramuscularly (into a muscle)	1½ H — IM
Sore throat all day	Sore throat [enter at the top of the days' column]
Went to dentist	Dentist

UNUSUAL OR UNEXPECTED BLOOD SUGAR VALUES

Once your blood sugars have been fine-tuned on one of the regimens described in this book, we expect that they will remain within narrow limits of your target value most of the time. There will, in all likelihood, be instances when your blood sugars will deviate from your target range.

Show What Caused Blood Sugars to Deviate

Sometimes you may stick precisely to your diet and medication plan, but find yourself in a restaurant and simply incapable of letting the dessert cart go by without partaking of its wonders. Your blood sugars will naturally show a precipitous rise. Or you may get some exercise that makes blood sugar go too low. To make it easy for both you and your physician to understand and evaluate this connection, circle the cause, then circle the resulting blood sugar value, and connect the two circles with a line. For example, a high morning blood sugar might be circled and connected to "chocolate mousse" at bedtime the previous night.

Circle Puzzling Blood Sugar Values

Sometimes, even though you stuck to your regimen with an iron will, your data will show an unexpectedly high or low blood sugar value. Circle this value, as it may require further investigation. There are several strange biologic phenomena that affect your blood sugar, which are detailed in the next chapter. Your physician or diabetes educator should help you figure out the cause of unexpected blood sugar readings so that you can prevent or anticipate them in the future.

Now that you have been exposed to blood sugar self-monitoring and the recording of data, you can begin using this knowledge to normalize your blood sugars.

6

Strange Biology:

PHENOMENA PECULIAR TO DIABETES
THAT CAN AFFECT BLOOD SUGAR

Sometimes, when you think you're doing everything right, your blood sugars may not respond as you expect. Often this will be due to one or more of the biologic curiosities that affect diabetics. The purpose of this chapter is to acquaint you with some real phenomena that can confound your plans, but which you can frequently circumvent if you are aware of them.

DIMINISHED PHASE I INSULIN RESPONSE

Figure 1-2, page 43, illustrates the normal, nondiabetic blood insulin response to a meal containing carbohydrate and protein. When glucose from dietary carbohydrate enters the bloodstream, beta cells of the pancreas respond — or should respond — immediately by releasing stored insulin granules. These granules may have been stored for many hours in anticipation of what is known as a glucose challenge. This rapid release is called phase I insulin response.

The nondiabetic body will utilize this immediate influx of insulin to prevent blood sugar from increasing significantly. As we discussed in Chapter 1, one of the hallmarks of Type II diabetes is the diminished ability to do this. Therefore, blood sugars will shoot up after eating (carbohydrates in particular) and will be brought back into line only slowly by phase II insulin response (the release of newly manufactured insulin). This blood sugar rise can be prevented, primarily by diet, if you understand what's happening and to what degree you're affected.

A possible but unproven explanation for this abnormality is that the beta cells are still capable of making insulin, but not capable of storing it. In this model, insulin would be released as soon as it is made. This inability to store insulin could also explain the inappropriate release of insulin that often occurs when blood sugar is already low in very early Type II diabetes. An alternate explanation is that the sensitivity of the beta cells to changes in the blood sugar diminishes, so that they respond inadequately to such changes.

GLUCONEOGENESIS, THE DAWN PHENOMENON, AND DELAYED STOMACH-EMPTYING

You may begin to notice as you regularly monitor your blood sugars that your fasting blood glucose on waking in the morning is considerably higher than it was when you went to bed, even though you didn't get up for a midnight snack. There are three common causes for this: gluconeogenesis, the dawn phenomenon, and gastroparesis (delayed stomach-emptying).

Gluconeogenesis

Gluconeogenesis, which we discussed briefly in Chapter 1, is the mechanism by which the liver converts amino acids into glucose. Dietary protein is not the only source of amino acids. Your muscles and other tissues continually receive amino acids from and return them to the bloodstream. This constant flux ensures that amino acids are always available in the blood for conversion to glucose by the liver or to protein by the muscles and vital organs. Some diabetics still make adequate insulin to prevent gluconeogenesis. However, once your insulin production drops below a certain level, your liver will inappropriately produce glucose and thus raise your blood sugar even while you're fasting.

In all likelihood, you won't be able to control this phenomenon by diet alone, particularly if you're a Type I diabetic or an obese Type II who's insulin-resistant. (Remember, high triglyceride levels in the bloodstream can make the liver insulin-resistant, and the more obese you happen to be, the more insulin-resistant you will be.) Appropriate weight loss and vigorous exercise may be the most help in improving the sensitivity of the liver to whatever insulin remains. The most reliable treatments will involve medication, either certain oral hypoglycemic agents or insulin. If you're obese, however, large doses of insulin can make you more obese and more resistant to insulin. So a primary goal should be to bring your weight into line.

The Dawn Phenomenon

As you know, I'm a Type I diabetic. I no longer make any insulin at all. If I decide to fast for 24 hours — eat absolutely nothing — I will need to inject 4 units of long-acting insulin in the morning to prevent gluconeogenesis for 18 hours. If I check my blood sugar every few hours, it will remain constant, confirming that the insulin is suppressing gluconeogenesis.

If, 18 hours after my first injection — and while still fasting — I inject another 4 units of insulin, common sense would maintain that this second dose should suppress gluconeogenesis overnight.

So I go to sleep and awaken 9–10 hours later. On arising, I check my blood sugar. Instead of being constant, as it was during my waking hours, it's now 20–100 mg/dl higher than it was at bedtime.

If I were to try the same experiment a week later, I'd experience about the same overnight rise in blood sugar. Why?

Although the mechanics of the dawn phenomenon aren't yet entirely clear, research suggests that the liver deactivates more circulating insulin during the early morning hours. It doesn't matter whether you made the insulin yourself or injected it; the liver has no preference.

Investigators have actually measured blood sugar every hour throughout the night under similar circumstances. They find that the entire blood sugar increase occurs about 6–10 hours after bedtime for most people who are so affected. That doesn't mean, however, that you should sleep only 5½ hours a night to try to avoid it. Both the time it takes for blood sugar to increase and the amount of the increase vary from one person to another. An increase may be negligible in some and profound in others. This is one of many reasons why any truly workable program for blood sugar normalization must be tailored to the individual.

Though it is more apparent in Type I diabetics, many Type II diabetics also show signs of the dawn phenomenon. As you will see, the treatments described in this book take this phenomenon into account.

Gastroparesis

This phenomenon has a chapter all its own (Chapter 21) and we will discuss it there in detail. However, it's important to mention it in any list of factors that can lead to puzzling blood sugar readings.

Most people who've had long-standing diabetes develop some degree of damage to the nerves that govern the muscles of the stomach and intestines. *Gastroparesis diabeticorum* (the weak or paralyzed stomach of diabetics) is caused by many years of elevated blood sugars. If you're Type I, or a Type II who isn't making significant amounts of insulin, it can have unpredictable effects on blood sugar.

Like diabetes itself, gastroparesis can be mild or severe. In extreme cases, people may walk around for days with constipation and bulging stomachs. More common, however, is mild gastroparesis in which physical symptoms are not apparent but blood sugars are affected.

The big problems with gastroparesis arise if you're taking medication that lowers blood sugar. If you take your insulin or pill before a meal to cover a rise in blood sugar, but the meal remains in your stomach and your blood sugar doesn't rise as predicted, the medication can take your blood sugar dangerously low. I know three individuals who experienced daily episodes of unconsciousness and seizures for several years before I met them and diagnosed this condition.

There are, however, ways of controlling blood sugars in spite of the unpredictability of this condition, and these are discussed in Chapter 21, "Delayed Stomach-Emptying."

STRESS AND BLOOD SUGAR

Sustained Emotional Stress

For years, many physicians have blamed stress for the frequent unexplained blood sugar variations that many patients experience. This is a problematic diagnosis: it puts the responsibility for unexplained variations in blood sugar on the patient's shoulders and leaves the physician with no obligation to examine the treatment regimen. Certainly there is no question that stress can have adverse effects on your health. I have reviewed hundreds of thousands of blood sugar entries from many patients, including myself. One common feature of all this data is that most emotional stress rarely has a *direct* effect upon blood sugar. This kind of stress can, however, have a secondary effect by precipitating overeating, binge eating, or indulgence in kinds of eating that will increase blood sugar.

I know many diabetics who've been involved in stressful marriages, divorces, loss of a business, death of a close relative, and the countless other sustained stresses of life we all must endure. These stresses have one thing in common: they aren't sudden but usually last many hours, days, or even years. I have yet to see such a situation directly cause blood sugar to increase — or, for that matter, decrease. An important thing to remember during sustained periods of life when everything seems out of control is that at least you *can* control one thing: your blood sugar.

Adrenaline Surges

Many patients have reported sudden blood sugar spurts after brief episodes of severe stress. Examples have included an automobile accident without physical injury; speaking in front of a large audience; taking very important exams in school; and having arguments that nearly become violent. I am occasionally interviewed on television, and I always check — and, if necessary, adjust — my blood sugar immediately before and after such appearances. My blood sugar inevitably increases 75–100 mg/dl, even though on the surface I may appear relaxed. As a rule of thumb, from personal experience and from observing my patients, I would say that if an acute event is stressful enough to start your epinephrine (adrenaline) flowing, as indicated by rapid heart rate and tremors, it is likely to raise your blood sugar. Epinephrine is one of the counterregulatory hormones that cause the liver to convert stored glycogen to glucose. This is part of what is often called the "fight or flight" response, your body's attempt to provide you with enough extra energy either to overcome an enemy or run like heck to get away. Type II diabetics who make a lot of insulin are less likely to have their blood sugar reflect acute stress than are those who make little or none.

An occasional blood sugar increase after a very stressful event may well have been brought on by the event. On the other hand, unexplained blood sugar increases extending for days or weeks can rarely be properly attributed to stress. I know of no instances where emotional stress caused abnormally *low* blood sugars in diabetic or nondiabetic individuals. Therefore, if you experience a prolonged unexplained change in your blood sugar levels after extended periods of normal blood sugars, it is wise to seek out a cause other than emotional stress.

Infection

A third important category of stress is infection, which can frequently raise blood sugar. A kidney infection, for example, can triple insulin requirements overnight. When blood sugar rises unexpectedly after weeks of normal values, it is wise to suspect infection. I have noted that my own blood sugars rise 24 hours before the onset of a sore throat or cold.

General Anesthesia

If not treated with special dosing of insulin, Type I and most Type II diabetics will experience a blood sugar increase during surgery that is accompanied by general anesthesia.

INSULIN RESISTANCE

Insulin's ability to facilitate the transport of glucose from the blood into liver, muscle, fat, and other cells is impaired as blood sugar rises. This reduced effectiveness of insulin, known as insulin resistance, has been attributed to a phenomenon called postreceptor defects in glucose utilization. If, for example, 1 unit of injected or self-made insulin will lower your blood sugar from 130 to 90 mg/dl, you may need 3 units to lower it from 430 to 390 mg/dl.

Consider again what might happen if I, a Type I diabetic, am fasting and inject just enough long-acting insulin to keep my blood sugar at 90 mg/dl for 12 hours. If I eat 8 grams of glucose — enough to raise my blood sugar to 130 mg/dl — the chances are that my blood sugar won't just rise to 130 mg/dl and remain there. It will continue to rise slowly throughout the day, so that 12 hours after I take the insulin, my blood sugar may actually be at 165 mg/dl. Insulin resistance, at least for Type I diabetics, occurs as blood sugar increases, and so elevated blood sugar should be corrected as soon as it's feasible. Delay will only permit it to rise higher. Because Type II's still produce some insulin, their bodies are more likely to correct the blood sugar rise automatically.

THE CHINESE RESTAURANT EFFECT

Many years ago a patient asked me why her blood sugar went from 90 mg/dl up to 300 mg/dl every afternoon after she went swimming. I

[handwritten margin note: insulin's effective-ness is impaired by high blood sugar values!]

asked what she ate before the swim. "Nothing, just a freebie," she replied. As it turned out, the "freebie" was lettuce. When I asked her just how much lettuce she was eating before her swims, she replied, "A head."

A head of lettuce contains about 10 grams of carbohydrate, which can raise a Type I adult's blood sugar about 50 mg/dl at most. So what accounts for the other 160 mg/dl rise in her blood sugar?

The explanation lies in what I call the Chinese Restaurant Effect. Often Chinese meals contain *large amounts* of protein or slow-acting, low-carbohydrate foods such as bean sprouts, bok choy, mushrooms, bamboo shoots, and water chestnuts, that can make you feel full.

How can these low-carbohydrate foods affect blood sugar so dramatically?

The upper part of the small intestine contains cells that release hormones into the bloodstream when they are stretched, as after a large meal. These hormones signal the pancreas to produce some insulin to prevent the blood sugar rise that might otherwise follow the digestion of a large meal. Since a very small amount of insulin released by the pancreas can cause a large drop in blood sugar, the pancreas simultaneously produces the less potent hormone glucagon to offset the potential excess effect of the insulin. If you're diabetic and deficient in producing insulin, you might not release insulin, but you will still release glucagon, which will cause gluconeogenesis and glycogenolysis and thereby raise your blood sugar. Thus, if you eat enough to feel stuffed, your blood sugar can go up even if you eat something undigestible, such as sawdust. The lesson here is: *Don't stuff yourself.*

THE EFFECTS OF EXERCISE UPON BLOOD SUGAR

Exercise can have varying effects upon blood sugar, depending upon a number of variables, including the type of exercise, how vigorously it's performed, and what type of medication you are using, if any. These effects are too varied and numerous to discuss in this brief space. Please see Chapter 13, "Using Exercise to Enhance Insulin Sensitivity," if you are embarking on an exercise program or find your blood sugars unpredictably affected by your existing exercise program.

THE HONEYMOON PERIOD

At the time they are diagnosed, Type I diabetics usually have experienced very high blood sugars that cause a host of unpleasant symptoms, such as weight loss, frequent urination, and severe thirst. These symptoms subside soon after treatment with injected insulin begins. After a few weeks of insulin therapy, many patients experience a dramatic reduction of insulin requirements, almost as if the diabetes were reversing. Blood sugars may become nearly normal, even with low insulin doses. This benign "honeymoon period" may last weeks, months, or even as long as a year. If the medical treatment is conventional, the honeymoon period eventually terminates and the well-known roller coaster of blood sugar swings ensues.

Why doesn't the honeymoon period last forever? My belief is that it can, *with proper treatment.* But there are several likely reasons why it does not with conventional treatment. At this writing, however, they still remain speculative.

- The normal human pancreas contains many more insulin-producing beta cells than are necessary for maintaining normal blood sugars. For diabetes to appear, at least 80 percent of the beta cells must have been destroyed. In early Type I diabetes, many of the remaining 20 percent have been weakened by constant high blood sugars and overwork. They can recover if given a rest with the help of injected insulin. Even if they recover, however, they still must work at least five times as hard to match the job of a normal pancreas working at 100 percent capacity. Eventually, with conventional treatment, this overwork causes them to break down.
- It is now believed that high blood glucose levels are toxic to beta cells. Even a brief blood sugar increase after a high-carbohydrate meal may take a small toll. Over a period of time, the cumulative effect may wipe them out completely.
- The autoimmune attack upon beta cells, the presumed cause of Type I diabetes, is focused upon several proteins. One is insulin, and another is present on the special vesicles — or bubbles — that are formed at the outer membrane of the beta cell. These vesicles contain insulin. Normally, they burst at the surface of the cell, releasing insulin granules into the bloodstream. The more vesicles

created and the more insulin manufactured, the greater the auto-immune attack upon the beta cell.

Based upon my experience with the fair number of Type I diabetics I've treated from the time of diagnosis, I'm convinced that the honeymoon period can be prolonged indefinitely. The trick is to assist the pancreas and keep it as quiescent as possible. With the meticulous use of small doses of injected insulin and with the essential use of a very low carbohydrate diet, the remaining capacity of the pancreas, I believe, can be preserved.

7

The Laws of Small Numbers

"**B**ig inputs make big mistakes; small inputs make small mistakes." That is the first thing my friend Kanji Ishikawa says to himself each morning on arising. It is his mantra, the single most important thing he knows about diabetes.

Kanji is the oldest surviving Type I diabetic in Japan (he is, by the way, younger than I, but afflicted with numerous long-term diabetic complications because of many years of uncontrolled blood sugars).

Many biological and mechanical systems respond in a predictable way to small inputs but in a chaotic and considerably less predictable way to large inputs. Consider for a moment traffic. Put a small number of automobiles on a given stretch of highway, and traffic acts in a predictable fashion: cars can maintain speed, enter and merge into open spaces, and exit with a minimum of danger. There's room for error. Double the number of cars, and the risks don't just double, they increase geometrically. Triple or quadruple the number of cars, and the unpredictability of a safe trip increases exponentially.

The name of the game for the diabetic in achieving blood sugar normalization is *predictability*. It's very difficult to use medications safely unless you can predict the effect they'll have. You can't normalize blood sugar unless you can predict the effects of what you're eating.

If you can't accurately predict your blood sugar levels, then you can't accurately predict your insulin needs. If the kinds of foods you're eating give you continuously unpredictable blood sugar levels, then it will be impossible to normalize blood sugars.

One of the prime intents of this book is to give you the information you need to learn how to predict your blood sugar levels, and to learn how to ensure that your predictions will be accurate. Here the Laws of Small Numbers are exceedingly important.

Predictability. How do you achieve it?

THE LAW OF CARBOHYDRATE ESTIMATION

The old ADA dietary recommendations allowed 150 grams of carbohydrate per meal. This, as you may know by now, is grossly excessive. Here is one reason why.

Typically, 150 grams of carbohydrate would be a good-sized bowl of cooked pasta. Let's say that you're a whiz at estimating the amount of carbohydrate in the pasta and can usually estimate it to within 20 percent from one day to the next. Twenty percent of 150 grams is 30 grams of carbohydrate. Now, if you're a nonobese Type I diabetic who makes no insulin, 1 gram of carbohydrate will raise your blood sugars by about 5 mg/dl. So, even with your finely tuned ability to "guesstimate" the amount of carbohydrate, your blood sugar is off by a whopping ±150 mg/dl for just this one meal. If your target blood sugar level is approximately 85 mg/dl, you've now got a blood glucose level of 235 mg/dl, or, alternately, 0 mg/dl. Either situation is clearly unacceptable. If a 20 percent margin of error is your average, then there will be some days you're off by only 10 percent, but others when you're off by 30 percent.

Let's try another example. Say you're a Type II diabetic, obese, and make some insulin of your own but also inject insulin. You've found that 1 gram of carbohydrate only raises your blood sugar by 3 mg/dl. Your blood sugar would be off by ±90 mg/dl. If your target blood sugar value is, say, 90 mg/dl, you're looking at a postmeal blood sugar level of anywhere from 180 mg/dl to 0 mg/dl.

That's the chief problem with the old ADA diet. Big inputs. But if you can eat food that will affect your blood sugar by one-tenth of that margin of error, then you're going to have a much simpler time of normalizing blood sugar levels. My diet plan, which we will get into in Chapters 9–11, aims to keep these margins in the realm of about 10–20 mg/dl. How do we accomplish this? Small inputs.

Eating only a half-cup of pasta is not the answer. Even small amounts of some carbohydrate can cause big swings in blood sugar. And anyway, who would feel satisfied after a meal of a half-cup of pasta? The key is to eat foods that will affect your blood sugar in a very small way.

Small inputs, small mistakes. Sounds so simple and straightforward, so elegant, it may make you want to ask why no one has told you about it before.

Say that instead of eating pasta as the carbohydrate portion of your meal, you eat salad. If you estimate 2 cups of salad at 12 grams of carbohydrate and are off not by your usual 20 percent but by 30 percent, that's still only four grams of carbohydrate — a maximum potential 20 mg/dl rise or fall in blood sugar. A bowl of pasta for a couple of cups of *salad?* Not much of a trade, you may say. Well, we don't intend that you starve. As you decrease the amount of fast-acting carbohydrate you eat, you can often simultaneously increase the amount of protein you eat. Protein can, as you may recall, also cause a blood sugar rise, but this takes place much more slowly, to a much smaller degree, and is more easily prevented with medication.

In theory, you could weigh everything you eat right down to the last gram and make your calculations based on information provided by the manufacturer or derived from some of the books we use. Still, there are problems with that approach. Say you weigh dried pasta — the manufacturer's estimate of how much carbohydrate exists in a serving is exactly that, an estimate, with a margin for error. The Food and Drug Administration allows for a margin of error in labeling. And there are other variables — some pastas are made with egg yolks and wheat flour, some with water and durum semolina flour. If the manufacturer's estimate proves to be off by 20 percent, and then your estimate is off by 20 percent, you're in a realm of complete unknown. You will have only a vague idea of what you're actually consuming, and of the effect it will have on blood sugar.

The idea here is to stick with low levels of carbohydrates. In addition, stick with foods that will make you feel satisfied without causing huge swings in blood sugar. Simple.

THE LAW OF INSULIN DOSE ABSORPTION

If you do not take insulin, you can skip this section.

Think again of traffic. You're driving down the road and your car drifts slightly toward the median. To bring it back into line, you make a slight adjustment of the steering wheel. No problem. But yank the steering wheel, and it could carry you into another lane, or could send you careening off the road.

When you inject insulin, not all of it reaches your bloodstream. Research has shown that there's a level of uncertainty as to just how much absorption of insulin takes place. The more insulin you use, the greater the level of uncertainty.

When you inject insulin, you're putting beneath your skin a substance that isn't, according to your immune system's way of seeing things, supposed to be there. So a portion of it will be destroyed as a foreign substance before it can reach the bloodstream. The amount that the body can destroy depends on several factors. First is how big a dose you inject. The bigger the dose, the more inflammation and irritation you cause, and the more of a "red flag" you send up to your immune system. Other factors include how deep you injected it, how fast you injected it, and where you injected it.

Your injections will naturally vary from one time to the next. Even the most fastidious person will unconsciously alter minor things in the injection process from day to day. So the amount of insulin that gets into your bloodstream is always going to have some variability. The bigger the dose, the bigger the variation.

A number of years ago, researchers at the University of Minnesota demonstrated that if you inject about 20 units of insulin into your arm, on average, you'll get a 39 percent variation in the amount that makes it into the bloodstream from one day to the next. They found that abdominal injections had only a 29 percent average variation, and so recommended that we use only abdominal injections. On paper that seems fine, but in practice the effects on blood sugar are intolerable.

Say you do inject 20 units of insulin at one time. Each unit lowers the blood sugar of a typical 150-pound adult by 40 mg/dl. A 29 percent variability will create a 7-unit discrepancy in your 20-unit injection, which means a 280 mg/dl blood sugar uncertainty (40 mg/dl x 7 units). The result is totally haphazard blood sugars and complete unpredictability, just by virtue of the different amounts of insulin absorption.

Research and my own experience demonstrate that the smaller your dose of insulin, the less variability you get. For Type I diabetics who are not obese, we'd ideally like to see doses anywhere from ½ unit to 6 units or at the most 7. Typically, you might take 3–5 units in a shot. At these lower doses, the uncertainty of absorption approaches zero.

I have a very obese patient who requires 27 units of long-acting insulin at bedtime. He's so insulin-resistant that there's no way to keep his blood sugar under control without this massive dose. In order to ameliorate the unpredictability of large doses, he splits his bedtime insulin into four small shots given into four separate sites using the same disposable syringe. As a rule, I recommend that a single insulin injection not exceed 7 units.

THE LAW OF INSULIN TIMING

Again, it's very difficult to use any medication safely unless you can predict the effect it will have. With insulin, this is as true of *when* you take it as it is of how much you take. If you're a Type I diabetic, fast-acting (regular) insulin can be injected 30–40 minutes prior to a meal tailored to your diet plan to cover the ensuing rise in blood sugar. Regular, fast-acting insulin, despite the name, doesn't act very fast, and cannot come close to approximating the phase I insulin response of a nondiabetic. To a lesser degree this is also true of the new, faster-acting lispro insulin. Still, these are the fastest we have. Small doses of regular start to work in about 40 minutes and finish in about 5 hours; lispro starts to work in about 15 minutes and finishes in 4–5 hours. This is considerably slower than the speed at which fast-acting carbohydrate raises blood sugar.

If you eat a meal not specifically tailored to our restricted-carbohydrate diet, you'll get a postprandial increase in blood sugar, eventually followed by a decrease as the fast-acting insulin catches up. This means that you'll have high blood sugars after every meal, and you could still fall prey to the long-term complications of diabetes. If you try to prevent the inevitable postprandial blood sugar spike by waiting to eat until after the start-time of your insulin, you may easily make yourself hypoglycemic, which could in turn cause you to overcompensate and overeat — that is, presuming you don't lose consciousness first.

Type II diabetics have a diminished or absent phase I insulin response, and so they face a problem similar to that of Type I's. They have to wait hours for the phase II insulin to catch up if they eat fast-acting carbohydrate.

The key to timing insulin injection is to know how carbohydrates and insulin affect your blood sugar and to use that knowledge to minimize the swings. Since you can't approximate phase I insulin response, you have to eat foods that allow you to work within the limits of the insulin you make or inject. (If you think you'll miss out on the great high-carbohydrate, low-fat diet many have been raving about, there is considerable evidence that restricting carbohydrate is healthier not only for diabetics but for everyone. See *Protein Power,* by Michael and Mary Dan Eades, Bantam Books, 1996, for more details on this point.)

If you consume only *small amounts* of slow-acting carbohydrate, you can actually prevent postprandial blood sugar elevation even with injected regular insulin. In fact, by restricting carbohydrate intake, many Type II diabetics will be able to prevent this rise with their phase II insulin response, and will not need preprandial (premeal) injected insulin.

OBEYING THE LAWS OF SMALL NUMBERS

Essential to "obeying" the laws of small numbers is to eat only small amounts of slow-acting carbohydrate when you eat carbohydrate, and no fast-acting carbohydrate. Even the slowest-acting carbohydrate can outpace injected or phase II insulin if consumed in greater amounts than recommended later in this book (Chapters 10 and 11).

If you eat a small amount of slow-acting carbohydrate, you might get by with a very small postprandial blood sugar increase. If you double the amount of slow-acting carbohydrate, you'll double the potential increase in blood sugar (and remember that high blood sugar leads to even higher blood sugar). If you *fill up* on slow-acting carbohydrate, it will work as fast as a lesser amount of fast-acting carbohydrate, and if you feel stuffed, you'll compound it with the Chinese Restaurant Effect.

All of this not only points toward eating less carbohydrate, it also implies eating smaller meals 4 or 5 times a day rather than three large meals. If you're a Type II diabetic and require no medication, eating like this may work well for you. The difficulty with this sort of plan is its inconvenience, but some people don't mind and actually prefer to eat this way. I have one patient, a Type I diabetic who still makes some insulin. She eats a couple of bites of protein every 15 minutes and takes long-acting insulin. In a 16-hour day, that adds up to a lot of meals and a lot of clock-watching. This routine would drive a lot of people nuts, but it works for her. As long as she keeps up with her frequent little meals and covers the insulin, she's fine. If she misses a few "meals," there could be trouble.

For the Type II diabetic who doesn't need insulin injections, smaller meals throughout the day can be a very effective way of maintaining a constant level of blood sugar. Since this kind of diet would be tailored to work with a phase II insulin response, blood sugars should never go too high. It would, however, involve a certain amount of daily preparation and routinization that could be thrown off by changes in schedule — illness, travel, houseguests, and so forth. (People with gastroparesis, or delayed stomach-emptying, may *have* to eat this way. We discuss this phenomenon further in Chapter 21.)

PART TWO

Treatment

8

Establishing a Treatment Plan:

THE BASIC TREATMENT PLANS
AND HOW WE STRUCTURE THEM

Now that you know the different factors that can affect blood sugar levels, we can begin to discuss treatment plans. Blood sugar normalization for most diabetics can be achieved through one of four basic plans. Although there are only two major types of diabetes — Type I and Type II — there are so many variations, particularly in Type II, that a treatment plan that works for one diabetic won't necessarily work for another. Each plan has to be tailored to the individual.

The basic treatment plans increase in complexity with the severity of the disease.

For Type II diabetes

Level 1: Diet (and appropriate weight loss)*
Level 2: Diet (and appropriate weight loss) *plus* exercise
Level 3: Diet (and appropriate weight loss) *plus* exercise *plus* an oral hypoglycemic agent
Level 4: Diet (and appropriate weight loss) *plus* exercise *plus* insulin injections, with or without an oral hypoglycemic agent

For Type I diabetes

Same as level 4 above, with the addition of multiple daily insulin injections, with questionable benefit from exercise in controlling blood sugars, and with rare benefit from oral hypoglycemic agents

---

* Since 80 percent or more of Type II diabetics are overweight, weight loss should be an important part of treatment for the majority.

STRUCTURING A TREATMENT PLAN

What are normal blood sugar levels? What range do we find in nondiabetics? The answers depend upon whom you ask. I've seen figures in the scientific literature over the years ranging anywhere from 60 to 140 mg/dl. My experience checking random blood sugar readings on nonobese nondiabetics, as well as figures from large population studies, tells me that for most nondiabetics, blood sugar levels cover a pretty narrow range of about 80–95 mg/dl (by finger stick), except after meals containing large amounts of sweets.

I usually select a target of 90 mg/dl for most of my patients who take insulin or oral hypoglycemic agents. This target is not an average, but one we try to maintain 24 hours a day. If your blood sugars are bouncing back and forth between 60 and 140 mg/dl, you're still on the roller coaster. Our object is to find a treatment plan that will get you off the roller coaster and keep you off.

For those who can be treated by diet or by diet and exercise alone, I set a target of 85–90 mg/dl. This assumes that you're comfortable at such levels, that is, not experiencing symptoms of low blood sugars.

One of the most important considerations in setting up an *initial* target is that people who have had high blood sugar levels for many months or years usually experience unpleasant symptoms of hypoglycemia as blood sugars approach normal. Someone who has grown accustomed to blood sugars consistently over 300 mg/dl may feel "shaky" at 100 mg/dl. In such a case, we might start with 160 mg/dl as the initial target. We'd then lower the target to its ultimate value over a period of weeks or months as treatment proceeds.

It's unusual when an initial meal plan and dosage of medication instantly results in the desired blood sugar profiles. Some people, a few days into their regimen, may find something objectionable, such as not enough to eat for a certain meal. Because of this, it's often necessary to experiment with a plan, making small changes based upon their feelings and blood sugar profiles.

People tend to become discouraged if they cannot see rapid improvement, and so, where warranted, I try to make adjustments to the regimen every few days in order to demonstrate that our efforts are accomplishing positive results. To this end, I ask patients to bring or to fax to my office their blood sugar profiles about one week after their final training visit, if initial treatment is by diet alone. If I've prescribed oral hypoglycemic pills or insulin, I like to see profiles within one or two days. I certainly try to make sure that no blood sugars are below 70 mg/dl during this trial period. I ask all new patients to phone me at any time of the day or night if they experience a blood sugar under 70 or become confused about their instructions. Additional repeat visits or phone calls may be necessary every few days or weeks, depending upon how rapidly blood sugar profiles reach our target.

Many new patients come to my office from out of town, sometimes traveling distances of several thousand miles. Clearly, frequent office visits would be impractical in such cases. For these patients, I often schedule follow-up "telephone visits" instead of office visits. Patients will either fax or read their blood sugar data to me.

These subsequent office or telephone interactions enable me to fine-tune the original plan, and also to reinforce the training program by catching any mistakes that a patient may inadvertently make. This interactive training is much more effective for patients than just reading a book or hearing a few lectures.

BEGINNING TREATMENT WITH YOUR DOCTOR OR DIABETES EDUCATOR

Although the protocol will likely differ at every doctor's office, in the next several pages, I'll try to give you an idea of how things work at our Diabetes Center. This way, you'll get a general notion of how a comprehensive diabetes treatment program should work.

In my experience, most patients will cooperate with a treatment plan that shows them concrete results. Greatly improved blood sugars, weight normalization, halting or reversing diabetic complications, and a sense of improved overall health can go a long way toward convincing an individual to stick with a treatment program.

Much is written in the diabetes literature about the key role of patient "compliance." Treatment failures are often blamed upon "lack of compliance." I think it's unreasonable to expect you to comply with a treatment that explains little and isn't really effective. What we must do is set up a rational plan that you understand and agree with. I'm not just going to have my staff hand you a photocopied diet and expect you to abide by it. This is something that has to be negotiated, worked out, so you understand and agree. Only then can we expect your cooperation. For cooperation to continue, however, you must see positive results.

Not all people are able to follow a given treatment plan. For example, someone who's been overeating carbohydrate for a lifetime may find it next to impossible to begin to follow a restricted diet immediately. Some absolutely resist exercise. But for most people we are able to develop a treatment plan that works. If, for example, someone whose blood sugar can be controlled with diet and exercise refuses to exercise, I prescribe medication instead.

YOUR FIRST FEW VISITS

When seeing new patients, my preference is an introductory visit followed later by a series of treatment/training visits lasting 2–3 hours each.* The continuity of time is invaluable to showing rapid results. However, most insurance companies don't like to pay for lengthy office visits — especially for "unnecessary" diabetes training — and so it may be necessary to break down the initial workup and training into multiple brief visits. Although I don't like to, I may do this with local patients but not with patients who come from out of town. With out-of-town patients, it's simply not workable to have successive short visits.

My preferred procedure for the first few days of treatment is to break down visits into three sessions. For some patients, these three lengthy visits may be, for purposes of insurance coverage, stretched out into as many as nine or twelve brief visits.

Introductory Visit
Since blood glucose profiles are so essential to formulating a treatment plan, at the introductory visit I usually ask a new patient to procure blood glucose testing supplies. I provide guidelines for blood glucose self-monitoring (like those you have seen in Chapter 4), and ask the patient to learn how to use the equipment so that, later, on the first treat-

---

* My training program consists essentially of the material covered in this book. It's my hope that physicians who have little time to educate patients will use this book to assist in that purpose.

ment/training visit, I can look over that week's blood glucose profiles. I also give the patient a large bottle so that a 24-hour urine specimen can be collected for a subsequent visit.

First Treatment/Training Visit

If I haven't done so in the introductory visit, I take a medical history and begin a physical exam geared toward uncovering long-term complications of diabetes. This will include some of the tests described in Chapter 2. We check to ensure the patient has purchased the right supplies. If we haven't done so already, we provide a supply list (Chapter 3) with appropriate items checked off.

We discuss plans for treatment of medical problems other than blood glucose control. These may include conditions the patient already knows about, but also anything uncovered by blood testing or by the physical exam. If the patient has already acquired supplies and begun measuring blood sugars, I review his or her technique and correct it if necessary.

Second Treatment/Training Visit

Many of my patients come from out of town, and so the second visit may take place the day after the first. Usually, however, it will be approximately a week later. At this visit we finish the physical examination. I also use this visit to give verbal instructions and a printed handout regarding foot care (see Appendix E). We also recheck the patient's blood glucose measurement technique.

If I feel that the patient should be taking insulin, I give instructions for insulin doses to be taken the night before and the morning of the third visit. I also provide training in self-injection (Chapter 15) to patients who have never injected before. For those who are veteran insulin users, I evaluate self-injection technique and correct it if necessary. It's my experience that most insulin-using patients have previously been taught improper techniques for filling syringes and injecting insulin.

Third Treatment/Training Visit

This visit may take place anytime after the second. We ask the patient to come in fasting and bring a 24-hour urine collection. At this visit I draw blood for baseline studies and continue training. I also enter all the "data to remember" at the top of a GLUCOGRAF data sheet (Chapter 5).

Patients to be treated with insulin are kept fasting until supper on the day of this visit in order to determine if the small dose of long-acting insulin that was injected that morning is adequate to maintain blood glucose at a fixed level. On this day, if the patient arises with a blood glucose above our target value, she'd have instructions to take a trial dose of fast-acting insulin to bring blood sugar down to the target value. If blood sugar on awakening is below the target, she'd use glucose tablets to increase blood glucose to target. By this means, we confirm or correct my estimation of how much a given amount of insulin or glucose will lower or raise the individual's blood sugar.

To this visit the patient is expected to bring the blood sugar data he or she has collected over the prior week(s), together with a list of everything eaten during the past week. This information is important in that it enables me to estimate if the patient will need medication for blood glucose control. The blood glucose profile also provides a snapshot of the patient's status before beginning the new treatment regimen. We can review this at a later date to evaluate progress.

SETTING GOALS OF TREATMENT

On the third visit, it's generally appropriate to prepare a list of treatment goals. Exactly what are we going to accomplish, how, and over what time frame? The patient and I discuss a list of goals to make sure that he or she understands and agrees. The following list is typical of the things I want to see any given patient accomplish. (Remember, the training I provide to my patients is the substance of this book, so if you don't entirely understand all of these goals right now, don't be discouraged. Mark this chapter and come back to it when you've finished the book. By then you should understand the whole philosophy of my approach and the goals will make perfect sense. You may also by that time have developed — if you haven't already — conscious goals of your own.)

- Normalization of blood glucose profiles.
- Normalization of hemoglobin A_{1C} values.
- Attainment of ideal weight (where appropriate).
- Full or partial reversal of diabetic complications, including pain or numbness in feet, diabetes-related retinal or kidney problems, gas-

troparesis, cardiac autonomic neuropathy, neuropathic erectile impotence, postural hypotension, and so on. If blood sugar levels are kept normal, some of these improvements will appear within weeks to years, depending upon the particular problem and its severity.

- Reduction in frequency and severity of hypoglycemic episodes (where appropriate).
- Relief of chronic fatigue and mild dementia associated with high blood sugars.
- Improvement or normalization of the following laboratory tests that respond to blood glucose control (Chapter 2): lipid profile, thrombotic risk profile, renal profile, red blood cell magnesium, and hemoglobin A_{1C}.
- Reduction of demand upon beta cells. If fasting C-peptide was present (that is, if your pancreas is producing insulin), glucose tolerance should improve if a regimen is pursued that minimizes the demand upon the beta cells. This is a very important goal. Remember that small sacrifices now can prevent the need for 5 daily insulin doses down the road. Beta cell burnout (see page 89) can frequently be prevented.
- Increased strength, endurance, and feeling of well-being.

The patient may wish to add some personal goals. The doctor should respect these if at all possible. For example, I have several patients who are willing to do whatever I ask, provided I do not put them on insulin. I consider this a reasonable preliminary goal, for some, even though it may increase the risk of beta cell burnout. After all, if we cannot enlist a patient's cooperation, we achieve nothing.

9

The Basic Food Groups,

OR MUCH OF WHAT YOU'VE BEEN TAUGHT ABOUT DIET IS PROBABLY WRONG

I n Chapter 1 we discussed generally how diabetics and nondiabetics might react to a particular meal. Here we'll talk about how the specific kinds of foods can affect your blood sugar.

Perhaps the most curious fact about diet, nutrition, and medication is that while we can make accurate generalizations about how most of us will react to a particular diet or medical regimen, each individual will react somewhat differently to a given food.

The foods we consume, once you take away the water and undigestible contents, can be grouped into three major categories: protein, carbohydrate, and fat. Seldom is food from one of these major groups solely one type of nutrient. Protein foods often contain fat; carbohydrate foods frequently contain some protein and fat. The only foods that are virtually 100 percent fat are oils, butter, and margarine.

Since our principal concern here is blood sugar control, we'll concentrate on how the three major types of nutrients affect blood sugar. If you're a long-standing diabetic and have followed the standard ADA diet for years, you'll find that much of what you're about to read is radically at odds with the ADA's dietary guidelines — and with good reason, as you'll soon learn.

When we eat, the digestive process breaks down the three major food groups into their building blocks. These building blocks are then absorbed into the bloodstream and reassembled into the various products our bodies need in order to function.

PROTEIN

Proteins are chains of building blocks called amino acids. Through digestion, dietary proteins are broken down by enzymes in the digestive tract into their amino acid components. These amino acids can then be reassembled not only into muscle, nerve fiber, and vital organs, but also into hormones, enzymes, and neurochemicals.

We acquire dietary protein from many sources, but the foods that are richest in it are egg whites, cheese, and meat (including fish and fowl). Protein is available in much lower amounts from vegetable sources such as legumes (beans), seeds, and nuts, which also contain the other nutrients, fat and carbohydrate.*

As stunning as it sounds — and unbelievable, given the popular media's recent love affair with a high "complex" carbohydrate, low-fat diet — you can quite easily survive on a diet in which you would eat *no* carbohydrate. Furthermore, by sticking to a diet that contains no carbohydrate, but high levels of fat and protein, you can reduce your cardiac risk profile — serum cholesterol, blood lipids, et cetera — though you'd deprive yourself of all the "fun foods" that we crave most. We've all been trained to think that carbohydrates are our best, most benign source of food, so how can this be?

Protein is the second of our two dietary sources of blood sugar. Protein foods are only about 20 percent protein by weight (6 grams per ounce), the rest being fat, water, or undigestible "gristle." The liver, instructed by the hormone glucagon, can *very slowly* transform as much as 52 percent of the above 6 grams per ounce into glucose† if blood sugar descends too low or the body's other amino acid needs have been met. Neither carbohydrate nor fat can be transformed into protein.

---

* Phosphate, a by-product of protein digestion, requires calcium in order to be eliminated from the body — about 1 gram of calcium for every 10 ounces of protein foods. If you don't eat much cheese, milk (too high in carbohydrate), yogurt, or bones, all good sources of calcium, it would be wise to take a calcium supplement. This will prevent slow loss of calcium from your bones. I recommend calcium citrate, which is available at pharmacies in 315 mg tablets.

† This amounts to about 10 percent of the total *weight* of a protein food. Say you eat a 3-ounce (85 grams) hamburger, no bun, for lunch — the protein in it can slowly be transformed by the liver into about 9 grams of glucose.

In the 1920s, Arctic explorer Vilhjalmur Stefansson noted in his travels that Eskimos seemed to fare quite nicely on a zero-carbohydrate diet (the Arctic being not exactly the ideal climate for cultivating fruits, grain, or vegetables). Under the watchful eyes of physicians from New York's Cornell University Medical College and Bellevue Hospital, Stefansson and a colleague submitted themselves to a meat-only diet for a year. They ate 2,500 calories a day, of which 75 percent was fat. As reported in the *Journal of the American Medical Association,* on July 6, 1929, the two men finished out their year of a no-carbohydrate diet not only slimmer — each had lost 6 pounds — but with reduced (and completely normal) cholesterol. It's worth repeating that the men were eating a diet with 75 percent of the calories coming from fat. Current recommendations are to eat no more than 30 percent of calories as fat — which very few people can maintain — and there are some recommendations for even lower percentages than that.

This is almost precisely the opposite of the prevailing "wisdom," which says that if you want to lose weight and get your cholesterol down, you need to eat lots of fruit, vegetables, and grain products, and cut out meat as much as possible. Despite this prevailing "wisdom," many contemporary dietary researchers exploring this phenomenon have begun to arrive at the conclusion that a high-carbohydrate diet is not so benign. In fact, it has been shown — and it is my own observation — that such a diet can increase body weight, increase blood insulin levels, and raise most cardiac risk factors. Why?

The answer is really quite simple. The advent of our agricultural society is comparatively recent in evolutionary terms — that is, it began only about 10,000 years ago. For the millions of years that preceded the constant availability of grain and vegetable products, our ancestors were hunter-gatherers, and ate what was available to them in the immediate environment, primarily meat, fish, nuts — food that was present year-round, and predominantly protein and fat. In the summers they may have eaten fruits and berries that were available locally in some regions, but if they stored away fat during those seasons, that fat was quickly burned up during the winter. Although for the past two centuries, fruit, grain, and vegetables have, in one form or another, been available to us in this country year-round, our collective food supply has historically been interrupted often by famine — in some cultures more than others. The history of the planet as best as we can determine is one of feast and famine, and suggests that famine will strike again and again. The recent famines in Ethiopia and Somalia are examples.

Curiously, the genetic predisposition toward obesity, or what *today* seems in our society to be a predisposition toward obesity, functioned during the famines of prehistory as an effective method of survival. Ironically, the ancestors of those who today are most at risk for Type II diabetes were, during prehistory, not the sick and dying, but the *survivors*. If famine struck today in the United States, guess who would survive most easily? The same people who are most at risk for Type II diabetes.

You can take this knowledge and make it work *for* you rather than against you.

If you give it some thought, it makes perfect sense: If a farmer wants to fatten up his pigs or cows, he doesn't feed them meat or butter and eggs, he feeds them grain. If you want to fatten yourself up, just start loading up on bread, pasta, potatoes, cake, and cookies — all high-carbohydrate foods. If you are already obese, you know and I know that you crave — and consume — these foods and probably avoid fats.

In many respects — and going against the grain of a number of the medical establishment's accepted notions about diabetics and protein — protein will become the most important part of your diet if you are going to control blood sugars.

If you are a long-standing diabetic and are frustrated with the care you've received over the years, you have probably been conditioned to think that protein is more of a poison than sugar and is the cause of kidney disease. I was conditioned the same way — many years ago, as I mentioned, I had laboratory evidence of advanced proteinuria, signifying potentially fatal kidney disease — but in this case, the conventional wisdom is just a myth.

Nondiabetics who eat a lot of protein don't get diabetic kidney disease. Diabetics with normalized blood sugars don't get diabetic kidney disease. High levels of dietary protein do not cause kidney disease in diabetics or anyone else. There is no higher incidence of kidney disease in the cattle-growing states of the United States, where many people eat steak every day, than there is in the states where beef is more expensive and consumed to a much lesser degree. Similarly, the incidence of kidney disease

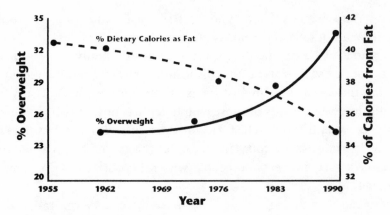

Fig. 9-1. *From 1955 to 1990, even as the percentage of calories consumed as fat declined, the percentage of overweight Americans increased by nearly half.*

in vegetarians is the same as the incidence of kidney disease in nonvegetarians. *It is the high blood sugar levels that are unique to diabetes, and to a much lesser degree the high levels of insulin required to cover them (causing hypertension), that cause the complications associated with diabetes.*

FAT

Call it the Big Fat Lie. Fat has, through no real fault of its own, become the great demon of the American dietary scene. It is no myth that one-third of Americans are overweight. It *is*, however, a myth that Americans are overweight due to excessive fat consumption.

The body acquires fat in two ways. The primary source of body fat for most Americans is not dietary fat but carbohydrate, which is converted to blood sugar and then, with the aid of insulin, to fat by fat cells. Remember, insulin is our main fat-building hormone. Eat a plate of pasta. Your blood sugar will rise and your insulin level (if you have Type II diabetes or are not diabetic) will also rise in order to cover the jump in blood sugar. All the blood sugar that is not burned as energy or stored as glycogen is turned into fat. So you could, in theory, acquire more body fat from eating a high-carbohydrate "fat-free" dessert than you would from eating a tender steak nicely marbled with fat.

The other manner in which your body acquires fat is by eating it. Fat by itself doesn't taste particularly good. Pour yourself a tall, frosty mug of cooking oil and you'll likely gag trying to get it down. Take that same oil and french-fry potatoes in it, or drizzle some olive oil on your salad with vinegar, and suddenly it's delicious. The effect dietary fat has is to enhance flavor.

When you eat food that contains fat (triglycerides), your digestive system breaks it down into fatty acids. These your body can burn or store, or convert into other compounds, depending on what it requires. Consequently, fat is always in flux in the body, being stored, appearing in the blood, and being converted to energy. The amount of triglycerides in your bloodstream at any given time will be determined by your heredity, your level of exercise, your blood sugar levels, your diet, your ratio of lean body mass (muscle) to visceral (abdominal) fat, and *especially by your recent consumption of carbohydrate.* The slim and fit tend to be very sensitive (i.e., responsive) to insulin and have low serum levels not only of triglycerides but insulin as well. But even *their* triglyceride levels will increase after a high-carbohydrate meal, as excess blood sugar is converted to fat. The higher the ratio of lean body mass to abdominal fat, the more sensitive to insulin you'll tend to be. In the obese, triglycerides tend to be present at high levels in the bloodstream all the time. (This is sometimes exaggerated during weight loss because fat is appearing in the bloodstream as it comes out of storage to be converted into energy.) Not only are high triglyceride levels a direct cause of insulin resistance, but they also contribute to fatty deposits on the walls of your blood vessels (atherosclerosis), which are a frequent factor in heart disease, strokes, and amputations not caused by injury. Research demonstrates that if you injected high concentrations of triglycerides into the blood supply of the liver of a well-conditioned athlete, someone very sensitive to insulin, she would become insulin-resistant until the excess triglyceride had been cleared from the bloodstream. (The most important thing to note here is that insulin resistance, as well as other risk factors for the diabetic complications I just mentioned, can be reversed by eating less carbohydrate, normalizing blood sugars, and slimming down, which we'll discuss in greater detail later on.)

If you become overweight, you'll produce more insulin, become insulin-resistant (which will require you to produce yet more insulin), and become yet more overweight because you'll create more fat and store more fat. You'll enter the vicious circle depicted in Figure 1-1.

Consider that steak I mentioned earlier. As you know, the body can convert protein to blood sugar, but it does so at a very slow rate, and inefficiently. Serum insulin levels derived from the phase II insulin response or even from insulin injected before a meal are thus sufficient to prevent a blood sugar rise from protein consumption. Fat cannot be converted to blood sugar, and therefore doesn't cause serum insulin levels or requirements for injected insulin to increase. Say you eat an 8-ounce steak with no carbohydrate side dish — this won't require much insulin to keep your blood sugar steady, and the lower insulin level will cause only a small amount of the fat to be stored.

Now consider what would happen if you ate the caloric equivalent of that steak as a "fat-free" dessert. Your insulin level has to jump dramatically in order to cover the carbohydrate in the dessert. Remember, insulin is *the* fat-building and fat-storage hormone. Since it's dessert, you probably won't be going out to run a marathon after eating, so the largest portion of your blood sugar won't get burned. Instead much of it will be turned into fat and stored.

Interestingly enough, eating fat with carbohydrate can actually slow the digestion of carbohydrate, so the jump in your insulin level might thereby be slowed down. This would probably be relatively effective if you're talking about eating salad with vinegar-and-oil dressing. But if you're eating a regular dessert, or a baked potato with your steak, the slowdown in digestion would not prevent blood sugar elevation in a diabetic.

Much of the reason Arctic explorer Stefansson and his colleague came out of their year-long meat-only diet thinner and with lowered cholesterol levels was that their blood sugar wasn't getting kicked up by carbohydrate — since they ate none.

Despite what the popular media would have us believe, fat is not evil. In fact, many researchers are becoming quite concerned about the dangerous potential of "fat substitutes." Fat is absolutely necessary for survival. Much of the brain is constructed from fatty acids. Without essential fatty acids — which, like essential amino acids, cannot be manufactured by the body and must be eaten — you would die. Fat substitutes such as the recently FDA-approved Olestra bring about the spectre of people trying to subsist on a no-fat diet, a diet that could kill them. (Olestra actually robs the body of important vitamins and fats, and the FDA has required that it contain additives of those vitamins. In test markets, some consumers have been made quite ill by the product, while others don't see any effect. I don't recommend it — it's completely unnecessary.)

Diabetics are affected disproportionately by diseases such as atherosclerosis. This has led to the long-standing myth that diabetics have abnormal lipid profiles because they eat more fat than nondiabetics.* It was likewise thought that dietary fat *caused* all the long-term complications of diabetes. For many years, this was taken as gospel by most in the medical community. In truth, however, the high lipid profiles in many diabetics with uncontrolled blood sugar have nothing to do with the fat they consume. Most diabetics consume very little fat — they've been conditioned to fear it. High lipid profiles are a symptom not of excess dietary fat, but of high blood sugars. Indeed, even in most nondiabetics, the consumption of fat has little if anything to do with their lipid profiles.

On the other hand, high consumption of carbohydrate, as we will discuss shortly, *can* cause nondiabetics to develop some of the complications usually associated with diabetes.

When I was on a very low fat, high-carbohydrate diet thirty years ago, I had high triglycerides (usually over 250 mg/dl) and high serum cholesterol (usually over 300 mg/dl), and I developed a number of vascular complications. When I went onto a very low carbohydrate diet and did not restrict my fat, the same thing happened to me that happened to Arctic explorer Stefansson, but more so — my lipids plummeted. Now, at sixty-three, I have the lipid profile of an Olympic athlete, apparently from eating a low-carbohydrate diet in order to normalize my blood sugars. That I exercise regularly probably doesn't hurt my lipid profile, either — but I was also exercising when my lipid profile was abnormal.

Dare your physician. Ask him or her if his lipid profile on a low-fat diet can remotely compare to mine, on a high-fat, low-carbohydrate diet:

- LDL — the "bad" cholesterol — 83 (below 130 is considered normal)
- HDL — the "good" cholesterol — 110 (above 30 is considered normal)

---

* A lipid profile is the measurement of cholesterol, HDL (good cholesterol), LDL (bad cholesterol), and triglyceride levels in the blood (see Chapter 2).

- Triglycerides — 45 (below 150 is considered normal)
- Lipoprotein(a) — undetectable (below 60 is considered normal)

Contrary to popular myth, fat is not a demon. It's the body's way of storing energy. Without essential fatty acids, your body would cease to function.

CARBOHYDRATE

I've saved carbohydrate for last because it's the food group that affects blood sugar most profoundly — both by eating it and by *not* eating it. If you're like most diabetics — or even most Americans — you probably eat a diet that's mostly carbohydrate. Breakfast cereal. Grains. Fruit. Bread. Cake. Beans. Snack foods. Rice. Potatoes. Pasta.

No doubt you've heard the endless talk in the popular media about carbohydrate. Books tout the value of a high "complex carbohydrate" diet. Athletes "carbo-load" before big games or marathons. TV and radio commercials extol the virtues of Brand X sport drink over Brand Y because it contains more "carbos."

What if I, a physician, told you, a diabetic, to eat a diet that consisted of 60 percent sugar, 20 percent protein, and 20 percent fat? More than likely, you'd think I was insane. *I'd* think I was insane, and I would never make this suggestion to a diabetic (nor, in reality, would I even make it to a nondiabetic). But this is just the diet to which I was subjected for many years. The ADA made this recommendation to diabetics for decades. On the surface, these recommendations seemed to make sense because of kidney disease, heart disease, and our elevated lipid profiles. But this is what is known as single-avenue thinking. It *seemed* logical to insist that dietary intake of protein and fat be reduced because no one had looked at elevated blood sugars and the high levels of insulin necessary to bring them down as the possible culprits.

So if you eat very little fat and protein, what's left to eat? Carbohydrate.

As I discovered in my years of experimentation on myself, and then in my medical training and practice, the real dietary problem for diabetics is fast-acting or large amounts of carbohydrate, which result in high blood sugars requiring large amounts of insulin to try to contain them.

So what are carbohydrates?

The technical answer is that carbohydrates are chains of sugar molecules. The carbohydrates we eat are mostly chains of glucose molecules. The shorter the chain, the sweeter the taste. Some chains are longer and more complicated (hence, simple and complex carbohydrates), having many links and even branches. But simple or complex, carbohydrates are composed entirely of sugar.

Sugar? you might ask, holding up a slice of coarse-ground, seven-grain bread. This is sugar?

In a word, yes, at least after you digest it.

With some important exceptions, carbohydrates, or foods derived primarily from plant sources, such as vegetables, grains, and fruits, have the same effect on blood glucose levels that table sugar does. (The ADA has recently recognized officially that, for example, bread is as fast-acting a carbohydrate as table sugar. But instead of issuing a recommendation against eating bread, its response has been to say that table sugar is therefore okay, and can be "exchanged" for other carbohydrates. To me, this is nonsense.) Whether you eat a piece of the nuttiest whole-grain bread, drink a Coke, or have a dollop of mashed potatoes, the effect on blood glucose levels is the same — blood sugar rises, *fast.*

How can this be?

As noted in the introduction to this chapter, the digestion process breaks each of the major food groups down into its basic elements, and these elements are then utilized by the body as needed. The basic elements of most carbohydrates are glucose molecules. We usually think of simple carbohydrates as sugars and complex carbohydrates as fruits and grains and vegetables. In reality, most fruit and grain products, and some vegetables, are what I prefer to talk about as "fast-acting" carbohydrates. Our saliva and digestive tract contain enzymes that can rapidly chop the longer chains down into the shorter, sweeter chains. We haven't the enzymes to break down some carbohydrates, such as cellulose, or "undigestible fiber." Still, even our saliva can break down starches into the shorter chains on contact.

Pasta, which is often made from durum wheat flour and water (but can also be made from plain white flour and egg yolks, or other variants), has been touted as a dream food — particularly for runners carbo-loading before marathons — but it quickly becomes glucose, and can raise blood sugar very rapidly.

In the Type II diabetic with impaired phase I insulin response, it takes hours for the pancreas to catch up with the levels of sugar in the blood, and day after day, during that time, the high blood sugars can wreak havoc. In the diabetic who injects insulin, there is a tremendous amount of guesswork involved in finding the proper dosage of insulin and timing it to cover a carbohydrate-heavy meal, and the injected insulin doesn't work fast enough (see Chapter 7, "The Laws of Small Numbers").

Some carbohydrate foods, like fruit, consist of high levels of simple, fast-acting carbohydrates. Maltose and fructose — malt sugar and fruit sugar — are slower-acting than sucrose — table or cane sugar — but they will cause the same increase in blood sugar levels. It may be the difference between nearly instant elevation and elevation in 2 hours, but the elevation is still high, and still requires a lot of insulin to bring it into line. Despite the old admonition that an apple a day keeps the doctor away, I haven't had fruit in more than twenty-five years, and I am considerably healthier for it. Some foods, like broccoli, contain lots of cellulose, or undigestible fiber, which slows the digestion and dilutes the small amount of digestible carbohydrate they contain.

As noted previously, most Americans who are obese are overweight not because of dietary fat, but because of excessive dietary carbohydrate. Much of this obesity is due to "pigging out" on carbohydrate-rich snack food or junk foods, or even supposed healthy foods like bread and pasta. It's my belief that this pigging out has little to do with hunger and nothing at all to do with being a pig.

I'm convinced that people who crave carbohydrate have inherited this problem. To some extent, we all have a natural craving for carbohydrate — it makes us feel good. The more people gorge on carbohydrates, the more people will become obese, even if they exercise a lot. But certain people have a natural, *overwhelming* desire for carbohydrate that doesn't correlate to hunger. These people in all likelihood have a genetic predisposition toward carbohydrate craving, as well as a genetic predisposition toward insulin resistance and diabetes. This craving can be reduced for some by embarking upon a low-carbohydrate diet.

SOME WORDS ABOUT ALCOHOL

Alcohol can provide calories, or energy, without directly raising blood sugar, but if you're an insulin-dependent diabetic, you need to be cautious about drinking. Ethyl alcohol, which is the active ingredient in hard liquor, beer, and wine, has no direct effect on blood sugar. In the case of distilled spirits and very dry wine, the alcohol generally isn't accompanied by high enough amounts of carbohydrate to affect your blood sugar very much. For example, 100 proof gin has 83 calories per ounce. These extra calories can indirectly increase your weight slightly, but not your blood sugar. Different beers — ales, stouts, and lagers — can have varying amounts of carbohydrate, which is slow enough in its action that if you figure it into your meal plan, it won't raise your blood sugar too much. Mixed drinks and dessert wines can be loaded with sugar, so they're best avoided. Exceptions would be mixed drinks that can be made with a sugar-free mixer, such as sugar-free tonic water.

However, ethyl alcohol can indirectly lower blood sugar of a Type I diabetic if consumed at the time of a meal. It does this by paralyzing the liver and thereby inhibiting gluconeogenesis so that it can't convert the protein of the meal into glucose. For the average adult, this appears to be a significant effect with doses greater than 1.5 ounces, or one standard shot glass. If you have two 1.5-ounce servings of gin with a meal, your liver may be partially unable to convert protein into glucose. If you're insulin-dependent, and your calculation of how much insulin you'll require to cover your meal is based on, say, two hot dogs, and those hot dogs don't get 10 percent converted to glucose, the insulin you've injected will take your blood sugar too low. You'll have hypoglycemia, or low blood sugar.

The problem of hypoglycemia itself is a relatively simple matter to correct — you just eat some glucose and your blood sugar will rise. But this gets you into the kind of messy jerking up and down of your blood sugar that can cause problems. It's best if you can avoid hypo- and hyperglycemia (high blood sugar) entirely.

Another problem with alcohol and hypoglycemia is that if you consume much alcohol, you'll have symptoms that could indicate either alcohol intoxication or hypoglycemia — light-headedness, confusion, and slurring of speech. The only way you'll know the cause of your symptoms is if you've been monitoring your blood sugar throughout your meal. This is unlikely. So you could find yourself with dangerously low blood sugar and just think you've consumed too much alcohol. Remember, that early blood sugar–measuring device I got was developed in order to help emergency room staffs tell the difference between unconscious alcoholics and unconscious diabetics. Don't make yourself an unconscious diabetic. A simple oversight could turn fatal.

Many of the symptoms of alcohol intoxication mimic those of ketoacidosis, or the extreme high blood sugar and ketone buildup in the body that can result in diabetic coma. The buildup of ketones causes the diabetic to have a sweet aroma, rather like someone who's been drinking. If you don't die of severe hypoglycemia, then you might easily die of embarrassment when you come to and your friends are aghast and terrified that the emergency squad had to be called to bring you around.

In small amounts, alcohol is relatively benign — one glass of dry wine or a light beer with dinner — but if you're the type who can't limit drinking, it's best to avoid it entirely. For the reasons already discussed, alcohol can be more benign between meals than it is at meals.

10

Diet Guidelines:

BASIC TREATMENT FOR ALL DIABETICS

Perhaps someday there will be a miraculous replacement for the burned-out beta cells of your pancreas, but until then, if you're going to control your diabetes and get on with a normal life, you will have to change your diet. No matter how mild or severe your diabetes, the key aspect of all treatment plans for normalizing blood sugars and preventing or reversing complications of diabetes is diet. In the terms of the Laws of Small Numbers, the single largest "input" you can control is what you eat.

THE FUNDAMENTAL IMPORTANCE OF A
RESTRICTED-CARBOHYDRATE DIET

The next several pages may well be the most difficult pages of this book for you to accept — as well as some of the most important. They're full of the foods you're going to have to restrict or eliminate from your diet if you're going to normalize your blood sugars. You may see some of your favorite foods on our No-No list, but before you stop reading, keep in mind a few important things. First, toward the end of this chapter we discuss the foods you *can* safely eat. Second, while you will have to eliminate certain foods, there are some genuinely sugar-free alternatives.

One purpose of blood glucose self-monitoring is to learn through your blood sugar profiles how particular foods affect you. Over years of examining these profiles, I've observed that some people are more tolerant of certain foods than other people. For example, bread makes my own blood sugar rise very rapidly. Yet some of my patients eat a sand-wich of thin bread every day with only minor problems. This is in-evitably related to delayed stomach-emptying (see Chapter 21). In any case, you should feel free to experiment with food and then perform blood sugar readings. It's likely that for most diabetics all of our restric-tions will be necessary.

Patients often ask, "Can't I just take my medication and eat whatever I want?" It almost seems logical, and would be fine if it worked. But, as explained earlier, it doesn't work, so we have to find something that does. We have.

Many diabetics can be treated with diet alone, and if your disease is relatively mild, you could easily fall into this category. Some patients who have been using insulin or oral hypoglycemic agents find that once on our diet they no longer need blood sugar–lowering medication. Even if you require insulin or other agents, diet will still constitute the most essential part of your treatment.

Think small inputs. You may recall from prior chapters that the im-pairment or loss of phase I insulin response makes normalizing blood sugars impossible for at least a few hours after a high-carbohydrate meal. Even eating small amounts of fast-acting carbohydrate raises blood sugar so rapidly that any remaining phase II insulin response can-not promptly compensate. This is true if you're injecting insulin or if you're still making your own insulin.

Any sensible meal plan for normalizing blood sugar takes this into account and follows these basic rules:

- First, eliminate all foods that contain simple sugars. As you should know by now — but it bears repeating — "simple sugar" does not mean just table sugar. Most breads and other starchy foods, such as potatoes and grains, become simple sugars so rapidly that they can cause serious postprandial increases in blood sugar.
- Second, limit your total carbohydrate intake to an amount that will work with your injected insulin or your body's remaining phase II insulin response. In this way, you avoid a postprandial blood sugar increase, and avoid overworking any remaining insulin-producing beta cells of your pancreas (research has demonstrated that beta cell burnout can be slowed or halted by normalizing blood sugars).

- Third, stop eating when you no longer feel hungry, *not* when you're stuffed. There's no reason for you to leave the table hungry, but there's also no reason to be gluttonous. Remember the Chinese Restaurant Effect (page 87).

TESTING FOR GLUCOSE OR SUCROSE IN FOODS

Sometimes you'll find yourself at a restaurant, hotel, or reception where you cannot predict if foods have sugar or flour in them. Your waiter may have no idea what's in a given recipe. I've found that the easiest way to make certain is to use the Clinistix or Diastix that should have been checked off on your supply list (Chapter 3). These are manufactured to test urine for glucose. We use them to test food. If, for example, you want to determine if a soup or salad dressing contains table sugar (sucrose) or a sauce contains flour, just put a small amount in your mouth and mix it with your saliva. Then spit a tiny bit onto a test strip. Any color change indicates the presence of sugar. Saliva is essential to this reaction because it contains an enzyme that releases glucose from sucrose or flour in the food, permitting it to react with the chemicals in the test strip. This is how I found that one restaurant in my neighborhood uses large amounts of sugar in its bouillon while another restaurant uses none.

Solid foods can also be tested this way, but you must chew them first. The lightest color on the color chain label of the test strip indicates a very low concentration of glucose. Any color paler than this may be acceptable for most foods. The Clinistix/Diastix method works on nearly all the foods on our No-No list except milk products, which contain lactose. It will also not react with fructose. If in doubt, assume the worst.

NO-NO FOODS: ELIMINATING SIMPLE SUGARS

Named below are many of the common foods that contain simple sugars, which rapidly raise blood sugar or otherwise hinder blood sugar control and should be eliminated from your diet. Virtually all grain products, for example — from the flours in "sugar-free" cookies to pasta — are converted so rapidly into glucose by the enzymes in saliva that they are, as far as blood sugar is concerned, essentially no different than table sugar. There are plenty of food products, however, that contain tiny amounts of simple sugars and will have a negligible effect on your blood sugar. One gram of carbohydrate will not raise blood sugar more than 5mg/dl for most adults. A single stick of chewing gum or a single tablespoon of salad dressing made with only 1 gram of sugar certainly poses no problems. In these areas, you have to use your judgment and your blood sugar profiles. If you're the type who, once you start chewing gum, has to have a new stick every 5 minutes, then you should probably avoid chewing gum. If you have delayed stomach-emptying, chewing gum may help facilitate your digestion.

Powdered Artificial Sweeteners

Sweet'n Low, Equal, The Sweet One, Sugar Twin, and similar powdered products in paper packets usually contain about 96 percent glucose and about 4 percent artificial sweetener. They are sold as low-calorie sweeteners because they contain only 1 gram of glucose as compared to 3 grams of sucrose in a similar paper packet labeled "sugar." More suitable for diabetics are tablet sweeteners such as saccharin, cyclamate, and aspartame (Equal in the United States). Note that the same brand name can denote two different products: Equal is a powder containing 96 percent glucose and also a tablet containing no glucose. Stevia powder and liquid (sold in health food stores) contain no sugar of any kind.

So-Called Diet Foods and Sugar-Free Foods

Because U.S. food-labeling laws have permitted products to be called "sugar-free" if they do not contain common table sugar (sucrose), the mere substitution of another sugar for sucrose permits the packager to deceive the consumer legally. Most so-called "sugar-free" products were, for many years, full of sugars that may not promote tooth decay but most certainly will raise your blood sugar. If you've been deceived, you're not alone. I've been in doctor's offices that have candy dishes full of "sugar-free" hard candies especially for their diabetic patients! Sometimes the label will disclose the name of the substitute sugar.

Here is a partial list of some of the many sugars you can find in "sugar-free" foods. All of these will raise your blood sugar.

carob	honey	saccharose
corn syrup	lactose	sorbitol
dextrin	levulose	sorghum
dextrose	maltose	treacle
dulcitol	mannitol	turbinado
fructose	mannose	xylitol
glucose	molasses	xylose

Some, such as sorbitol and fructose, raise blood sugar more slowly than glucose but still too rapidly to prevent a postprandial blood sugar rise in people with diabetes.

Other "diet" foods contain either sugars that are alternates to sucrose, large amounts of rapid-acting carbohydrate, or both. Many of these foods are virtually 100 percent rapid-acting carbohydrate (e.g., sugar-free cookies), so that even if they were to contain none of the above added sugars, consumption of a small quantity would easily cause rapid blood sugar elevation.

There are exceptions — most diet sodas, sugar-free Jell-O brand gelatin desserts, and No-Cal brand syrups (available in the New York metropolitan area). All of these are made without sugar of any kind. These you need not restrict. See the "So What's Left to Eat?" section later in this chapter.

Candies, Including "Sugar-Free" Brands
A tiny "sugar-free" hard candy containing only 2½ grams of sorbitol can raise blood sugar almost 13 mg/dl. Ten of these can raise blood sugar 125 mg/dl. Are they worth it?

Honey and Fructose
In recent years a number of "authorities" have claimed that fructose (which is now sold as a powdered sweetener) and honey are useful to diabetics because they are "natural sugars." Well, *glucose* is the *most* natural of the sugars, since it is present in all plants and all but one known species of animal. These substances will raise blood sugar far more rapidly than either phase II insulin release, injected insulin, or oral hypoglycemic agents can bring it down. Just eat a few grams of honey or

fructose and check your blood sugar every 15 minutes. You will readily prove that "authorities" can be wrong.

Desserts and Pastries

With the exception of sugar-free Jell-O and similar gelatin products marked "carbohydrate — 0" on the nutrition label, virtually every food commonly used for desserts will raise blood sugar too much and too fast. This is not only because of added sugar, but also because flour, milk, and other components of desserts are very high in rapid-acting carbohydrate.

Bread and Crackers

One average slice of white, rye, or whole wheat bread contains about 12 grams carbohydrate. The "thin" or "lite" breads now available in U.S. supermarkets are usually cut at half the thickness of standard bread slices and contain half the carbohydrate. So-called high-protein breads contain only a small percentage of their calories as protein and are not significantly reduced in carbohydrate unless they are thinly cut. Brown bread, raisin bread, and corn bread all contain as much or more fast-acting carbohydrate as rye, white, or whole wheat. Some diabetics with gastroparesis (Chapter 21) can tolerate the inclusion of 1–2 slices of thin bread or a few crackers as part of their low-carbohydrate meal limits. Unfortunately, most of us experience very rapid increases of blood sugar after eating any product made from any grain (bread, crackers, pastry shells, et cetera).

Rice and Pasta

Although pasta is made from flour, much pasta is derived from a different kind of wheat (durum semolina) than is used in bread. Both pasta and wild rice (which is actually not a true variety of rice but another grain entirely) are claimed by some nutrition authorities to raise blood sugar quite slowly. Just check your blood sugar levels after eating them and you'll prove these "authorities" wrong. Alternately, you might try the Clinistix/Diastix test described on page 123. Like wild rice and pasta, white and brown rices also raise blood sugar quite rapidly for most of us and should be avoided.

Breakfast Cereals

All cold cereals, like snack foods, are virtually 100 percent carbohydrate. Many contain large amounts of added sugars. Since they are made from grain, small amounts, even of whole-grain cereals, will cause a rapid rise in blood sugar.

Cooked cereals generally contain about 10–25 grams of fast-acting carbohydrate per half-cup serving. I find that even small servings make blood sugar control impossible.

Snack Foods

These are the products in cellophane bags that you find in vending machines and supermarkets. They include not just cookies and cakes, but pretzels, potato chips, taco chips, tiny crackers, and popcorn. These foods are virtually 100 percent carbohydrate and frequently have added sucrose, glucose (the label may say dextrose), corn syrup, et cetera.

Milk and Cottage Cheese

Milk contains a considerable amount of the simple sugar lactose and will rapidly raise blood sugar. Skim milk actually contains more lactose per ounce than does whole milk. One or 2 teaspoons of milk in a cup of coffee will not significantly affect blood sugar, but ¼ cup of milk will make a considerable difference to most of us. (Cream, which you have probably been avoiding, is okay. One tablespoon has only 0.4 gram of carbohydrate.) The powdered lighteners for coffee contain relatively rapid-acting sugars and should be avoided if you use more than a teaspoonful at a time or drink more than 1 cup of coffee at a meal. An excellent coffee lightener is Westsoy brand soybean milk, which is sold in health food stores throughout the United States. Although several Westsoy flavors are marketed, only the one marked "unsweetened" is unsweetened. It contains 4 grams of carbohydrate in 8 ounces. Soybean milk can be stored in the unopened container for up to one year without refrigeration. Once opened, however, it must be refrigerated. One catch — it curdles in very hot coffee or tea.

Cottage cheese also contains a considerable amount of lactose because, unlike most other cheeses, which are okay, it is only partly fermented. I was unaware of this until several patients showed me records of substantial blood sugar increases after consuming a small container of cottage cheese. It should be avoided except in very small amounts, say about 2 tablespoons.

Fruits and Fruit Juices

These contain a mixture of simple sugars and more complex carbohydrates. A few experiments with blood sugar measurements will show you how rapidly these foods can raise your levels. Bitter-tasting fruits such as grapefruit and lemon contain considerable amounts of simple sugars. They taste bitter because of the presence of bitter chemicals, not because sugar is absent. Although deleting fruit from the diet can be a big sacrifice for many of my patients, they usually get used to this rapidly, and they appreciate the effect upon blood sugar control. I haven't eaten fruit in twenty-five years, and I haven't suffered in any respect. Some people fear that they will lose important nutrients by eliminating fruit, but that shouldn't be a worry. Nutrients found in fruits are also present in the vegetables you can safely eat.

Vegetables

Beets. Like most other sweet-tasting vegetables, beets are loaded with sugar. Sugar beets are a source of table sugar.

Carrots. After cooking, carrots taste sweeter and appear to raise blood sugar much more rapidly than when raw. This probably relates to the breakdown of complex carbohydrates into simpler sugars by heat. Even raw carrots should be avoided. If, however, you are served a salad with a few carrot shavings on top for decoration, don't bother to remove them. The amount is insignificant, just like a teaspoon of milk.

Corn. Nearly all of the corn grown in the United States is used for two main purposes. One is the production of sweeteners. Most of the sugar in Pepsi-Cola, for example, comes from corn. The other purpose is animal feed, e.g., fattening up hogs, cattle, and chickens. Corn for consumption by people, as a vegetable or as snack foods, comes in third. Diabetics should avoid eating corn, whether popped, cooked, or in chips — even 1 gram of corn will rapidly raise my blood sugar by about 5 mg/dl.

Potatoes. For most people, cooked potatoes raise blood sugar almost as fast as pure glucose, even though they may not taste sweet. Giving up potatoes is a big sacrifice for many people, but it will also make a big difference in your postprandial blood sugars. Raw potatoes, if you happen to like them, as well as sweet potatoes or yams, should also be on your nix list.

Tomatoes, Tomato Paste, and Tomato Sauce. Tomatoes are actually a fruit, not a vegetable, and as with citrus fruits, their tang can conceal just how sweet they are. The prolonged cooking necessary for the preparation of tomato sauces releases a lot of glucose, and you would do well to avoid them. If you're at someone's home for dinner and are served meat or fish covered with tomato sauce, just scrape it off. The small amount that might remain should not significantly affect your blood sugar. If you are having them uncooked in salad, limit yourself to one slice or a single cherry tomato per cup of salad.

Commercially Prepared Soups. Believe it or not, most commercial soups marketed in this country can be as loaded with added sugar as a soft drink. The taste of the sugar is frequently masked by other flavors — spices, herbs, and particularly salt. Even if there were no added sugar, the prolonged cooking of vegetables can break down the long chains of complex, slow-acting carbohydrates and cellulose, turning them into simple sugars. There are still some commercial soup possibilities that fit into our scheme. See the corresponding heading in the "So What's Left to Eat?" section on page 132.

Health Foods. Of the hundreds of packaged food products that you see on the shelves of the average health food store, perhaps 1 percent are low in carbohydrate. Many are sweetened, usually with honey or other so-called natural sugars. Since the health food industry shuns artificial (nonsugar) sweeteners like saccharin or aspartame, if a food tastes sweet, it probably contains a sugar. There are a few foods carried by these stores that are unsweetened and low in carbohydrate. You'll find some of these listed later in this chapter.

SO WHAT'S LEFT TO EAT?

It's a good question, and the same one I asked myself twenty-five years ago as I discovered that more and more of the things I had been eating made blood sugar control impossible. In the following pages, I'll give you a broad overview of the kinds of food my patients and I usually eat. Please remember that with the exception of the no-calorie beverages and moderate portions of sugar-free Jell-O, there are no "freebies." Virtually everything we eat will have some effect upon blood sugar if

No-No's in a Nutshell

Below is a concise list of foods to avoid that are discussed in this chapter. You may want to memorize it or copy it, as it is worth learning.

Sweets and Sweeteners
- Powdered sweeteners (other than stevia)
- Candies, including so-called sugar-free types
- Honey and fructose
- Most "diet" and "sugar-free" foods (except sugar-free Jell-O gelatin and diet sodas that do not contain fruit juices)
- Desserts (except Jell-O) and pastries: cakes, cookies, pies, tarts, et cetera
- Foods containing, as a significant ingredient, products whose names end in -*ol* or -*ose* (dextrose, glucose, lactose, mannitol, mannose, sorbitol, sucrose, xylitol, xylose, et cetera); also, corn syrup, molasses, et cetera

Sweet or Starchy Vegetables
- Beans (chili beans, chickpeas, lima beans, lentils, sweet peas, et cetera; string beans are okay, as are many soybean products)
- Beets
- Carrots
- Corn
- Onions, except in small amounts
- Packaged creamed spinach containing flour
- Parsnips
- Potatoes
- Tomatoes, tomato paste, tomato sauce, and raw tomatoes except in small amounts
- Winter squash

Fruit and Juices
- All fruits (except avocados)
- All juices (including tomato and vegetable juices)

Certain Dairy Products
- Milk
- Sweetened and low-fat yogurts
- Cottage cheese (except in very small amounts)
- Powdered "milk substitutes" and "coffee lighteners"

Grains and Grain Products
- Wheat, rye, barley, corn
- White, brown, or wild rice
- Pasta
- Breakfast cereal
- Pancakes and waffles
- Bread, crackers, and flour products

Prepared Foods
- Most commercially prepared soups
- Most packaged "health foods"
- Snack foods (virtually anything that comes wrapped in cellophane)
- Balsamic vinegar (compared to wine vinegar, white vinegar, or cider vinegar, balsamic contains considerable sugar)

enough is consumed. You may discover things I've never heard of that have a benign effect on your blood sugar. If so, feel free to include them in your meal plan (and let me know about them).

Vegetables

Most vegetables, other than those listed in the No-No section, are acceptable — such as asparagus, avocado, broccoli, brussels sprouts, cabbage and sauerkraut, cauliflower, eggplant, onions (in small amounts), peppers (any color), mushrooms, spinach, string beans, summer squash, and zucchini. As a rule of thumb, ⅔ cup of cooked vegetable or 1 cup of mixed salad acts upon blood sugar as if it contains about 6 grams of carbohydrate. Remember that cooked vegetables tend to raise blood sugar more rapidly than raw vegetables. On your self-measurements, note how your favorite vegetables affect your blood sugar. Raw vegetables can present digestive problems to people with gastroparesis.

Meat, Fish, Fowl, Seafood, and Eggs

These are usually the major sources of calories in the meal plans of my patients. The popular press is currently down on meat and eggs, but my personal observations and recent research implicate *carbohydrates* rather than dietary fat in the heart disease and abnormal blood lipid profile of diabetes. If you are frightened of these foods, you can restrict them, but depriving yourself will be unlikely to buy you anything. Appendix A details the current controversy and the shaky science behind the present, faddish high-carbohydrate dietary recommendations, and lays out my concerns and opinions.

Tofu, and Soybean Substitutes for Bacon, Sausage, Hamburger, Fish, Chicken, and Steak

About half the calories in these products come from vegetable fat, and the balance from equal amounts of protein and slow-acting carbohydrate. They are easy to cook in a skillet or microwave Protein and carbohydrate content should be read from the labels and counted in your meal plan. Their principal value is for people who are vegetarian or want to avoid red meat. Health food stores stock many of these products.

Certain Commercially Prepared and Homemade Soups

Although most commercial and homemade soups contain large amounts of simple sugars, you can learn how to buy or prepare low- or zero-carbohydrate soups. Many but not all packaged bouillon preparations have no added sugar and only small amounts of carbohydrate. Check the labels or use the Clinistix/Diastix test as described on page 123. Plain consommé or broth in some restaurants may be prepared without sugar. Again, check with Clinistix/Diastix.

Homemade soups, cooked without vegetables, can be made very tasty if they are concentrated. You can achieve this when making stock by barely covering the meat or chicken with water while cooking. Do not fill the entire pot with water, as is the customary procedure. Alternately, let the stock cook down (reduce) so you get a more concentrated, flavorful soup. You can also use herbs and spices, all of which have negligible amounts of carbohydrates, to enhance flavor. See "Mustard, Pepper, Salt, Herbs, Spices," below. Clam broth (not chowder) is usually very low in carbohydrate. In the United States you can also buy Snow's Clam Juice (not Clamato), which contains only 2 grams of carbohydrate in 3 fluid ounces.

Cheese, Butter, and Cream

Most cheeses (other than cottage cheese) contain approximately equal amounts of protein and fat and small amounts of carbohydrate. The carbohydrate and the protein must be figured into the meal plan, as I will explain in Chapter 11. For people who want to avoid animal fats, there are some special soybean cheeses. Cheese is an excellent source of calcium. Every ounce of cheese contains 1 gram carbohydrate, except cottage cheese, which contains more.

Butter will not affect your blood sugar significantly, and shouldn't be a problem as far as weight is concerned if you're not consuming a lot of carbohydrate along with it. One tablespoon of cream has only 0.4 gram carbohydrate — it would take 8 tablespoons to raise my blood sugar 16 mg/dl.

Yogurt

Although personally I don't enjoy yogurt, many of my patients feel they cannot survive without it. For our purposes the plain whole-milk yogurt, without fruit, is a reasonable food. A full 8-ounce container of plain, Erivan brand, unflavored whole milk yogurt contains only 11 grams of carbohydrate and 2 ounces of protein. You can even throw in some chopped vegetables and not exceed the 12 grams of carbohydrate limit we suggest for lunch. Do not use nonfat yogurt. The carbohydrate goes up to 17 grams per 8-ounce container. Yogurt can be flavored with cinnamon, with No-Cal brand syrups mentioned below, with baking flavor extracts, or with the powder from sugar-free Jell-O brand gelatin without affecting the carbohydrate content. It can be sweetened with stevia liquid or powder. Erivan brand yogurt is available at health food stores throughout the United States. If you read labels, you may find other brands, such as Summerfield Farms, equally low in carbohydrate.

Soy Milk

There are any number of valuable soy products that can be used in our diet plan, and soy milk is no exception. It's a fine lightener for coffee and tea, and one of my patients adds a small amount to diet sodas. Others drink it as a beverage, either straight or with added flavoring such as the flavor extracts used for baking. Personally, I find the taste too bland to drink without flavoring. When used in small amounts (up to 1 ounce), soy milk need not be figured into the meal plan. It will curdle if you put it into very hot drinks.

As noted in the No-No foods section, of the many brands of soy milk on the market, the Westsoy "unsweetened" flavor is the only unsweetened one I have been able to find. Other unsweetened brands are available in various parts of the country.

Soybean Flour

If you or someone in your home is willing to try baking with soybean flour, you will find a neat solution to the pastry restriction. One ounce of full-fat soybean flour (about ¼ cup) contains only 7.5 grams of slow-acting carbohydrate. You could make chicken pies, tuna pies, and even Jell-O or chocolate mousse pies. Just remember to include the carbohydrate in your meal plan.

Soybean flour usually must be blended with egg to form a batter suitable for breads, cakes, and the like. Some recipes using soy flour appear in Appendix D.

Bran Crackers

Of the dozens of different crackers that I have seen in health food stores and supermarkets, I have found only two brands that are truly low in carbohydrate.

No-Cal Brand Syrups

These artificially sweetened liquid flavors are sold by many supermarkets in the New York metropolitan area. (They are distributed by H. Fox and Co., Inc., Brooklyn, NY 11212.) The available flavors include strawberry, raspberry, black cherry, chocolate, and pancake/waffle topping. This product contains no calories, no carbohydrate, no protein, and no fat. It takes a bit of imagination to put it to good use. For example, I sometimes spike my coffee with the chocolate flavor, or my tea with fruit flavors. I put the pancake/waffle topping on my eggs in the morning after heating it in a skillet.

Flavor Extracts

There are numerous flavor extracts often used in baking that you can use to make your food more exciting. They usually can be found in small brown bottles in the baking supply aisles of supermarkets. Read carbohydrate content from the label. Usually it's zero and therefore won't affect your blood sugar.

Mustard, Pepper, Salt, Spices, Herbs

Most commercial mustards are made without sugar and contain essentially no carbohydrate. This can readily be determined for a given brand by reading the label or by using the Clinistix/Diastix test. Pepper and salt have no effect upon blood sugar. Hypertensive individuals with *proven* salt sensitivity should, of course, avoid salt and highly salted foods (see page 318).

Most herbs and spices have very low carbohydrate content and are used in such small amounts that the amount of ingested carbohydrate would be insignificant. Watch out, however, for certain combinations such as powdered cinnamon with sugar. Just read the labels.

Low-Carbohydrate Salad Dressings

Most salad dressings are loaded with sugars and other carbohydrates. The ideal dressing for someone who desires normal blood sugars would therefore be oil and vinegar, perhaps with added spices, mustard, grated cheese, or even bacon bits. There are now available some commercial salad dressings with only 1 gram carbohydrate per 2-tablespoon serving. This is low enough that such a product can be worked into our meal plans. Be careful with mayonnaise. Most brands are labeled "carbohydrate —

0 grams," but may contain up to 0.4 grams per tablespoon. This is not a lot, but it adds up if you eat large amounts. Some imitation mayonnaise products have 5 grams of carbohydrate per 2-tablespoon serving.

Nuts

Although all nuts contain carbohydrate (as well as protein and fat), they usually raise blood sugar slowly and can therefore be worked into meal plans. As with most other foods, you will want to look up your favorite nuts in one of the books listed in Chapter 3 in order to obtain their carbohydrate content. By way of example, 10 (small, not jumbo) pistachio nuts contain only 1 gram carbohydrate, versus 10 cashew nuts, which contain 5 grams of carbohydrate. Although a few nuts may contain little carbohydrate, the catch is in the word "few." Very few of us can eat only a few nuts. In fact, I don't have a single patient who can count out a preplanned number of nuts, eat them, and then stop. So unless you have unusual will power, beware. Also beware of peanut butter — another deceptive addiction. One tablespoon of natural, unsweetened peanut butter contains only 3 grams of carbohydrate, but imagine the effect on blood sugar of downing the contents of a jar.

Sugar-Free Jell-O Gelatin

This is one of the few foods that in reasonable amounts will have no effect upon blood sugar. It is fine for snacks and desserts. A ½-cup serving contains no carbohydrate, no fat, and only 1 gram of protein. Just remember not to eat so much that you feel stuffed (see "The Chinese Restaurant Effect" in Chapter 6). You can enhance the taste by pouring a little heavy cream over your portion. One of my patients discovered that it becomes even tastier if you whip it in a blender with cream when it has cooled, just before it sets. If you add No-Cal chocolate syrup or chocolate-flavored baking extract and some stevia before whipping, you will have a delicious chocolate mousse. Of the many flavors of sugar-free Jell-O that are available, I like apple, Hawaiian pineapple, and watermelon. Unfortunately, very few supermarkets seem to carry the apple flavor, and I wonder if it still exists.

Sugar-Free Jell-O Puddings

Available in chocolate, vanilla, pistachio, and butterscotch flavors, these make a nice dessert treat. Unlike Jell-O gelatin, they contain a small amount of carbohydrate (about 6 grams per serving), which should be counted in your meal plan. Instead of mixing the powder with milk, use water or cream diluted with water.

Chewing Gum

Gum chewing can be a good substitute for snacking. The carbohydrate content of one stick of chewing gum varies from about 1 gram in a stick of sugar-free Trident to about 7 grams per piece for some liquid-filled chewing gums. The 7-gram gum will rapidly raise my blood sugar by about 35 mg/dl. The carbohydrate content of a stick of chewing gum can usually be found on the package label. "Sugar-free" gums all contain small amounts of sugar — the primary ingredient of Trident "sugarless" gum is sorbitol, a corn-based sugar alcohol. It also includes mannitol and aspartame.

Frozen Diet Soda Pops

Many supermarkets and toy stores in the United States sell plastic molds for making your own ice pops. If these are filled with sugar-free sodas, you can create a tasty snack that has no effect upon blood sugar. Do not use the commercially made "sugar-free" or "diet" ice pops that are displayed in supermarket freezers. They contain fruit juices and other sources of carbohydrate.

Very Low Carbohydrate Desserts

Appendix D of this book consists of low carbohydrate recipes, prepared and tested by chefs. It includes easy recipes for some low-carbohydrate desserts that are truly delicious.

Coffee, Tea, Seltzer, Mineral Water, Club Soda, Diet Sodas

None of these products should have significant effect upon blood sugar. The coffee and tea may be sweetened with liquid or powdered stevia, or with *tablet* sweeteners such as saccharin, cyclamate, and aspartame (Equal tablets). Remember to avoid the use of more than 2 teaspoons of cow's milk as a lightener. Try to use cream (which has much less carbohydrate). Read the labels of "diet" sodas, as a few brands contain sugar in the form of fruit juices. Many flavored mineral waters, bottled "diet" teas, and seltzers also contain added carbohydrate or sugar, as do many powdered beverages. Again, read the labels.

Alcohol, in Limited Amounts

Ethyl alcohol (distilled spirits), as we discussed in Chapter 9, has no direct effect upon blood sugar. Moderate amounts, however, can have a rapid effect upon the liver, preventing the conversion of dietary protein to glucose. If you are following a regimen that includes insulin or a pancreas-stimulating oral hypoglycemic agent, you're dependent upon conversion of protein to glucose in order to maintain blood sugar at safe levels. The effects of *small* amounts of alcohol (i.e., 1½ ounces of spirits for a typical adult) are usually negligible. Most "light" beers contain only about 3 grams of carbohydrate per can or bottle. (See Chapter 9.)

INCREASE YOUR AWARENESS OF FOOD CONTENTS

Read Labels

Virtually all packaged foods bear labels that reveal something about the contents. The FDA now requires that labels of packaged foods list the amount of carbohydrate, protein, fat, and fiber in a serving. Be sure, however, to note the size of the "serving." Sometimes the serving size is so small that you wouldn't want to be bothered eating it.

Beware of labels that say "lite," "light," "sugar-free," "dietetic," "diet," "reduced-calorie," "low-calorie," et cetera. "Fat-free" desserts may be the most dangerous of all. Even if you're losing weight, carbohydrate intake will impede your efforts much more than fat (see Chapter 9). These foods frequently but not always contain more carbohydrate than the foods they replace. The only way you can determine the carbohydrate content is to read the amount stated on the label. But even this can be deceptive. For example, one popular brand of "sugar-free" strawberry preserves has a label that states "carbohydrate — 0." Yet anyone can see the strawberries in the jar, and common sense would tell you strawberries contain carbohydrate. So deceptive labeling occurs, and, in my experience, is fairly prevalent in the "diet" food industry.

Use Food Value Manuals

In Chapter 3 a number of books are listed that show the carbohydrate contents of various foods. These manuals are recommended but not essential tools for creating your meal plan. The guidelines and advice set forth in Chapters 9–11 of this book, plus perhaps the recipes in Appendix D, are all you really need to get started.

If you want the potential for considerable variety in your meals, get all the books listed in Chapter 3. *Food Values of Portions Commonly Used* has been the dietitian's bible for over fifty years. It is updated every few years. Be sure to use the index at the back to locate the foods of interest. Note that on every page in the main section, carbohydrate and fat content are listed in the same column. The carbohydrate content of food always appears below the fat content. Do not get the two confused. Also, be sure to note the portion size in all these books. Another book on the list, *Kosher Calories,* is not just for people whose diets are restricted to kosher foods. Over 10,000 common brand-name foods available in the United States are listed.

VITAMIN AND MINERAL SUPPLEMENTS

It is common practice to prescribe supplementary vitamins and minerals for diabetics. This is primarily because most diabetics have chronically high blood sugars and therefore urinate a lot. Excessive urination causes a loss of water-soluble vitamins and minerals. If you can keep your blood sugars low enough to avoid spilling glucose into the urine (you can test it with Clinistix/Diastix), and if you eat a variety of vegetables, and red meat once or twice a week, you should not require supplements. Note, however, that major dietary sources of B-complex vitamins include breads and grains. If you're following a low-carbohydrate diet and exclude these from your meal plan, you should eat some bran crackers, bean sprouts, spinach, broccoli, brussels sprouts, or cauliflower each day. If you do not like vegetables or bran crackers, you might take a B-complex capsule or a multivitamin/mineral capsule each day. See pages 153–154 for a discussion of calcium supplementation for certain people who follow high-fiber or high-protein diets.

Supplemental vitamins and minerals should not ordinarily be used in excess of the FDA's recommended daily requirements. Large doses can inhibit the body's synthesis of some vitamins and intestinal absorption of certain minerals. Large doses are also potentially toxic. Doses of vitamin C in excess of 500 mg daily appear in the blood and may interfere with the chemical reaction on your blood sugar strips. As a result, your blood sugar readings can appear erroneously low. Vitamin E has been shown to reduce one of the destructive effects of high blood sugars (glycosylation of the body's proteins), in a dose-dependent fashion —

up to 1,200 IU (international units) per day. It has recently been shown to lower insulin resistance. I therefore recommend 400–1,200 IU per day to a number of my patients.

CHANGES IN BOWEL MOVEMENTS

A new diet often brings about changes in frequency and consistency of bowel movements. This is perfectly natural and should not cause concern unless you experience discomfort. Increasing the fiber content of meals, as with salads, bran crackers, and soybean products, can cause softer and more frequent stools. More dietary protein can cause less frequent and harder stools. Normal frequency of bowel movements can range from 3 times per day to 3 times per week. If you notice any changes in your bowel habits other than these, discuss them with your physician.

HOW DO PEOPLE REACT TO THE NEW DIET?

Most of my patients initially feel somewhat deprived, but also grateful because they feel more alert and healthier. I fall into this category myself: my mouth waters whenever I pass a bakery shop and sniff the aroma of fresh bread, but I am also grateful simply to be alive and sniffing.

11

Creating a Customized Meal Plan

Now that you have the essentials of what you should eat and what you should avoid, it's time to take you through the steps of customizing a meal plan that will get you on your way to blood sugar normalization.

A NOTE BEFORE YOU EMBARK UPON THE DIET

If you found yourself thinking as you went through the No-No foods section of the prior chapter that all of this information goes against conventional thinking — you're right. No doubt as you embark upon a meal and treatment plan to normalize your blood sugars, well-meaning but ill-informed friends and relatives will urge you to try more "fun" foods, or to eat less fat and more "complex" carbohydrates. I suggest that you read Appendix A, which provides some possible explanations as to why conventional wisdom may have taken a wrong turn. Or you can pass this book along to those friends and relatives. Perhaps they'll change their own diets.* The ultimate evidence will be how you feel and the improvement in your test results (Chapter 2).

---

* Before-and-after lipid and thrombotic risk profiles would answer the question for any nondiabetics who want to try our diet.

GENERAL PRINCIPLES FOR TAILORING A MEAL PLAN

If you use blood sugar–lowering medications such as insulin or oral hypoglycemic agents, the first rule of meal planning is *don't change your diet unless your physician first reviews the new meal plan and reduces your medications accordingly.* Most people who begin our low-carbohydrate diet show an immediate and dramatic drop in postprandial blood sugar levels, as compared to blood sugars on their prior, high-carbohydrate diets. If at the same time your medications are not reduced, your blood sugars can drop dangerously low.

The initial meal plan should be geared toward blood sugar control, and toward keeping you content with what you eat. So with those things in mind, if I sat down with you to "negotiate" your meal plan, I would have to have before me a GLUCOGRAF data sheet (Chapter 5) showing blood sugar profiles and blood sugar–lowering medications (if any) taken during the preceding week. Keyed to each day's blood sugar levels on the reverse side of the page would be a separate list of everything you ate and when. This information would give me an idea of what you like to eat, what effect particular doses of blood sugar–lowering medications have on your blood sugars, and the nuances of how your blood sugars are affected by particular foods. I also must know your current weight and about any other factors — such as delayed stomach-emptying and medications for other ailments — that might affect your blood sugar. In negotiating the meal plan, I'd try wherever possible to incorporate foods you like.

Changes for the purpose of weight reduction (or gain), as we will discuss in Chapter 12, can be made after observing the effects of the initial diet for a month or so.

If you've tried dieting to lose weight or to control your blood sugar, you may have found that simply cutting back on calories according to preprinted tables or fixed calculations can be frustrating and can even have the opposite effect. Say you have a supper that's too small to satisfy you. Later you're so hungry you feel you must have a snack. If you're like most people, your snack will likely be something loaded with carbohydrate, so you end up with high blood sugars and more calories than you would have consumed if you'd started with a sensible meal. My experience is that it's always best to start with a plan that allows you to get up from the table feeling comfortable but not stuffed.

If you've ever followed the old "exchange" system for preparing diabetic meal plans, you'll find that keeping track of grams of carbohydrate and ounces of protein (we always estimate carbohydrate in grams and protein in ounces) requires considerably less effort. Not only is it easier than the exchange approach, it's more effective, because it places the focus on carbohydrate, the nutrient that has the greatest effect upon blood sugar.

Since all of my patients bring me glucose profiles, over the years it has not been very difficult to develop guidelines for carbohydrate consumption that make blood sugar control relatively easy without causing too great a feeling of deprivation, even for those trying to lose weight.

My basic approach in negotiating a meal plan is that I first set carbohydrate limits for each meal. Then I ask my patient to tell me how many ounces of protein we should add to make him/her feel satisfied. For example, I usually advise patients to restrict their carbohydrate intake at breakfast to about 6 grams of *slow-acting* carbohydrate, 12 grams for lunch, and 12 grams for supper. (These guidelines also apply to children. Despite what the popular press might have you believe, carbohydrate is *not* essential to normal development, but protein and fat are.) Very few people would be willing to eat less than these amounts of carbohydrate. This is the main reason I don't recommend even smaller amounts of carbohydrate. Ideally, your blood sugar should be the same after eating as it was before. If blood sugar increases by more than 20 mg/dl after a meal, even if it eventually drops to your target value, either the meal content should be changed or blood sugar–lowering medications should be used before you eat.

What does 6 or 12 grams of carbohydrate look like?

SLOW-ACTING CARBOHYDRATE

The foods on the following list consist of slow-acting carbohydrate. These can constitute the building blocks of the carbohydrate portion of each meal. Of course you needn't limit your foods to these — many other such building blocks can be created. Read labels on packaged foods, consult nutrition tables for carbohydrate values of foods you like, check your blood sugars, and find out which foods work for you.

Equivalent to approximately 6 grams of carbohydrate per serving

- 6 Worthington Stripples or Morningstar Farms Breakfast Strips (meatless bacon) (contains 1 ounce protein)
- 3 Morningstar Farms Breakfast Links (meatless sausage) (contains 2 ounces protein)
- 2 Bran-a-Crisp crackers
- 3 G/G crispbreads
- 4½ ounces Erivan whole-milk unflavored yogurt (8 ounces contains 11 grams carbohydrate) (contains 1 ounce protein)
- 1 cup mixed salad with oil-and-vinegar dressing
- ⅔ cup cooked green vegetable, zucchini, mushrooms, eggplant, et cetera
- 1 serving Jell-O sugar-free pudding made with water or water and 1 tablespoon cream
- ½ medium avocado (3 ounces)

Equivalent to approximately 12 grams of carbohydrate per serving

- 1 cup mixed salad with oil-and-vinegar (not balsamic) dressing, plus ⅔ cup cooked green vegetable
- 1 cup mixed salad prepared with 4 tablespoons packaged dressing (if each tablespoon contains 1.5 grams of carbohydrate)
- 8 ounces Erivan whole-milk unflavored yogurt (contains 11 grams of carbohydrate plus 2 ounces protein), plus 1 Stripple

These lists slightly exaggerate the carbohydrate content of salad and cooked vegetables, but because of their bulk and the Chinese Restaurant Effect, the net effect upon blood sugar is approximately equivalent to the amounts of carbohydrate shown. To this slow-acting carbohydrate, we'd add an amount of protein that would allow you to leave the table feeling comfortable but not stuffed.

PROTEIN

It is wise to keep the size of the protein portion at a particular meal constant from one day to the next, so if you eat 6 ounces at lunch one day, you should have 6 ounces at lunch the next. This is especially important if you're taking blood sugar–lowering medications. Remember that about 10 percent of the cooked weight of most protein foods can be converted to glucose by the liver. If you are using tables of food values, keep in mind that 1 ounce of a protein food typically contains only 6 grams of actual protein. To estimate by eye, a cooked portion the size of a deck of playing cards weighs about 3 ounces (red meats weigh about 3.7 ounces because of their greater density).

Protein foods with virtually no carbohydrate

- Beef, lamb, veal
- Chicken, turkey
- Eggs
- Fish and shellfish (fresh or canned)
- Frankfurters
- Pork (ham, chops, bacon, et cetera)

Protein foods with a small amount of carbohydrate (1 gram/ounce)

- Cheeses (other than cottage cheese); the gram of carbohydrate per ounce found in most cheeses should be included when computing the carbohydrate portion of that meal

Soy products (6 grams carbohydrate/ounce of protein — check nutrition label on package)

- Veggi burgers
- Tofu
- Meatless bacon
- Meatless sausage
- Other soy substitutes (for fish, chicken, and so on)

If you have a rare disorder called familial dyslipidemia, restrictions on the amounts and types of dietary fats may be appropriate.

THE TIMING OF MEALS AND SNACKS

Meals need not follow a rigidly fixed time schedule, provided, in most cases, that you do not begin eating within 3½ hours of the end of the prior meal. This is so that the effect of the first meal upon blood sugar won't overlap with that of the next meal. For those who inject insulin, it's very important that meals should be separated by at least 5 hours. This is also ideally but not always true of snacks covered by insulin.

Snacks are permitted for some diabetics but certainly not required. The carbohydrate content of snacks may duplicate but should not exceed that allocated for lunch or supper. So if you ate lunch at noon, you might tolerate a snack that didn't exceed 12 grams of carbohydrate at about 3:30–4:00. You would then eat supper at about 7:30. Snacks are discussed in greater detail later in the chapter.

You need not be restricted to only three daily meals if you prefer four or more similar meals on a regular basis. The timing, again, should ideally be at least 3½ hours (5 hours for those who inject insulin) after the end of the prior meal or snack. For most diabetics, it can be far easier to control blood sugar, with or without medication, after smaller meals than after only one or two large meals.

Remember that there are no restrictions on coffee and tea used without milk or cream and with tablet (not powdered, except for stevia) sweeteners.

Let's now attempt to translate our guidelines into some practical examples.

BREAKFAST

With or without blood sugar–lowering medications it is usually more difficult to prevent a blood sugar rise after breakfast than after other meals. Therefore, for the reasons discussed under "The Dawn Phenomenon" in Chapter 6, I usually suggest half as much carbohydrate at breakfast as at other meals. Your body will probably not respond as well to either the insulin it makes or to injected insulin for about 3 hours after you rise in the morning because of the dawn phenomenon.

It is wise to eat breakfast every day, especially if you're overweight. In my experience, most obese people have a history of either skipping or eating very little breakfast. Then they become hungry later in the day and overeat. Nevertheless, for most of us, any meal can be skipped without adverse complications.

A typical breakfast on our meal plan would include 6 grams carbohydrate and an amount of protein to be determined initially by you. There are numerous possible sources of appetizing ideas for the carbohydrate portion of your breakfast. The best place to start is with what you currently eat, as long as it's not on the No-No list (see pages 130–131). You can also sample recipes from Appendix D. You can experiment with foods in the "So What's Left to Eat?" section, on page 129. There are many soybean products, such as the foods mentioned on page 132. Despite restrictions, with a little creativity you can find any number of satisfying things to have for breakfast.

Suppose that, like many of my new patients, you've been eating for breakfast a bagel loaded with cream cheese and 2 cups of coffee with skim milk and Sweet'n Low powdered sweetener (totaling about 40 grams of rapid-acting carbohydrates). As we negotiate, I might propose that you substitute other sweeteners for the Sweet'n Low and 1 ounce Westsoy soy milk (0.5 gram carbohydrate) for the skim milk in each cup of coffee (or use a small amount of cream). Then I'd recommend that instead of a bagel you eat a G/G cracker (2 grams carbohydrate) with 2 ounces of cream cheese (2 grams carbohydrate). This adds up to 5 grams of carbohydrate. Finally, I'd suggest that you add a protein food to your meal to make up for the calories and "filling power" that disappeared with the bagel.

Let's say you eat eggs for breakfast (or egg whites or Egg Beaters). I'd ask how many eggs it would take to make you feel satisfied after giving up the bagel. If you're unnecessarily afraid of egg yolks, you might use only egg whites. If you find the taste of egg whites bland, you could add spices, or soy or Tabasco sauce, or some mushrooms or a small amount of onion or cheese, or even cinnamon or chili powder, to enhance the taste.

In the past, I'd try to help my patients who love cold cereal to include a small amount in their breakfast meal plan, but blood glucose profiles showed consistently that this just didn't work. Grain products, with the exception of the bran products I've mentioned, contain too much fast-acting carbohydrate to allow us to keep blood sugar under control, and so we've had to eliminate breakfast cereals entirely. An alternative might be the bran cracker cereal described on page 135.

The good news is that there are lots of other tasty, filling things to eat.

If you don't want eggs, you might try some smoked fish, tuna fish, or even a hamburger. I have one patient who eats two hot dogs for breakfast — her favorite food. The quantity of fish or hamburger would be up to you, but it would have to be kept constant from one day to the next. You can either weigh the protein portion on a food scale or estimate it by eye. The rule of thumb is, again, that a cooked portion of poultry or fish the size of a standard deck of playing cards will weigh about 3 ounces (3.7 ounces for red meat). One egg has the approximate protein content of 1 ounce of poultry or fish.

You can take any of the foods in the 6 grams of carbohydrate list on page 146 and add protein to them (cheese, eggs, et cetera) to make a satisfying breakfast.

LUNCH

Follow the same guidelines for lunch as for breakfast, with the exception that the carbohydrate content may be doubled, to 12 grams.

Say, for example, that you and your friends go to lunch every day at the "greasy spoon" around the corner from work and are served only sandwiches. You might try discarding the slices of bread and eating the filling — meat, turkey, cheese, or other protein food — with a knife and fork. (If you choose cheese, remember to count 1 gram carbohydrate per ounce.) You could also order a hamburger without the bun. And instead of ketchup, you could use mustard, soy sauce, or other carbohydrate-free condiments. You then might add a bottle of regular beer (13 grams of carbohydrate) *or* 2 cups of salad with vinegar-and-oil dressing (12 grams of carbohydrate) to round out your meal.

If you want to create a lunch menu from scratch, use your food value guides to look up foods that interest you. The following building blocks may be helpful in giving you a start.

For the protein portion

- A small can of tuna fish contains 3¼ ounces by weight in the United States. If you're packing your lunch, these can be quite convenient if you like tuna. The next larger size can contains 6 ounces.
- 4 standard slices of packaged pasteurized process American cheese weigh about 3 ounces. This will contain 3 ounces of protein and 3 grams of carbohydrate.

For about 12 grams carbohydrate

- 1⅓ cups cooked green vegetables (green beans, zucchini, spinach, broccoli; *not* green peas)
- 2 cups mixed green salad, with 1 slice of tomato and vinegar-and-oil dressing
- 1½ cups salad, as above, but with 3 tablespoons of commercial salad dressing (other than simple vinegar-and-oil) containing 1 gram of carbohydrate per tablespoon. Check the label.

You might decide that 2 cups of salad with vinegar-and-oil dressing is fine for the carbohydrate portion of your lunch. You then should decide how much protein must be added to keep you satisfied. One person might be happy with a 3¼-ounce can of tuna fish, but another might require 2 large chicken drumsticks or a small packet of lunch meat weighing 6 ounces. For dessert, you might want some cheese (in the European tradition) or perhaps some sugar-free Jell-O pudding covered with Westsoy or heavy cream or whipped up in a blender with a little cream plus No-Cal chocolate syrup or a baking flavor extract to make a zero-carbohydrate chocolate mousse. You might consider some of the desserts described in Appendix D. The possible combinations are endless; just use your food value books or read labels for estimating protein and carbohydrate. Some people, after having routinely eaten the same thing for years, discover that their new meal plan opens up culinary possibilities they never knew existed. Our patients, as well as readers, are always looking for recipes, so if you come up with a recipe that you think is tasty, please feel free to send it to me at the Diabetes Center, 1160 Greacen Point Road, Mamaroneck, NY 10543-4696.

SUPPER

Supper should follow essentially the same approach as lunch. There is, however, one significant difference that will only apply to those taking insulin who are affected by delayed stomach-emptying, or gastroparesis. As we've discussed briefly, this can cause unpredictable shifts in blood sugar levels because food doesn't always pass into the intestines at the same rate from meal to meal. The difficulty with supper is that you can end up with high or low blood sugars while you are sleeping and unable to monitor and correct them. Sustained exposure to high blood sugars while sleeping — even if they are normalized during the day — can lead to long-term diabetic complications. For certain affected people, a viable approach to this problem is to facilitate stomach-emptying by substituting cooked vegetables for salads at supper and reducing protein content. For these people, the amount of protein at supper would be less than that eaten at lunch — just the opposite of what has become customary for most of us. A more complete analysis of this problem appears in Chapter 21.

If you like cooked green vegetables for supper, remember that most can be interchanged with salads as near equivalents — ⅔ cup of cooked green vegetable and 1 cup of salad each have the blood sugar effect of about 6 grams carbohydrate.

If you like wine with dinner, choose a very dry variety and limit yourself to 1 glass (see pages 118–120 for further details). An average bottle of beer will use up your entire carbohydrate allocation (about 13 grams), so you may want to use a "light" beer, which typically contains only 3 grams of carbohydrate per bottle (read the label). Still, don't drink more than one.

SNACKS

For most people with diabetes, snacks should be neither mandatory nor forbidden. They do, however, pose a problem for people who take fast-acting insulin before meals, for reasons we will discuss in Chapter 18. Snacks should be a convenience, to relieve hunger if meals are delayed or spaced too far apart for comfort. If your diabetes is severe enough to warrant the use of rapid-acting blood sugar–lowering medication before meals, such medication may also be necessary before snacks.

The carbohydrate limit of 6 grams during the first few hours after arising and 12 grams of carbohydrate thereafter that applies to meals also applies to snacks. Be sure that your prior meal has been fully digested before your snack starts (this usually means waiting 3½–4 hours). This is so that the effects upon blood sugar will not add to one another. You needn't worry if the snack is so sparse (say, a bit of toasted nori) as to have negligible effects on blood sugar. Sugar-free Jell-O can be consumed pretty much whenever you like, provided you don't stuff yourself and provoke the Chinese Restaurant Effect. As a rule, snacks limited to small amounts of protein will have less effect upon blood sugar than those containing carbohydrate. Thus 2–3 ounces of cheese or cold cuts might be reasonable snacks for some people.

If you're being treated with only longer-acting blood sugar–lowering agents, the question of random or even preplanned snacking is best answered by experimentation using blood sugar measurements (see Chapter 18).

OTHER CONSIDERATIONS

Meal and Medication Adjustments

Although your blood sugars will respond best if you adhere to our restrictions on carbohydrate, you'll find that you have considerable leeway when it comes to planning the amount of *protein* for each meal. At the initial meal-planning session with your physician or other health care provider, you may estimate that you will require perhaps 6 ounces protein to satisfy your appetite at lunch. When you actually try eating such a lunch, you may conclude that this amount of protein is either too much or too little. This can readily be changed, provided that you advise your health care provider, so that dosage of any medication you may be taking is changed accordingly. Once a comfortable amount of protein has been established for a meal, it should not change from day to day but, like the carbohydrate, be held constant. The predictability of blood sugar levels under this regimen depends, in part, upon the predictability of your eating pattern.

Carbohydrate Juggling

Many patients ask me if they can juggle carbohydrate or protein from one meal to another, keeping the totals for the day constant. Such an approach doesn't work, for reasons that should be obvious by now, and can be downright dangerous if you're taking medications that lower blood sugars.

Calcium Concerns

Some people who follow my dietary guidelines consume considerable amounts of fiber. Slow-acting carbohydrate foods that are especially high in fiber include salads, broccoli, cauliflower, bran, and soybean products. Fiber binds dietary calcium in the gut, causing a reduction of calcium absorption and potential depletion of bone mineral, which contains 99.5 percent of our calcium reserves. The phosphorus present in proteins also may bind calcium slightly. Since I discourage the use of milk and milk products (except cheese, yogurt, and cream), which are good sources of dietary calcium, the potential for bone mineral depletion is indeed real. This is a special problem for women, who tend to lose bone mass at an increased rate after menopause. I recommend a calcium supplement to anyone who follows our diet and doesn't eat cheese or use cream, especially women. Since some women rapidly lose calcium from their bones after menopause, it makes sense to build up calcium stores earlier in life, and to offset high-fiber and high-protein diets with extra calcium. Calcium supplementation, by the way, is most important for growing teenagers who follow such diets. I recommend calcium citrate (Citracal, from Mission Pharmacal Company) because it is well absorbed in the gut and, unlike other calcium formulations, does not predispose to formation of kidney stones. Each tablet contains 315 mg of elemental calcium. Appropriate daily doses are 2–6 tablets for men and 4–8 tablets for women. One study of calcium supplementation suggests the equivalent of at least 3 Citracal tablets for every 10 ounces of protein consumed. Calcium supplements should be taken with meals. Calcium tablets taken at bedtime are often effective in reducing the frequency of nocturnal muscle cramps in the legs. Sedentary people lose more bone calcium over a lifetime than do physically active people. Exercise builds bone just as it builds muscle.

SOME PROTOTYPE MEAL PLANS

The guidelines set forth in this chapter should be adequate for you to create your own meal plan, but I don't want to leave you with any uncertainty as to how it is done. I have, therefore, listed below 3 days' worth of breakfasts, lunches, and suppers to give you an idea of how I do it. These meals should serve as a starting point. You may want to overhaul them entirely to reflect your favorite foods. If, for example, you prefer canned salmon to frankfurters, just substitute a small can (3¼ ounces) of salmon for the frankfurters in the lunch of Day One.

The carbohydrate content of each meal reflects our 6-12-12 guidelines. If you're going to maintain normal blood sugars, then these amounts of carbohydrate must remain rigid and really should reflect maximum amounts. That said, however, exceeding or diminishing carbohydrate allocations by 1–2 grams per meal will not make a great difference in your blood sugars — remember the Laws of Small Numbers. Aside from these constraints, you are otherwise limited only by your imagination. The protein content of meals, on the other hand, is completely up to you. For the following examples, I've arbitrarily assumed certain amounts of protein that may be too much or too little to satisfy your desires; you will want to experiment to determine your own preferences. Remember, however, that protein, like carbohydrate, should be kept constant from one day to the next for any given meal.

Let's asume that you've negotiated a meal plan, and the amounts of assigned carbohydrate and amounts of protein that you think will satisfy you are as follows:

Breakfast: 6 grams carbohydrate, 3 ounces protein
Lunch: 12 grams carbohydrate, 4 ounces protein
Supper: 12 ounces carbohydrate, 5 ounces protein

Note that only one of the nine meals to follow adds up precisely to these guidelines for total carbohydrate and protein, yet all of them are quite close and thus acceptable. Note also that I usually don't list beverages. This is simply because most acceptable beverages other than beer and dry wine contain neither carbohydrate nor protein and may therefore be ignored in our computations. Remember, however, that every tablespoon of cream for your coffee or tea contains 0.4 grams of carbohydrate.

Day One

Breakfast	Carbohydrate (grams)	Protein (ounces)
Mushroom Omelet with Bacon (page 337)	3.1	2.8
1 Bran-a-Crisp with butter	<u>3.0</u>	=
	6.1	2.8

Lunch		
2 servings Asparagus and Artichoke Salad (page 342)	8.0	0.6
2 frankfurters	<u>3.0</u>	<u>3.4</u>
	11.0	4.0

Supper		
⅔ cup mixed salad with oil, vinegar, and spices	4.0	—
2 tablespoons crumbled blue cheese on salad	0.4	0.7
Pan-Fried Swordfish with Ginger Scallion Butter (page 351)	<u>7.3</u>	<u>4.5</u>
	11.7	5.2

Day Two

Breakfast	Carbohydrate (grams)	Protein (ounces)
Pancakes (page 340)	5.0	1.1
2 sausage patties, 1 ounce each	<u>0.6</u>	<u>1.8</u>
	5.6	2.9

Lunch		
1 small can tuna (3¼ ounces) mixed with 1 tablespoon each mayonnaise and chopped celery	0.3	3.25
1 slice American cheese (place on top of tuna and heat in microwave for tuna melt)	0.75	0.75
12-ounce bottle Blatz Cream Ale	<u>11.1</u>	<u>0.18</u>
	12.15	4.18

Supper		
Quiche Lorraine (page 354)	9.7	3.6
Chocolate Soufflé (page 357)	<u>2.9</u>	<u>1.8</u>
	12.6	5.4

Day Three

Breakfast	Carbohydrate (grams)	Protein (ounces)
2 ounces Nova Scotia salmon	—	2.0
1 ounce cream cheese	1.0	1.0
2 Bran-a-Crisp crackers	<u>6.0</u>	<u>=</u>
	7.0	3.0

Lunch		
Leek Soup (page 341)	9.8	0.2
3½ ounces hamburger meat	—	3.5
1 tablespoon Bacos brand soy bacon bits (knead into hamburger before cooking)	<u>2.0</u>	<u>0.5</u>
	11.8	4.2

Supper		
1 medium artichoke, boiled, served with melted butter	12.4	0.5
4½ ounces any meat, fish, or poultry, cooked as you like	=	<u>4.5</u>
	12.4	5.0

To nearly any one of these meals you could add as a dessert a serving of sugar-free Jell-O brand gelatin, which would not appreciably affect your carbohydrate allocations. Again, you are limited only by your imagination, and there are countless different meals you can create that add up to 6 or 12 grams of carbohydrate, and 3, 4, 5, or more ounces of protein.

12

Weight Loss — If You're Overweight

Weight loss can significantly reduce your insulin resistance. You may recall from Chapter 1 that obesity, specifically abdominal (truncal, or visceral) obesity, causes insulin resistance and thereby can play a major role in the development of both impaired glucose tolerance and Type II diabetes. If you have this kind of obesity, it is important that weight loss become a goal of your treatment plan. Weight reduction can also slow down the process of beta-cell burnout by making your tissues more sensitive to the insulin you still produce, allowing you to require (and therefore produce or inject) less insulin.

It may even be possible, under certain circumstances, to completely reverse your glucose intolerance. Long before I studied medicine, I had a friend, Howie, who gained about 100 pounds over the course of a few years. He developed Type II diabetes and had to take a large amount of insulin (100 units daily) to keep it under control. His physician pointed out to him the likely connection between his diabetes and his obesity. To my amazement, during the following year, he was able to lose 100 pounds. At the end of the year, he had normal glucose tolerance, no need for insulin, and a new wardrobe. This kind of success may only be possible if the diabetes is of short duration, but it is certainly worth keeping in mind — weight loss can sometimes work miracles.

Before we talk about weight loss, it makes sense to talk about obesity.

THE THRIFTY GENOTYPE

When I see a very overweight person, I don't think, "He ought to control his eating." I think, "He has the thrifty genotype."

What is the thrifty genotype?

The hypothesis for the thrifty genotype was first proposed by James V. Neel in 1962 to explain the high incidence of obesity and Type II diabetes among the Pima Indians of the southwestern United States. Evidence for a genetic determinant of obesity has increased over the years. Photographs of the Pimas from a century ago show a lean and wiry people. They did not know what obesity was and in fact had no word in their vocabulary to identify it.

Their food supply diminished in the early part of this century, something that had occurred repeatedly throughout their history. Now, however, they weren't faced with famine. The Bureau of Indian Affairs took over feeding them, and an astonishing thing happened. These lean and wiry people developed an astronomical incidence of obesity — 100% of adult Pima Indians today are grossly obese, with a staggering rate of diabetes. Fully 60 percent of adults are Type II diabetics.

What happened to the Pimas? How did such apparently hardy and fit people become so grossly obese? Though their society was at least in part agrarian, they lived in the desert, where drought was frequent and harvests could easily fail. During periods of famine, those of their forebears whose bodies were not thrifty or capable of storing enough energy to survive without food died out. Those who survived were those who somehow could survive without food. How did they do it? Although it may be simplifying somewhat, the mechanism essentially works like this: Those who naturally craved carbohydrate and consumed it whenever it was available, even if they weren't hungry, would have made more insulin and thereby stored more fat. Add to this the additional mechanism of the high insulin levels caused by inherited insulin resistance, and serum insulin levels would have become great enough to induce fat storage sufficient to enable them to live through famines. (See Figure 1-1.) Truly survival of the fittest — provided famines would continue.

A strain of chronically obese mice created in the early fifties demonstrates quite vividly how valuable thrifty genes can be in famine. When these mice are allowed an unlimited food supply, they balloon and add as much as half again the body weight of normal mice. Yet deprived of food, these mice can survive a mind-boggling 40 days, versus 7–10 days for normal mice.

Recent research on these chronically obese mice provides some tantalizingly direct evidence of the effect a thrifty genotype can have upon physiology. In ordinary mice, a hormone called leptin is produced in the fat cells (also a hormone the human body produces, with apparently similar effect). The hormone tends to inhibit overeating, speed metabolism, and act as a modulator of level of body fat. A genetic "flaw" causes the obese mice to make a less effective form of leptin. In recent experiments, when injected with the real thing they almost instantly slimmed down. Not only did they eat less but they lost as much as 40 percent of their body weight, their metabolism sped up, and they became much more active. Many were diabetic, but their loss of weight (and the change in the ratio of fat to lean body mass) reversed or even "cured" their diabetes. Ordinary mice injected with leptin also ate less, became more active, and lost weight, though not as high a percentage. Research on humans has not advanced sufficiently to provide conclusive evidence that the mechanism is the same in obese humans, but researchers believe it is at least equivalent and probably related to more than one gene, and to different gene clusters in different populations.

In a full-blown famine, the Pima Indian's ability to survive long enough to find food is nothing short of a blessing. But when satisfying carbohydrate craving is suddenly just a matter of going to the grocery, what was once an asset becomes a very serious liability.

Although about 30 percent of the overall population of the United States is chronically obese, there is considerable reason to be concerned, because the number has been increasing by 1 percent each year. Some researchers attribute rising obesity in the United States at least in part to increasing numbers of former smokers. Others attribute it to the recent increase in carbohydrate consumption by those trying to avoid dietary fat. Whatever the reasons, obesity can lead to diabetes.

The thrifty genotype has its most dramatic appearance in isolated populations like the Pimas, which have recently been exposed to an unlimited food supply after millennia of intermittent famine. The Fiji Islanders, for example, were another lean, wiry people, accustomed to the rigors of paddling out against the Pacific to fish. Their diet, high in protein and low in carbohydrate, suited them perfectly. After the onset of the tourist economy that followed World War II, their diet changed to our high-carbohydrate western diet, and they too began (and continue) to suffer from a high incidence of obesity and Type II diabetes. The same is true of the Australian Aborigines after the Aboriginal Service began to provide them with grain. Ditto for South African blacks who migrated from the bush into the big cities. Interestingly, a study that paid obese, diabetic South African blacks to go back to the countryside and return to their traditional high-protein, low-carbohydrate diet found that they experienced dramatic weight loss and regression of their diabetes.

It's clear that thrifty genotypes work in isolated populations to make metabolism supremely energy-efficient, but what happens when the populations have unrestricted access to high-carbohydrate foods?

It would appear that the mechanism of the thrifty genotype works something like this: Certain areas of the brain associated with satiety — that sensation of being physically and emotionally satisfied — have lower levels of certain chemicals known as neurotransmitters. A number of years ago, Drs. Richard and Judith Wurtman at the Massachusetts Institute of Technology (MIT) discovered that the level of the neurotransmitter serotonin is raised in certain parts of the hypothalamus of the animal brain when the animal eats carbohydrate, especially fast-acting concentrated carbohydrate like bread. Serotonin is a neurotransmitter that seems to reduce anxiety as it produces satiety. Other neurotransmitters such as dopamine and norepinephrine can also affect our senses of satiety and anxiety, euphoria and dysphoria. There are now seventy-five known neurotransmitters, and many more of them may affect mood and food in ways that are just beginning to be researched and understood.

In persons with the thrifty genotype, deficiencies of these neurotransmitters (or diminished sensitivity to them in the brain) causes both a feeling of hunger and a mild dysphoria — often a sensation of anxiety, and the opposite of euphoria. Eating carbohydrates temporarily causes the individual to feel not only less hungry but also more at ease.

A frequent television sitcom scenario is the woman just dumped by her boyfriend who plops down on the couch with a pie or half a gallon of ice cream, a spoon, and the intention of eating the whole thing. She's not really hungry. She's depressed and trying to make herself feel better. She's indulging herself, we think, rewarding herself in a way for enduring one of life's traumas, and we laugh because we understand the feeling. But there is a very real biochemical mechanism at work here. She craves the sugar in the pie or the ice cream not because she's hungry but because she knows, consciously or not, that it *really will* make her feel better. Contrary to popular belief, the fat in the ice cream or in the crust of the pie doesn't make much of a difference. It's the carbohydrate that will increase the level of certain neurotransmitters in her brain and make her feel better temporarily. The side effect of the carbohydrate is that it also causes her blood sugar to rise and her body to make more insulin; and, as she sits on the couch, the elevation in her insulin will turn the sugar she eats into fat.

On television the actress never gets fat. But for the real-life woman, high serum insulin levels from eating high-carbohydrate foods will cause her to crave carbohydrate again. If she is a Type I diabetic making no insulin, she'll have to inject a lot of insulin to get her blood sugar down, with the same effect — more carbohydrate craving and building up of fat reserves.

TOOLS FOR WEIGHT LOSS

Because of the diversity of the population of the United States, and the likelihood of there being more than one genetic mechanism that causes us to conserve body fat, there may be many genetic mechanisms that result in obesity. The most common overt cause of obesity is overeating carbohydrate, usually over a period of years. Unfortunately, this can be a very difficult type of obesity to treat.

If you're overweight, you're probably unhappy with your appearance, and no less with your high blood sugars. Perhaps in the past you've tried to follow a restricted diet, without success. Generally, overeating follows two patterns, and frequently they overlap. First is overeating at meals. Second is normal eating at mealtime but with episodic binge eating. Binge eating can be anything from nibbling and snacking between meals to eating everything that does not walk away. Many of the people who follow our low-carbohydrate diet find that their carbohydrate craving ceases almost immediately, possibly because of a reduction in their serum insulin levels. The addition of muscle-building exercise sometimes enhances this effect. Unfortunately, these interventions don't work for everyone.

Medications

If you're a compulsive overeater, if you just can't stop yourself from eating, and are addicted to carbohydrate, you may not be able to adhere to our diet without some sort of medical intervention. Carbohydrate addiction is just as real as drug addiction, and in the case of the diabetic, it can have equally disastrous results. (In actual fact, obesity kills more Americans annually from its related complications than all drugs of abuse combined, including alcohol.)

You need not despair of ever losing weight, however. I have seen a number of "diet-proof" patients over the years get their weight down and blood sugars under control. Over the last several years, as medical science has gained a much more sophisticated understanding of the biological mechanisms that contribute to emotional states such as hunger and mood, many relatively benign medications have been successfully applied to the treatment of compulsive overeating. There is no doubt that when used *properly*, many appetite suppressants are quite effective in helping people to lose weight. If you simply cannot lose weight, discuss with your physician medicines that may be of use to you. I have used more than forty different medications with my patients and have found many of them to be of great value for treating carbohydrate addiction. Their proper application, however, requires considerable specialized knowledge.

Reducing Serum Insulin Levels

Another group of Type II diabetics has a common story: "I was never fat until after my doctor started me on insulin." Usually these people have been following high-carbohydrate diets and so must have large doses of insulin to effect a modicum of blood sugar control.

Insulin, remember, is the principal fat-building hormone of the body. Although a Type II diabetic may be resistant to insulin-facilitated glucose transport (from blood to tissues), that resistance doesn't diminish insulin's capacity for fat-building. In other words, insulin can be great at making you fat, even though it may be inefficient at lowering your blood sugar. Since excess insulin *causes* insulin resistance, the more you take, the more you'll need, and the fatter you'll get. This is not an argument against the use of insulin; rather it supports our conclusion that high levels of dietary carbohydrate — which, in turn, require large amounts of insulin — make blood sugar control (and weight reduction) unworkable.

I have witnessed, over and over, dramatic weight loss and blood sugar improvement in people who have merely been shown how to reduce their insulin doses and carbohydrate intake.

Metformin, troglitazone, and similar agents, which we will discuss in detail in Chapter 14, "Oral Hypoglycemic Agents," can also be valuable tools in weight loss. They work by making the body's tissues more sensitive to injected or self-made insulin. As it takes less insulin to accomplish our goal of blood sugar normalization, you'll have less of this fat-building hormone circulating in your body. I have patients using these unique medications who are not diabetic, and they work in a similar way: the body is more sensitive to insulin, so it needs to produce less, and there is, again, less of it present to build fat. One may also have less of a sense of hunger, and less loss of control.

Increasing Muscle Mass

All the above suggests what we have been advocating all along — a low-carbohydrate diet. But what do you do if this plus one of the above medications does not result in weight loss? Another step is muscle-building exercise (see next chapter). This is of value in weight reduction for several reasons. Increasing lean body weight (muscle mass) upgrades insulin sensitivity, enhancing glucose transport and reducing insulin requirements for blood sugar normalization. Lower insulin levels facilitate loss of stored fat. Chemicals produced during exercise (endorphins) tend to reduce appetite, as do lower serum insulin levels. People who have seen results from exercise tend to invest more effort in looking even better (e.g., by not overeating, and perhaps exercising more). They know it can be done.

HOW TO ESTIMATE YOUR REAL FOOD REQUIREMENTS

Now suppose you have been following our low-carbohydrate diet, have been conscientiously "pumping iron" every day, and are, in effect, "doing everything right." What else can you do, if you have not lost weight? Well, everyone has some level of caloric intake below which they will lose weight. Unfortunately, the "standard" formulas and tables commonly used by nutritionists set forth caloric guidelines for theoretical individuals of a certain age, height, and sex, but not for real people like you. The only way to find out how much food *you* need in order to maintain, gain, or lose weight is by experiment. Here is an experimental plan that your physician may find useful. This method usually works, and without counting calories.

Begin by setting an initial target weight and a time frame in which to achieve it. Using standard tables of "ideal body weight" is of little value, simply because they give a very wide target range. This is because some people have more muscle and bone mass for a given height than others. The high end of the ideal weight for a given height on the Metropolitan Life Insurance Company's table is 30 percent greater than the low end for the same height.

Instead, estimate your target weight by looking in the mirror after weighing yourself. (It pays to do this in the presence of your health care provider, because he/she probably has more experience in estimating the weight of your body fat.) If you can grab handfuls of fat at the underside of your upper arms, around your thighs, around your waist, or over your belly, it is pretty clear that your body is set for the next famine. Your estimate at this point need not be terribly precise, because as you lose weight your target weight can be reestimated. Say, for example, that you weigh 200 pounds. You and your physician may agree that a reasonable target would be 150 pounds. By the time you reach 160 pounds, however, you may have lost your visible excess fat — so settle for 160 pounds. Alternately, if you still have fat around your belly when you get down to 150 pounds, it won't hurt to shoot for 145 or 140 as your next target, before making another visual evaluation. Gradually you home in on your eventual target, using smaller and smaller steps.

Once your initial target weight has been agreed upon, a time frame for losing the weight should be established. Again, this need not be utterly precise. It's important, however, not to "crash diet." This may cause a "yo-yo" effect by slowing your metabolism and making it difficult to keep off the lost bulk. Bear in mind that if you starve yourself and lose 10 pounds without adequate dietary protein and an accompanying exercise regimen, you may lose 5 pounds of fat and 5 pounds of muscle. If you gain back that 10 pounds from eating carbohydrate and still are not exercising, it may be 100 percent fat. After crash dieting, once you've reached your target, you may go right back to overeating. I like to have my patients follow a gradual weight-reduction diet that matches as closely as possible what they'll probably be eating after the target has been reached. In other words, once you reach your target, you stay on the same diet you followed while losing weight. This way you've gotten into the habit of eating a certain amount, and you stick to this amount, more or less, for life.

To achieve this, weight loss must be gradual. If you are targeted to lose 25 pounds or less, I suggest a reduction of 1 pound per week. If you're heavier, you may try for 2 pounds per week. If just cutting the carbohydrate, as suggested in prior chapters, results in a more rapid weight loss, don't worry — just enjoy your luck. This has happened to a number of my patients.

Weigh yourself once weekly — stripped, if possible, on the same scale, and before breakfast. Pick a convenient day, and weigh yourself on the same day each week at the same time of day. It's counterproductive and not very informative to weigh yourself more often. Small, normal variations in body weight occur from day to day and can be frustrating if you misinterpret them. Generally speaking, you won't lose or gain a pound of body fat in a day. Continue on your low-carbohydrate diet, with enough protein foods to keep you comfortable.

Let's say that your goal is to lose 1 pound every week. Weigh yourself after one week. If you've lost the weight, don't change anything. If you haven't lost the pound, reduce the protein at any one meal by one-third. For example, if you've been eating 6 ounces of fish or meat at dinner, cut it to 4 ounces. You can pick which meal to cut back at. Check your weight one week later. If you have lost a pound, don't change anything. If you haven't, cut the protein at another meal by one-third. If you haven't lost the pound in the subsequent week, cut the protein by one-third in the one remaining meal. Keep doing this, week by week, until you are losing at the target rate. Never add back any protein that you have cut out even if you subsequently lose 2 or 3 pounds in a week.

If you've managed to lose at least 1 pound weekly for many weeks, but then your weight levels off, this is a good time for your physician to pre-scribe the special insulin resistance–lowering agents described in Chapter 14. Alternately you can just start cutting protein again. Continue this until you reach your initial target or until your visual evaluation of ex-cess body fat tells you that further weight loss isn't necessary. Most adults require at least 5 ounces of high-quality protein daily to prevent certain forms of malnutrition. It is therefore unwise to cut your protein intake below this level. Some authorities recommend double this amount. Once you've reached your target weight, do not add back any food. You will probably have to stay on approximately this diet for many years, but you'll easily become accustomed to it. If you required some of the appetite-reducing medications mentioned earlier in the chapter, do not discontinue them. About six months after you reach your target weight, your physician may want to taper off the medication(s) gradually. If you start eating more than your final meal plan calls for, the medication(s) will have to be tapered up again.

REDUCE DIABETES MEDICATIONS WHILE CUTTING PROTEIN OR LOSING WEIGHT

While you're losing weight, keep checking blood sugars at least 5 times daily, at least two days a week. If they consistently drop below your target value for even a few days, advise your physician immediately. It will probably be necessary to reduce the doses of any blood sugar–lowering medications you may be taking. Keeping track of your blood sugar levels as you lose weight and eat less is essential for the prevention of dangerously low blood sugar levels.

INCREASED THROMBOTIC ACTIVITY DURING WEIGHT LOSS

During weight loss, many people unknowingly experience increased clumping of the small particles in the blood (platelets) that form clots (thrombi). This can increase the risk of heart attack or stroke. Your physician may therefore want you to take an 80 mg enteric coated aspirin once daily after a meal to reduce this tendency.

13

Using Exercise to Enhance Insulin Sensitivity

Strenuous, prolonged exercise is the next level of our treatment plan after diet, and should ideally accompany any weight-loss program. Before we go into our specific recommendations for exercise, all of which should be approved by your physician, it's important that you understand the benefits exercise can bring.

WHY EXERCISE?

While many people may begin exercising out of a sense of responsibility — the way children eat vegetables they don't like — the main reason they *keep* exercising is that it feels good. Whether it's the intense competition of a fast and furious basketball game, or cycling alone in the countryside, exercise brings many rewards — physical, psychological, and social.

People who aren't diabetic and exercise strenuously and regularly tend to live longer, are healthier, *look* healthier and younger, have lower rates of debilitating and incapacitating illnesses such as osteoporosis, heart disease, high blood pressure — and the list goes on. Overall, people who exercise regularly are better equipped to carry on day-to-day activities as they age.

Many Type I diabetics have been ill for so long with the complications of the disease that they are often depressed about their physical health. Numerous studies have established the link between good health and a positive mental attitude. If you're a Type I diabetic, as I am, strenuous exercise will not have the profound effect on your diabetes that it will for Type II's (which we'll discuss shortly), but it can have a profound effect on your self-image. It's possible, if you keep your blood sugars normal and exercise regularly and strenuously, to be in better health than your nondiabetic friends. Also, it's been my experience that Type I diabetics who engage in a regular exercise program tend to take better care of their blood sugars and diet.

Think of exercise as money in the bank — every 30 minutes you put into keeping in shape today will not only leave you better off right now, it will pay continual dividends in the future. If going up the stairs yesterday left you huffing and puffing, in a while you'll bound up the steps. Your strength will likely make you feel younger, possibly more confident. There is evidence that exercise actually does make you look younger: the skin of those who exercise regularly gets more oxygen and tends not to age as rapidly.

After working out for a few months, you'll look better, and people will mention it. With this kind of encouragement, you may be more likely to stick to other aspects of our regimen.

In addition to these important psychological and social aspects, exercise has, as I've mentioned, important benefits for your overall physical health. It has long been known that strenuous exercise raises the levels of serum HDL (good cholesterol) and lowers triglycerides in the bloodstream. Recent studies suggest that body-building exercise (anaerobic rather than aerobic exercise) also lowers serum levels of LDL ("bad" cholesterol). There is even evidence that atherosclerosis (hardening of the arteries) may be reversible in some individuals by major improvements in serum lipid profiles. I'm in my sixties, I exercise strenuously on a daily basis, I don't eat fruit, I've had Type I diabetes for over fifty years, and I have three eggs for breakfast many days. Where's my cholesterol? It's in a very healthy range that nondiabetics one-third my age rarely attain. Part of that's due to my diet, but part of it is due to my daily exercise program.

Frequent strenuous exercise has been shown to reduce significantly the likelihood of heart attack, stroke, and sudden blockage of blood vessels by lowering serum fibrinogen levels. Long-term strenuous exercise lowers resting heart rate and blood pressure, further reducing the risk of heart attacks and stroke.

Weight-bearing or resistance exercise slows the loss of bone mineral content associated with aging. Ever hear the slogan, "Use it or lose it"? In a very real sense, if we don't use our bones, we lose them.

Although exercise does make weight control easier, it does not — at least not as much as we may wish — "burn fat." Unless you work out at very strenuous levels for several hours each day, exercise isn't going to have a significant *direct* effect upon your body fat. The effects of exercise are broader and more indirect. One of the great benefits is that many people find that when they exercise, they have less desire to overeat. The reasons for this are probably related to the release in the brain of neuro-transmitters such as endorphins. (Endorphins are "endogenous opiates" manufactured in the brain. They can elevate mood, reduce pain, and reduce carbohydrate craving. Brain levels of endorphins are reduced in poorly controlled diabetes.) It might be said that the same way that obesity leads to further obesity, fitness leads to further fitness.

Even though your fat won't "melt away," exercise, particularly if you're a Type II diabetic, is still of value in a weight-reduction program because muscle building reduces insulin resistance. Insulin resistance, remember, is linked to your ratio of abdominal fat to lean body mass. The higher your ratio of abdominal fat to muscle mass, the more insulin-resistant you're likely to be. As you increase your muscle mass, your insulin needs will be reduced — and having less insulin present in your bloodstream will reduce the amount of fat you pack away. If you remember my old friend Howie from Chapter 12, his insulin resistance went away when he lost 100 pounds and radically changed his ratio of abdominal fat to lean body mass ratio.

Long-term, regular, strenuous exercise also reduces insulin resistance independently of its effect upon muscle mass. This makes you more sensitive to your own and injected insulin. As a result, your own insulin production gradually becomes more effective at lowering blood sugar. If you inject insulin, your dosage requirements will drop, and the fat-building effects of large amounts of insulin will likewise drop. In my experience, it takes about two weeks of daily strenuous exercise to bring about a steady, increased level of insulin sensitivity. This effect continues for about two weeks after stopping an exercise program. Awareness of this is especially important for those of us who inject insulin and must increase our doses after two weeks without our usual exercise. If you go out of town for only a week and cannot exercise, your increased insulin sensitivity will probably not suffer.

Although increased muscle bulk also increases insulin sensitivity, independently of the above effect, this is very gradual and may require many months of bodybuilding before becoming noticeable.

HOW DOES EXERCISE AFFECT BLOOD SUGAR?

Exercise does affect blood sugar, and for that reason it can make your efforts at blood sugar control slightly more difficult if you're taking blood sugar–lowering medications. The benefits, however, are so great compared to any added difficulty, that if you're a Type II diabetic, you'd be foolish not to get involved in an exercise program.

For years, guidelines for the treatment of diabetes have repeated the half-truth that exercise always lowers blood sugar levels. In reality, physical exertion can lower blood sugar via increased production of glucose transporters in muscle cells. Certain conditions, however, must be present: exertion must be adequately prolonged, serum insulin levels must be adequate, and blood sugar must not be too high.

Moderate to strenuous exercise such as swimming, running, weight lifting, or tennis — as opposed to more casual exercise such as walking — causes an immediate release of "stress," or counterregulatory, hormones (epinephrine, cortisol, et cetera). These signal the liver and muscles to return glucose to the bloodstream by converting stored glycogen into glucose. The nondiabetic response to the additional glucose is to release small amounts of stored insulin to keep blood sugars from rising. Blood sugar may therefore rise slightly and then normalize. If a Type II diabetic without phase I insulin response were to exercise for a few minutes, his blood sugar might increase for a while, but eventually it would return to normal, thanks to phase II insulin response. Thus, *brief* strenuous exercise can *raise* blood sugar, while *prolonged* exercise can *lower* it. For this reason, Dr. Elliot P. Joslin told a group of us (fifty years ago): "Don't run a block for a bus, run a mile."

When insulin is nearly absent in the blood, the glucose released in response to stress hormones cannot readily enter muscle and liver cells. As a result, blood sugar continues to rise, and the muscles must rely upon stored fat for energy. On the other hand, suppose that you have injected just enough long-acting insulin within the previous 12 hours to keep your blood sugar on target without exercise, and then you run a few miles. You will have a higher serum insulin level than needed, because exercise facilitates the action of the insulin already present. Blood sugar may therefore drop too low. The same effect may occur if you are using oral hypoglycemic agents (OHAs). Furthermore, if you have injected insulin into tissue that overlies the muscle being exercised, or perhaps into the muscle itself, the rate of release of insulin into the bloodstream may be so great as to cause severe hypoglycemia. Nondiabetics and Type II's not on insulin or sulfonylureas (a class of OHAs) can automatically turn down their insulin in response to exercise.

It may be unwise for you to exercise if your blood sugar exceeds about 200 mg/dl. This number varies with the individual, the medications you're taking, and any complications you might have, such as gastroparesis. This is because elevated blood sugars will tend to rise even further with exercise. This effect will be less dramatic if you're making a lot of insulin, and is most dramatic for a Type I diabetic who doesn't take extra insulin to cover the high blood sugar. I have one Type I patient who keeps her blood sugars essentially normal. She still makes a little insulin and dislikes insulin injections so much that she works out every day after lunch to save herself a shot to cover the lunch. In her case, the exercise plus the small amount of insulin she still makes together work very well.

One great benefit of regular, strenuous exercise in Type II diabetes, as mentioned earlier, is that it can bring about a long-term reduction of insulin resistance, by increasing muscle mass. Long-term muscle development, therefore, can facilitate blood sugar control and weight loss. It also reduces the rate of beta cell burnout, because the increased ratio of muscle mass to abdominal fat reduces insulin resistance and thus reduces the demand for insulin.

THE DAWN PHENOMENON AND EXERCISE

Several of my Type I patients must take additional fast-acting insulin when they exercise in the morning, but not when they exercise in the afternoon. This is a dramatic example of how the dawn phenomenon reduces even injected serum insulin levels. In the afternoon their blood sugar drops with exercise, but in the morning it actually goes up if they do not first inject some rapid-acting insulin.

RESTRICTIONS ON EXERCISE

Despite the benefits that exercise can have, an exercise program that isn't sensibly put together can have disastrous results. Even if you think you're perfectly fit, your physician should be consulted before you proceed. Keep in mind that there are certain physical conditions that may restrict the type and intensity of exercise you should attempt. Your current age, your cardiac and strength fitness, the number of years you've had diabetes, the average level of your blood sugars, whether or not — and how much — you're overweight, and what sort of diabetic complications you have developed: all these must be considered to determine what kind of exercise you should undertake, and at what intensity.

Before You Start

Following are several different aspects of your health you should consider and discuss with your physician before embarking upon an exercise program.

Heart. Everyone over the age of forty, and diabetics over the age of thirty, should be tested for significant coronary artery disease before beginning a new exercise program. At the very least, an exercising electrocardiogram or thallium scan is usually advised. An abnormal test may not necessarily rule out exercise, but it may suggest restraint or close supervision while exercising. Again, seek your doctor's advice before starting any new exercise program.

High blood pressure. Although long-term exercise helps to lower resting blood pressure, your blood pressure can rise while you are exercising. If you're subject to wide pressure swings, there may be risk of stroke and retinal hemorrhages during strenuous exercise. Again, first contact your physician.

Eyes. Before beginning any exercise program, you should have your eyes checked by a physician, ophthalmologist, or retinologist experienced in evaluating diabetic retinal disease (retinopathy). Certain types of retinopathy are characterized by the presence of very fragile blood vessels growing from the retina. If you strain too much, assume a head-down position, or land hard on your feet, these can rupture and hemorrhage, causing blindness. If your physician or ophthalmologist identifies such vessels, you'll probably be warned to avoid exercises requiring exertion of strong forces (e.g., weight lifting, chinning, push-ups, sit-ups) and sudden changes of motion (e.g., running, jumping, falling, diving). Bicycling and surface swimming are usually acceptable alternatives, but first check with your physician.

Fainting. A form of nerve damage called vascular autonomic neuropathy (caused by chronically high blood sugars) can lead to lightheadedness and even fainting during certain types of extreme exertion, such as weight lifting and sit-ups. Such activities should therefore be embarked upon gradually and only after instruction by your physician.

If you take blood sugar–lowering medications. If you take insulin or oral hypoglycemic agents, it is wise to make sure your blood sugars are stabilized before you begin a strenuous exercise program. As previously noted, exercise can have significant effects upon blood sugars and introduce another variable that can confuse anyone reviewing your blood sugar data. It's much easier to readjust your diet and/or medications to accommodate physical activity *after* blood sugars are under control.

Sympathetic autonomic neuropathy. If you're unable to sweat below your waist, there is a possibility that prolonged exercise may cause undue elevation of your body temperature.

Proteinuria. Elevated levels of urinary protein are usually exacerbated by strenuous exercise. This in turn can accelerate the kidney damage that you may already have.

Ongoing Concerns for Exercising Diabetics

Following is a list of aspects of health you should consider on an ongoing basis as you pursue your exercise program.

Recent surgery. A history of recent surgery usually warrants restraint or abstinence until you receive clearance from your surgeon.

Blood sugar changes. Even after blood sugars are reasonably well controlled, illness, dehydration, and even transient blood sugar values over 200 mg/dl are reasons for you to refrain from exercise. For many people, blood sugars above 200 mg/dl will increase further with exercise, due to the production of stress hormones that we discussed previously.

Blood sugars below target values. If you take blood sugar–lowering medications, do not exercise if blood sugar is below your target value. Bring it up to target first with glucose tablets (see the next section, and Chapter 19, "How to Prevent and Correct Low Blood Sugars").

Possible foot injury. If you've had diabetes for a number of years, there is a good chance that your feet are especially susceptible to injury while exercising. There are several reasons for this:

- The circulation to your feet may be impaired. With a poor blood supply, the skin is readily damaged and heals poorly. It also is more likely to be injured by freezing temperatures.
- Injury to nerves in the feet caused by chronically high blood sugars leads to sensory neuropathy, or diminished ability to perceive pain, pressure, heat, cold, and so on. This enables blisters, abrasions, and the like to occur and continue without warning.
- The skin of the feet can become dry and cracked from another form of neuropathy that prevents sweating. Cracks in heels are potential sites of ulcers.
- A third form of neuropathy, called motor neuropathy, leads to wasting of certain muscles in the feet. The imbalance between stronger and weaker muscles leads to a foot deformity very common among diabetics, which includes flexed or claw-shaped toes, high arches, and bumps on the sole of the foot due to prominence of the heads of the long metatarsal bones that lead to the toes. These prominent metatarsal heads are subject to high pressure during certain types of weight-bearing exercise. This can lead to calluses and even skin breakdown or ulcers. The knuckles of the claw-shaped toes are subject to pressure from the upper surface of your shoes or sneakers. The overlying skin can therefore blister and ulcerate.
- Another form of neuropathy makes it difficult to perceive joint position in the feet. This, in turn, can lead to orthopedic injuries (e.g., bone fractures) while exercising the lower body.

All of this implies that feet must be carefully protected during exercise. Your physician or podiatrist should be consulted before you start any new exercise, as some restrictions may be necessary. Even prolonged swimming can cause maceration of the skin. You should also be thoroughly trained in foot care. Please see Appendix E, "Foot Care for Diabetics."

You or a family member should examine your feet daily for any changes, abrasions, pressure points, pink spots, blisters, and so on. Be sure to check the soles of your feet, using a hand mirror if necessary. If you find any changes, see your physician immediately. Bring with you all the shoes and sneakers that you currently use, so that he can track down the cause of the problem. At the very least he may recommend the use of flexible orthotic inserts and deep toe box sneakers while exercising.

FOR DIABETICS WHO USE BLOOD SUGAR–LOWERING MEDICATIONS: COVERING EXERCISE WITH CARBOHYDRATE

People who do not take medications that lower blood sugar are usually able to "turn off" their insulin secretion in response to a drop in blood sugar brought about by exercising. You cannot, however, turn off sulfonylurea OHAs or injected insulin once you've taken them. (This is one of the reasons I rarely prescribe sulfonylureas.) To prevent the occurrence of dangerously low blood sugars, it is wise to cover the exercise with glucose tablets (e.g., Dextrotabs; see page 261) or another source of carbohydrate, in *advance* of a drop in blood sugar.

Some Type I diabetics try to use "treats," such as fruit or candy, to cover an anticipated blood sugar drop. I don't ordinarily recommend this approach, because it's not as precise as using glucose tablets. My experience with patients who've taken raisins or grapes or candies to cover their exercise has been that they suffer subsequent elevated blood sugars. Say you eat an apple. It will contain some fast-acting sugars that enter the bloodstream almost immediately. It will also contain other, slower-acting sugars that may take several hours to find their way into the bloodstream. On the other hand, as we will discuss below, certain sustained activities — such as cross-country skiing or physical labor —

can keep your blood sugar dropping all day. For those, you'll need something longer-acting to help keep you from becoming hypoglycemic.

To discover how much carbohydrate you should take for a given exercise session requires some experimentation and the help of your blood sugar meter. One valuable guideline is that 1 gram of carbohydrate will raise blood sugar about 5 mg/dl for people with body weights in the range of 140 pounds. A child weighing 70 pounds would experience double the increase, or 10 mg/dl per gram, and an adult weighing 280 pounds would probably experience only half this increase (2.5 mg/dl).

My own preference is Dextrotabs, each of which contains 1.6 grams of glucose. Other brands of glucose tablets are available at most large pharmacies and diabetes mail-order suppliers (see Chapters 3 and 19). If you weigh 150 pounds, one Dextrotab will raise your blood sugar about 8 mg/dl. Since these glucose tablets start raising blood sugar in about 3 minutes and finish in about 40 minutes, they're ideal for relatively brief exercise periods.

Let's run through a hypothetical example to demonstrate how you'd go about determining how many tablets you ought to take. Let's assume you weigh 170 pounds, and 1 Dextrotab will likely raise your blood sugar about 7 mg/dl. You've decided to lift weights (or play tennis) for an hour.

- First, check your blood sugar before starting (ideally, you should *always* check blood sugar before starting to exercise). If it's below your target value, take enough Dextrotabs to bring it up. Wait 40 minutes for them to finish working. If you don't, you may be too weak to exercise. Record your blood sugar level upon starting. (I use GLUCOGRAF® data sheets for recording all exercise-related blood sugars.)
- When you begin your activity, take 1 Dextrotab, and then 1 again every 10 minutes thereafter.
- Halfway into your activity, check blood sugar again, just to make sure it's not too low. If it is, take enough Dextrotabs to bring it back up, and continue the exercise. If it's too high, you may need to skip the next few tablets, depending upon how high the value.
- Continue the exercise and the tablets (depending upon blood sugar levels).

- At the end of the exercise period, measure blood sugar again. Correct it with tablets if necessary. Remember to write down all blood sugar values and the time when each tablet was taken.
- About an hour after finishing your workout, check blood sugar again. This is necessary because it may continue to drop for at least 1 hour after finishing. Bring it back up with glucose tablets if necessary. (Very intense or prolonged exercise may keep blood sugars dropping for as many as 5 hours.)
- If you required, say, a total of 8 tablets altogether, this suggests that in the future you should take 8 tablets spread out over the course of your workout. If you only required 4 tablets, then you'd take 4 tablets the next time. And so on.
- Repeat this experiment on occasion, because your activity level is rarely exactly the same for every exercise period. If you required 3 tablets the first time and 5 tablets the second time, take the average, or 4 tablets, the next time. If your activity level increases — say you've been playing with a slow tennis partner and you find another who makes you sweat your butt off — you may find it necessary to increase the number of glucose tablets.

There are some activities where coverage with a slower-acting form of carbohydrate may be appropriate, and it's here, perhaps, that you could use the "treats" I would normally discourage. For example, I have two patients, both on insulin, who are housepainters. Neither works every day, and the hours of work vary from day to day. They rarely work for less than 4 hours at a time. The painter in Massachusetts finds that half a blueberry muffin every hour keeps his blood sugars level, while the painter in New York eats a chocolate chip cookie every hour.

Several patients find that their blood sugars drop when they spend a few hours in the shopping mall. I tell them to eat a slice of bread (12 grams carbohydrate) when they leave their car. The bread will start to raise blood sugar in about 10 minutes, and will continue to do so for about 3 hours. The cookies and blueberry muffins contain mixtures of simple and complex sugars, so they start working rapidly but also continue to raise blood sugar for about 3 hours. I discourage the use of fruits, which can raise blood sugar less predictably.

Whatever your plan for covering exercise with carbohydrate, *always carry glucose tablets with you!*

WHAT FORM OF EXERCISE IS BEST FOR YOU?

As you are by now aware, insulin resistance, which is the hallmark of Type II diabetes, is enhanced in proportion to the ratio of abdominal fat to lean body mass. One of the best ways to improve this ratio in order to lower your insulin resistance is to increase your lean body mass. Therefore, for most Type II diabetics, the most valuable type of exercise is muscle-building exercise. (It's good for Type I's too, because it makes you feel better, look better, and can improve your self-image.) There also is cardiovascular exercise, which benefits the heart and circulatory system, and is discussed later in the chapter.

First, what is muscle-building exercise? Resistance training, weight training (weight lifting), or gymnastics would all qualify. If done properly, weight-lifting has many attributes that make it superior to the so-called aerobic exercises. Aerobic exercise is exercise mild enough that your muscles are not deprived of oxygen. When muscles exercise aerobically, they don't increase much in mass and they don't require as much glucose for energy. Anaerobic exercise deprives the muscles of oxygen; it tires them quickly and requires about fourteen times as much glucose to do the same amount of work as aerobic exercise. When you perform anaerobic exercise, your muscles break down for the first 24 hours, but then they build up over the next 24 hours. I have little old ladies performing weight-lifting exercise. They're never going to look like Arnold Schwarzenegger — it's physically impossible because women haven't the hormones for it — but they feel much better and are certainly stronger because of it.

But what about aerobic exercise, such as jogging or biking? I don't think it's as valuable for diabetics — or for anyone really, for reasons we shall discuss. Still, I usually suggest that my patients engage in activities that they will enjoy and will continue to pursue in a progressive fashion. Progressive exercise is exercise that intensifies over a period of weeks, months, or years. Below are listed various characteristics of an appropriate exercise program:

- It should comply with any restrictions imposed by your physician.
- The cost should not exceed your financial limitations.
- It should maintain your interest, so that you'll continue to pursue it indefinitely.

- The location should be convenient, and you should have the time to work out at least every other day. Daily activity is very desirable.
- It should be of a progressive nature.
- It should ideally build muscle mass, strength, and endurance.

AEROBIC AND ANAEROBIC EXERCISE

You've often heard of aerobics, and now you've seen me mention "anaerobic" several times. What makes one of these types of exercise better for diabetics than the other?

Our muscles consist of long fibers that shorten, or contract, when they perform work like lifting a load or moving the body. All muscle fibers require high-energy compounds derived from glucose or fatty acids in order to contract. Some muscle fibers utilize a process called aerobic metabolism to derive high-energy compounds from small amounts of glucose and large amounts of oxygen. These fibers can move light loads for prolonged periods of time, and are most effective for "aerobic," noncompetitive activities such as jogging, nonsprint swimming, and moderate-speed bicycling. Other muscle fibers can move heavy loads, but only for brief periods. They demand energy at a very rapid rate, and so must be able to produce high-energy compounds faster than the heart can pump blood to deliver oxygen. They achieve this by a process called anaerobic metabolism, which requires large amounts of glucose and virtually no oxygen.

This is of interest to diabetics for two reasons. First, the blood sugar drop during and after continuous anaerobic exercise will be much greater than after a similar period of aerobic exercise. Second, to accomplish efficient transport of glucose into muscle cells, as muscle strength and bulk develop, glucose transporters in these cells will increase greatly in number. Glucose transporters also become more numerous in tissues other than muscle, including the liver. As a result, the efficiency of your own (or injected) insulin in transporting glucose and in suppressing glucose output by the liver becomes considerably greater when anaerobic exercise is incorporated into your program.

Anaerobic metabolism produces lactic acid, which accumulates in the active muscles, causing pain. Since the acid is cleared almost immediately when the muscles relax, the pain likewise vanishes upon relaxation. You can identify anaerobic exercise by the local pain and the accompanying weakness. This pain is limited to the muscles being exercised, goes away quickly when the activity stops, and does not refer to agonizing muscle cramps or to cardiac pain in the chest. Anaerobic activities can include weight lifting, sit-ups, climbing, chinning, push-ups, running up a steep incline, uphill cycling, gymnastics, using a stair climber, and so forth, provided that these activities are performed with adequate loads and at enough velocity to cause pain or transient discomfort (not heart attack, but the pain of "no pain, no gain").

BODYBUILDING: NEARLY CONTINUOUS ANAEROBIC EXERCISE

Continuous anaerobic activity, as you can well imagine, is really impossible. The pain caused by lactic acid in the involved muscles becomes intolerable, and the weakness that develops with extreme exertion leaves you limp. Nevertheless, you can approach this goal by using the special "inverted pyramid" technique described on page 183.

Bodybuilding, or resistance exercise — which includes weight lifting, sit-ups, chinning, and push-ups — focuses on one muscle group at a time and then shifts the focus to another muscle group. If you use the inverted pyramid technique you can achieve continuous anaerobic activity, but on a rotating basis. After you finish exercising certain of your abdominal muscles by doing sit-ups, for instance, you switch to push-ups, which focus on various arm and shoulder muscles. From there, you go to chinning. Similarly, different weight-lifting exercises also focus on different muscle groups. Anaerobic exercise also can increase the benefits of exercise in stimulating heart rate and thereby exercising the heart. To maintain an elevated heart rate, you switch immediately from one anaerobic exercise to another, without resting in between.

I personally prefer this type of activity for Type II or obese diabetics because — as I have said before and will say again — the buildup of muscle mass lowers insulin resistance and thereby facilitates both blood sugar control and weight loss. A number of my patients engage in bodybuilding exercises, including men and women over sixty years of age. They are all very pleased with the results.*

---

* Several years ago, a report from the human physiology lab at Tufts University disclosed that only twelve weeks of weight training tripled the strength of male subjects

Some Suggestions for a Bodybuilding Routine
Please refer back to the section "Restrictions on Exercise," page 173. These restrictions and cautions apply especially to bodybuilding.

Even if you have room in your home, and the finances, to equip your own private gym, I usually recommend that people go to a gym or health club to learn the different exercises before beginning an anaerobic exercise program. Then, if you want to buy dumbbells or a weight-lifting machine for use at home, that's fine. But it's important to learn good technique and good form first. You can also consult books on the subject, but at least a few sessions supervised by an experienced instructor is best.

Equipment. For your upper body, you're going to have to use weights. I don't recommend that you lift barbells — they can be dangerous, and you should have assistance if you're using them — but I do recommend dumbbells and weight-lifting machines, which for the most part are quite safe to use.* Whether you're using dumbbells at home or in the gym, they should be solid cast iron, usually painted black enamel or gray. They're inexpensive — usually 50–75 cents a pound, so a 10-pound dumbbell costs about $5–$7.50. Don't use dumbbells consisting of a bar with plates on either end that can be added or removed. These can be dangerous — the plates frequently slide off — and they also defeat the whole method that I advocate (see "Technique" below).

Exercises. If you're going to a health club or gym to learn the ropes, I suggest that you learn fifteen upper body exercises, and as many lower body exercises as you can. Upper body would be for the arms, shoulders, and back. If you're going to the gym every day, which I recommend, you'd do your upper body exercises on one day, and lower body exercises

---

ages 60–96. This was believed to improve their quality of life significantly. Subsequent studies showed a similar effect upon women.

* A number of inexpensive multiexercise machines are on the market that utilize thick rubber bands instead of weights. Beware of these: since you have to stop and change the bands to change resistance, they do not permit true anaerobic training. Hydraulic and pneumatic machines that utilize rotary knobs to adjust settings are usually excellent but can be quite costly.

the next. Why alternate days? Because of the muscle breakdown over the first 24 hours after exercise and the need for time to rebuild. So on the second day, while you're doing your lower body exercises, your upper body muscles are rebuilding.

As you can guess, there are more muscle groups that work in more ways in the upper body than in the lower body, so there are fewer sensible lower body exercises. By sensible, I mean if you're using a treadmill, a stair, a bike, and a cross-country ski machine all in the same day, you're exercising more or less the same muscles with each apparatus, which isn't sensible. The other types of lower body exercises that involve weight-lifting are few in number: leg extensions, leg curls, toe presses, knee/thigh presses. Some gyms have machines to exercise your legs as you spread them, but in all, there are only about seven leg exercises commonly available.

As a consequence, I always add some other exercises on the days I do lower body exercises: grip strengthening, side bends (which exercise the side muscles), and sit-ups, as well as what's called cardiovascular exercise. The instructor at your health club will be able to help you with all of these.

Form. To get the most out of your weight-lifting exercises it's important to have perfect form. This means that you isolate and use only the muscles that are targeted by a particular exercise. You don't use your back muscles to help perform an arm exercise, for example. This is where having good instruction can pay off. Your instructor can critique your form and help you select the right equipment for each exercise.

Technique: The Inverted Pyramid System

First, a word of warning: Don't embark upon this technique until you have demonstrated perfect form for each exercise. This will ensure maximum benefit and minimize the possibility of muscle strain.

The most productive way to perform an anaerobic exercise is to tire a particular group of muscles as quickly as possible, and keep them tired during the course of the exercise. This may sound a little strange, given that we're all accustomed to the idea that athletes work in precisely the opposite manner — warming up slowly and building to a fast finish. That may be fine for a sprint, but we're not talking about racing here, we're talking about building muscle mass. By placing maximum demands on your muscles at first, you put yourself into the anaerobic (or oxygen-deprived) state right off. Then by slowly progressing to lighter weights, you force your muscles to work continuously in the anaerobic state and thereby build them. This is what I call the inverted pyramid approach to weight lifting, and for the purpose of building muscle mass, it's far superior to the old system.

Many weight lifters follow a regimen that requires 10 repetitions ("reps") of a lift, followed by a rest, another 10 reps, another rest, and another 10 reps. The rest between each set of reps allows the heart to slow, replenishes oxygen to the muscles, and thereby defeats our central goals. Anaerobically, you must continually keep your muscles deprived of oxygen and force them to develop new metabolic pathways that demand less oxygen. The idea is quality, not quantity, and it's my belief than you can accomplish a more thorough and sensible workout in 15–30 minutes than you can in an hour and a half of conventional, less strenuous aerobic activity.

I use the inverted pyramid system, so called because I start out with as much resistance as I can handle, and then ease up.

This is how it works: Let's say you're performing curls. These involve sitting at the edge of a bench or chair and flexing your arms at the elbows with weights in each hand. You start with the *heaviest* weight that you can lift 3–4 times without losing good form. By the time you've lifted it 4 times, your muscles are tired and you can't lift it anymore. You immediately pick up the next lighter weight and do as many reps as you can (say, 3–4), and so on down through lighter and lighter weights until you get to a total of about 20 reps. You might find that you can get out 21, or maybe you can only manage 19 — that's fine. The idea is that after the first few repetitions, your muscles are tired and they're working while they're tired, which is what stimulates muscles to build more mass.

Once you've done your reps for a particular muscle group, you don't need to do that exercise again until the day after tomorrow. You immediately go on to the next exercise. In this way, you can accomplish considerably more in a shorter time frame.

The same system applies to an exercise like sit-ups. Whether you're doing sit-ups with your legs straight, bent, or with one of those sit-up boards, you start off with your hands behind your head. If you can't do a single sit-up with hands behind your head, try it with hands at your sides or even pressing them on the floor. With practice you'll eventually be strong enough to put your hands behind your head. If you're really experienced at sit-ups and have strong abdominal muscles, you hold a plate — a flat weight — behind your head. You do as many repetitions as you can. Maybe you'll only get 5–6, maybe only 2–3. Immediately put down your weight if you're holding one, or take your hands from behind your head and fold them across your chest. Now start doing the same sit-ups in this fashion. You do as many more reps as you can, then put your hands at your sides and do as many more additional repetitions as you can. If you get very experienced and find yourself doing 40 or more sit-ups, it can get pretty boring, and it is also a waste of time. When you find yourself doing dozens of sit-ups, you can get an inclined board or a Roman chair, which is like a sit-up board but is raised about four feet off the ground and permits you to begin with your head below your waist. Again, you follow the same tactic. You can also get an abdominal crunch machine with variable resistance, but they're expensive. Again, you'd start at high resistance and work down for a total of about 20 reps. It is humanly possible to do more than 4,000 sit-ups at one session, but what's the point?

CARDIOVASCULAR EXERCISE

Cardiovascular exercise is widely associated in the public mind with what the popular press calls aerobic exercise. However, aerobic exercise as many people practice it — a leisurely jog, a relaxing bike ride, even a brisk walk — is really of only limited benefit to your cardiovascular system, doesn't build muscles, and has relatively little impact on your stamina and capacity. The kind of cardiovascular exercise I recommend to my patients (and follow myself) is very strenuous, operates in the anaerobic range, and accomplishes tremendous things. For example, many years ago, before I became a physician, I used to go to diabetes conventions. There was always a group of doctors who would get up in the morning, don their running togs, and go running. These were people who ran every day. I'm not a runner; I work out in the gym every day with my weights. But I do a particular cardiovascular workout on an exercise bicycle that I will explain. And so I would go out with these doctors on their runs. After a few miles, people would start dropping out.

Eventually, I'd be the only one left — and then I'd go another five miles and come back. Clearly, although I was older than most of these people, and not a runner, I had much more stamina. The stamina was created by this anaerobic cardiovascular exercise.

Exercise Harder, Exercise Better

Cardiovascular workouts can be performed on a treadmill, a stair climber, or bicycle — if you're male, I recommend a recumbent bicycle rather than the standard upright bike. It's much more comfortable for men because the seat is like an ordinary chair. Ideally, your machine should have a meter that reads the amount of work that you're doing in calories per minute as well as total calories, but certainly you can get a good workout without such an output display. It is important to wear a pulse meter. The brand that I like best is called Polar; it costs about $120, and you wear it around your chest. If you belong to a health club that has a treadmill with a pulse meter in the handlebars, you won't have to put one on your chest, but some sort of pulse meter is essential. The degree of workout you're getting is measured by how fast your heart works. When you get evaluated by a cardiologist before you start your exercise program, you should ask him or her what your target pulse rate ought to be. Over time, you can increase it.

There's a formula that we use to specify maximum pulse rate: we take 220 and subtract from it your age. So if you're sixty years old, you'd have a theoretical maximum pulse rate of 160 — that is, in theory, you shouldn't be able to exercise at a faster pulse rate. Your doctor will decide based on your overall health and fitness level what percentage of this would be a good target rate for you — say, 75–80 percent. Rarely would a doctor start you out at 85 percent of maximum or higher. Eventually, you may find that you can get up to and beyond your theoretical maximum — I can exercise at 170 even though my theoretical maximum is 157. I can do this without having a heart attack in part because I've been exercising strenuously for thirty years. Don't expect — even after years of this kind of exercise — to get your heart rate up to or even near your theoretical maximum, or even to your target, right after you begin your daily workout. This takes time. I get to my target pulse rate toward the end of my workout.

To do a really effective anaerobic/cardiovascular workout, you use the same principles as you use lifting weights. Start out by selecting a safe, comfortable speed and setting the resistance of your machine to the point where your muscles are so tired after about 20 seconds that you can't go any further. As soon as you reach this point, you lower the resistance setting slightly, and keep going. For treadmills, the resistance will be the angle at which you're running uphill. So if you're using a treadmill, you need to be able to set the incline of your treadmill from the handlebars — you don't want to have to get off, reset the angle, then get back on. You'll lose your rhythm, regain some of the oxygen in your muscles, and defeat the point of the workout.

As with the weights, you lower the resistance a little at a time, and each time you lower it, shoot for 20 seconds of exercise until you can't go anymore. Nearly from the beginning you're wiped out, yet you keep doing it at lower and lower resistance. *This* is a real workout.

Your goal will be to get your heart rate up to (but not above) the training level recommended by your physician. If you can't reach the recommended rate within 10 minutes, increase your speed until you get there. Try to maintain this rate for at least 5 minutes. When you think you've had enough, lower the resistance to zero but keep your legs moving until your pulse has slowed to a value near your starting point. This slow exercise pumps blood back to your heart from your legs, thereby greatly reducing the hazard of a postworkout heart attack.

It's unnecessary to exercise at your target heart rate for more than 5–10 minutes. A cardiovascular workout of this kind for about 15 minutes should be plenty for most people, unless you're training for competition. However, I recommend that rather than watch the clock, you look at the calorie counter on the machine, if it has one, and decide on a particular number of calories that you want to shoot for. Calories are a measure of work done and therefore a reasonable gauge of your workout. Minutes or even miles don't take effort into account. I aim for about 80–100 calories. When it gets up to that range, I call it quits. But, the point of this kind of exercise isn't weight loss, so don't start looking at the calorie counter thinking that if you burn 10 more calories you'll lose another pound — exercise just doesn't work that way.

AN IMPORTANT CAUTION

If you're doing cardiovascular exercise of this type, you have to be very careful, especially if you're a long-term diabetic, or a recent-onset diabetic over the age of forty, or have a family history of coronary disease. One rule is that you *never finish a cardiovascular workout and stop cold.* I had an overweight nondiabetic cousin who started jogging when he was about fifty years old. He was in his second month of exercising, not doing anything more than a casual jog with his friend. One day, after they stopped jogging, he dropped dead of a heart attack. He and his jogging buddy were in the habit of stopping cold after their run to chat. Stopping cold is an extremely bad idea — if people are going to drop dead of heart attacks during exercise, it's most often immediately after the exercise that this happens. Why?

If you have compromised circulation to your heart — say your coronary arteries are narrowed by atherosclerosis — while you're exercising, your heart is beating very rapidly because it requires a lot of blood. By pumping your legs up and down, you're pumping blood from your legs back to your heart. The muscles that are using up a lot of oxygen and demanding a lot of blood are both in your legs and in your heart, but the blood's getting pumped back to your heart by running. If you stop cold, your muscles are still going to demand a lot of blood — they've been depleted of oxygen and glucose — and gravity is going to help them get the blood. The problem is, they're no longer pumping the blood back to the heart. Suddenly your heart is deprived and you're set up for a heart attack.

Whether you're on a treadmill, bike, or stair climber, cut the resistance setting to zero and slow down to a comfortable pace after your workout until your heart rate slowly comes down to no higher than about one-third above your initial starting rate. If your resting pulse is 72, you don't want to stop your biking, walking, or step climbing until your heart rate is 110 or below.

PROGRESSIVE EXERCISE

As your strength and endurance increase for any exercise, it will become progressively easier to perform. If it becomes too easy, you won't get any stronger. The key to getting progressively more strength and endurance is to make the exercise progressively more difficult. This can be done for almost any activity.

If you are lifting weights, for example, every few weeks (or months) you can add a very small weight (say 2½ pounds) to the weight stack for any exercise. When doing a cardiovascular exercise, you might try to increase your maximum heart rate by, say, 2 beats every 2 months, by increasing your resistance setting or your speed. A swimmer can assign a fixed time period, say 30 minutes, for doing laps. The goal would be to gradually increase the number of laps. Thus, after a month you might increase your speed to get 7¼ laps instead of 7 laps in 30 minutes, and so on. Of course, a waterproof wristwatch would be helpful.

Even walking can evolve into both an endurance and a bodybuilding activity. All you need is a wristwatch, a few lightweight dumbbells, and a pedometer. The pedometer is a small gadget from a sporting goods store that you clip onto your belt. It measures distance by counting your steps. Suppose you wish to set aside 30 minutes per session for walking. You begin by walking at a leisurely pace for 15 minutes and then returning at the same pace. Record your distance from the pedometer. Thereafter, try to walk at least that distance in the same time period. After ten sessions, you might try to increase distance by 5 percent over the same time. If you increase distance by this amount every ten sessions, you'll eventually find yourself running. You can then gradually increase your running speed in the same fashion.

Suppose your doctor has told you not to run because of a bad knee or fragile retinal blood vessels. Limit your speed to a fast walk, but start swinging your arms a little bit. Over time, try swinging them higher and higher. When you think they are going so high that you look silly, start with the dumbbells. You might begin with a pair of 1-pound dumbbells and short swings of the arms. Wear gloves if the dumbbells feel cold. Again, gradually increase the distance you swing. When you eventually feel you look silly, try 2-pound dumbbells. After a year or two, you may be going at a very fast walk, swinging 5-pound (or even heavier) dumbbells. Imagine what your physique will look like then. You'll also probably feel younger and healthier.

The exercises I've mentioned above are by no means the only ones. There are countless different ways you can exercise — volleyball, snowboarding, surf-kayaking, cross-country skiing, you name it. The most important considerations are keeping within the restrictions your physician might place on your activity, and then discovering what you like to do best — and sticking with it. After that, all you have to do is be able to monitor and correct your blood sugars, and keep exercising in a progressive fashion. The payoff — longer life, lower stress, and better overall health — is usually worth the time and effort.

14

Oral Hypoglycemic Agents

I f diet and exercise are not adequate to bring your blood sugar readings under control, the next level of treatment to consider is blood sugar–lowering pills, known as oral hypoglycemic agents (OHAs). For people who still have sufficient insulin-producing capacity, OHAs alone may provide the extra help they need to reach their blood sugar target. Some insulin-resistant individuals who produce little or no insulin on their own may find two particular OHAs useful in reducing their doses of injected insulin.

Although there are several OHAs currently on the market, at this writing I routinely prescribe only one of them — metformin. By the time you read this, however, a new agent, troglitazone, will be available.* I expect to prescribe it at least as much as I do metformin.

METFORMIN AND TROGLITAZONE — THE OHAS OF CHOICE

The great advantage of metformin and troglitazone over all other OHAs is that they help to reduce blood sugar by making the body's tissues more sensitive to insulin, whether it's the body's own or injected. This is a benefit that can't be underestimated. Not only is it a boon to those try-

---

* Metformin is sold as Glucophage by Bristol-Myers Squibb in the United States and by Lifa abroad. Troglitazone is sold as Rezulin by Parke-Davis.

ing to get their blood sugars under control, but it's also quite useful to those who are obese and simultaneously trying to get their weight under control. By helping to reduce the amount of insulin in the bloodstream at any given time, these two drugs can help in controlling the powerful fat-building properties of insulin. I have many patients who are not diabetic but have come to me for treatment of their obesity. Metformin has been a real plus to the weight-loss efforts of some because of its ability to curtail insulin resistance. I expect the same benefits from troglitazone.

Some obese diabetic patients come to me who are injecting very large doses of insulin because their obesity makes them highly insulin-resistant. These high doses of insulin cause a lot of fat-building to take place, and weight loss becomes proportionately more difficult. Metformin and troglitazone make these patients more sensitive to the insulin they're injecting. In one case I had a patient taking 27 units of insulin at bedtime, even though he was on our low-carbohydrate diet. After he started on metformin, he was able to cut the dose to about 20 units. This is still a very high dose, but the metformin facilitated the reduction.

Both OHAs have also been shown to improve a number of measurable cardiac risk factors, including lipid profile, serum fibrinogen, blood pressure, and even abnormal thickening of the heart muscle itself. In addition, metformin has been found to inhibit the destructive binding of glucose to proteins throughout the body — independent of its effect upon blood sugar.

Most of the other OHA drugs on the market, the old sulfonylureas, only work if you are still producing some insulin on your own. They operate by stimulating the pancreas to produce more insulin, which can directly cause your remaining pancreatic beta cells to break down over a period of years. The higher their doses, the more likely will be beta cell burnout. They do not decrease the body's requirements for — or increase its sensitivity to — insulin. They also stimulate insulin production whether the body needs it or not, so there's the constant risk of hypoglycemia. Therefore, the only case in which I still prescribe a sulfonylurea is if a patient's blood sugars cannot be controlled by diet alone and for some reason he's likely to live less than five years — *and* he is terrified of insulin injections. Otherwise, the harm that sulfonylureas can do simply outweighs any benefit. There's a new sulfonylurea OHA being marketed in the United States which the manufacturer and several published studies claim lowers insulin resistance and serum insulin levels. This product, glimepiride (Amaryl, Parke-Davis), also stimulates beta cells to produce insulin. It is therefore the only sulfonylurea I will prescribe for special situations. At present, I only have one patient who is a "special situation." Thus far, when given the choice, all my other patients have chosen insulin or insulin in combination with metformin.

WHO IS A LIKELY CANDIDATE FOR METFORMIN OR TROGLITAZONE?

Generally speaking, these OHAs are natural choices for a Type II diabetic who despite a low-carbohydrate diet cannot get his weight down or his blood sugars into normal ranges. The blood sugar elevation may be limited to a particular time of the day, it may be during the night, or it may entail a slight elevation all day. We base our prescription on the individual's blood sugar profiles. If even on our diet, blood sugar exceeds 300 mg/dl at any time of the day, I'll immediately prescribe insulin and won't even attempt to use these agents, except to eventually reduce doses of injected insulin. If your blood sugar is higher upon arising than at bedtime, we'd give you metformin or troglitazone at bedtime. If your blood sugar goes up after a particular meal, we'd give you the OHA about 2 hours before that meal. Since food enhances the absorption of troglitazone, we might give this drug with the meal.

GETTING STARTED: SOME TYPICAL OHA PROTOCOLS

Let's say you're a Type II diabetic and through weight loss, exercise, and diet, you pretty much have your blood sugars within your target range. Still, your blood sugar profiles show a regular elevation in the mornings after a low-carbohydrate breakfast, probably due to the dawn phenomenon.

In order to get your blood sugars into normal ranges, we'd start you out on a progressive dose. Overall, metformin has a very low side-effects profile, with the exception of gastrointestinal distress — queasiness, nausea, diarrhea, or a slight bellyache — in as many as a third of the people who try it. Most people who experience such distress, however, find that their discomfort diminishes as they become accustomed to the medication. Only a very few patients can't tolerate it at all. (Some patients, particularly obese patients who are anxious to achieve weight loss that metformin can facilitate, will ignore any initial gastrointestinal distress and use an antacid drug such as Pepcid or Tagamet for relief. Others, who may only experience relatively mild discomfort, are willing to tolerate it for a few weeks just to get things rolling.) Gastrointestinal side effects have not been reported for troglitazone.

In any case, metformin takes about 2 hours to start working. Although the literature says that it peaks 2 hours after that, we find that it literally lasts all night if you take it at bedtime. It comes in two dosage strengths — 500 mg and 850 mg unscored tablets. It's my practice always to start patients on the lowest possible dose — so in the above case we'd set you up with a pill cutter and have you take half a 500 mg tablet immediately after breakfast. Studies show that troglitazone starts working after 30 minutes, peaks in about 2–3 hours, and stops working after about 48 hours. Because it remains in the blood for so long, after dosing for a few days it will reduce insulin resistance all day long. It is supplied as 200 mg and 400 mg unscored, coated tablets that probably should not be broken with a pill cutter. The maximum recommended dose is 600 mg per day.

Note that even though it takes 2 hours for metformin to begin working, and your blood sugar elevation is *after* breakfast, we'd still start you off by having you take the medication immediately *after* breakfast. We do this in order to reduce the likelihood of gastrointestinal discomfort. Many people don't have any discomfort when they take metformin on a full stomach. Troglitazone, on the other hand, can be taken before meals from the start, without distress, but it may not be fully absorbed without food.

We'd then have you check your blood sugars before lunch. If your blood sugar was lower but still elevated, after a few days, we'd gradually increase the dosage by half a pill (if metformin) until we got your pre-lunch blood sugars into your target range. To do this, we could go as high as five 500 mg metformin tablets. (Metformin ceases having any cumulative effect after 2,500 mg.) If you were to experience gastrointestinal discomfort at any dose, we'd revert back to the prior dose for three or four weeks and then increase it more slowly.

Once we determined what dose of metformin got your blood sugar normalized, we'd start to shift the dose to *before* breakfast — immediately upon arising. In shifting doses, we'd again work in small increments. Let's say we had found that it took three 500 mg tablets to get your blood sugars to within your target range. You'd shift the dose by starting to take half a tablet immediately upon arising, and the other 2½ tablets immediately after eating. After a week, provided you didn't experience any intestinal distress, we'd shift another half a pill to immediately upon arising, and so on until you were taking all 3 when you got up.

If, after moving a portion of your dose — say, 1½ tablets — you started experiencing gastrointestinal distress, we'd shift half a tablet back to after breakfast. Some people can take several weeks to acclimate to metformin, so we'd let the regimen stand for a few days before we'd try moving it again. We've done this with numerous patients, and it works for most (though not all) without any undue discomfort. This cautious tapering up of dose is not necessary for troglitazone, which is unlikely to cause gastrointestinal side effects.

This is how we'd get your postbreakfast blood sugar elevation under control. Let's look at some other instances where these drugs can be useful.

Let's say you wake up in the morning with a higher blood sugar than when you went to sleep — not an especially elevated blood sugar, just higher than when you went to bed. This would tell me that you need some kind of help overnight. I have many patients whose blood sugars don't go up after meals but do go up overnight. The cause of the rise in blood sugars may be slow digestion of dinner while you're asleep, or may be due to the dawn phenomenon. Whatever the case, you'd still need something to help. Here we'd have you take metformin or troglitazone at bedtime. I'd prefer the troglitazone because it appears to be longer-acting. Again, it takes 2 hours for metformin to start working, 30 minutes for troglitazone, but both drugs appear to work for most of the night.

There's a good chance that your stomach will be empty at bedtime, so you stand a higher risk of developing gastrointestinal distress from metformin. As before, we'd start you with a low dose and bring it up slowly if you showed gastrointestinal distress, or rapidly if you didn't. Over time, as we discovered the proper dose, your blood sugar profiles would, we hope, show that your fasting blood sugar in the morning was the same as at bedtime because of the metformin or troglitazone.

Another instance when we'd start you on these drugs would be if you showed an elevated blood sugar at bedtime. This would reflect the effects of dinner, and to get that under control, we'd want you on one of them before dinner. Again, with metformin, we'd start you out on the smallest possible dose immediately *after* dinner and eventually shift the dose to precede the meal. If you were also showing overnight blood sugar rises, we'd first work on the dinner dose. Of course, the same protocol can be applied to lunch if blood sugars are routinely elevated before dinner. Many of my patients take metformin before each meal and at bedtime.

Certainly if metformin were to cause gastrointestinal distress, we now have the option of switching to troglitazone. It is very possible that for some individuals we'd use both medications — perhaps metformin before meals and troglitazone at bedtime, or vice versa.

WILL THESE MEDICATIONS CAUSE HYPOGLYCEMIA?

Some OHAs — specifically the sulfonylureas — carry the very real possibility of causing dangerously low blood sugars, but this is only remotely likely with troglitazone or metformin. This is because their mode of action is to *increase your sensitivity* to insulin. Neither agent interferes with the self-regulating system of a pancreas that can still make its own insulin. If your blood sugar drops too low, your body will just stop making insulin automatically. Sulfonylureas, on the other hand, because they stimulate insulin production *whether the body needs it or not,* can cause hypoglycemia.

Although the manufacturer and the scientific literature claim that metformin does not cause hypoglycemia, I did have a single patient who experienced hypoglycemia. She was very obese but only very mildly diabetic, and I was giving her metformin to reduce insulin resistance and facilitate weight loss. When I put her on metformin, her blood sugars went too low — down into the 60s. While it's possible for any drug to have nearly any effect on a given individual, this was the only case I've seen of hypoglycemia with metformin, and I was using it in a patient who was only mildly diabetic. Her insulin resistance was causing her to make a lot of insulin, but why the metformin brought her down so low I can't explain.

So there may be some very slight risk of hypoglycemia with troglitazone or metformin, but this is not at all comparable to the great risk with the sulfonylureas. One warning, however. The body cannot turn off injected insulin, so if you are taking insulin plus either of these agents, hypoglycemia is possible.

WHAT IF THESE AGENTS DON'T BRING BLOOD SUGARS INTO LINE?

If neither of these drugs is adequate to normalize blood sugars completely, chances are there is something awry in the diet or exercise portion of your treatment program. The most likely culprit for continued elevated blood sugars is that the carbohydrate portion of your diet is somehow not properly controlled. So the first step is to examine your diet again to see if that's where the problem lies. With many patients, this is a matter of carbohydrate craving, patients eating restricted foods. If this is the case, if your carbohydrate craving is so overwhelming, I'd recommend that you look at appetite-suppressing medication as a way of getting uncontrollable craving into line. If diet is not the culprit, then the next thing — no matter how obese or resistant to exercise you might be — would be to try to get you started on a strenuous exercise program. If even this doesn't do the trick, we'll certainly use injected insulin. Another far-out possibility (I say far-out because I haven't tried it yet) would be to use both metformin and troglitazone together.

15

Insulin:

THE BASICS OF SELF-INJECTION

A s you may recall from the preceding chapter, doses of metformin over 2,500 mg usually fail to have any added effect on blood sugar levels. If you're taking this much metformin or 600 mg of troglitazone (or both) and your blood sugars remain elevated — in spite of diet, exercise (where feasible), and weight loss — injected insulin will be essential to bringing your blood sugars down into normal ranges. Because science has yet to come up with an insulin that isn't destroyed in the digestive tract, insulin must be injected — and, generally speaking, you're the one who's going to have to do it. Although many patients initially balk at the idea of injecting insulin, you should look at this as an opportunity, not a curse, because *insulin injections will increase the likelihood that you can bring about a partial recovery of your pancreatic beta cell function.* This is especially true if you are slim.

If you're afraid of insulin because you imagine that once you start, you'll never be able to stop, you've fallen victim to a common myth. In reality, injected insulin is the *best* means we have at this writing for preventing beta cell burnout. Tests are even under way to see if injected insulin can prevent the development of Type I diabetes in susceptible individuals.

If the prospect of injecting yourself horrifies you, don't let it. Many people assume injections must be painful, but they needn't be. If you've already been using insulin for years and find the shots painful, the likelihood is you were taught to inject improperly.

HOW TO GIVE A PAINLESS INJECTION

If you have Type II diabetes, sooner or later you may require insulin injections, either temporarily (as during infections) or permanently. This
is nothing to be afraid of, even though many people with long-standing
Type II diabetes spend literally years worrying about it. I usually teach
all my patients how to inject themselves at our first or second meeting,
before there's any urgency. Once they give themselves a sample injection
of sterile saline (salt water), they find out how easy and painless it can
be, and they are spared years of anxiety. If you're anxious about injections, after you read this section, please ask your physician or diabetes
educator to allow you to try a self-administered injection.

Insulin is usually injected subcutaneously. This means into a layer of
fat under the skin. The regions of the body that usually contain appropriate deposits of fat are illustrated in Figure 15-1. Examine your body
to see if you have enough fat at the illustrated sites to comfortably grab
a big hunk between your thumb and first finger.

To show you how painless a shot can be, your teacher should give
him- or herself a shot and leave the syringe dangling in place, to illus-
trate that no pain is felt. Your teacher should next give you a shot of
saline to prove the point. Now it's time for you to give yourself an injec-

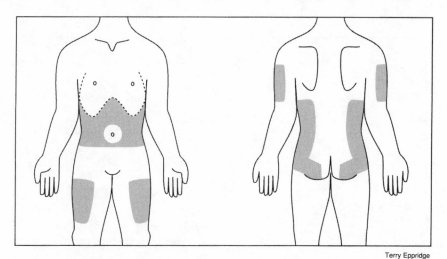

Terry Eppridge

Fig. 15-1. *Potential sites for subcutaneous injections.*

tion, using a syringe that's been partly filled for you with about 5 "units" of saline.

1. First, with your "nonshooting" hand, grab as big a chunk of skin plus underlying fat as you can hold comfortably. If you have a nice roll of fat around your waist, use this site. If not, select another site from those illustrated in Figure 15-1. Nearly everyone has enough subcutaneous buttocks fat to inject there without grabbing any flesh. Just locate a fatty site by feel. To inject into your arm, use the top of a chair, the outside corner of two walls, or the edge of a door to push the loose flesh from under your arm to a forward position that you can easily see and reach with the needle.

2. Hold the syringe like a dart, with the thumb and first three fingers of either hand.

3. Now comes the most important part. *Penetration must be rapid. Never* put the needle against the skin and push. That's the method still taught in many hospitals, and it's often painful. If you can find only a small amount of flesh to hold, the needle should pierce the skin at a 45-degree angle, as in Figure 15-2, or even better, use one of the new insulin syringes with a short needle (5/16 inch). If you can grab a hefty handful, you should plunge the needle straight in, perpendicular to the skin surface, or at any angle between 45 degrees and 90 degrees, as shown in Figure 15-3.

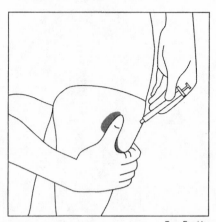

Terry Eppridge

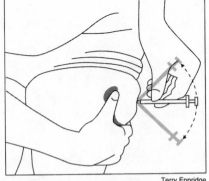

Terry Eppridge

Fig. 15-2. *If you are skinny, pierce the skin at a 45-degree angle, or use a short (5/16-inch) needle.*

Fig. 15-3. *If you're chunky, pierce the skin at any angle between 45 degrees and 90 degrees.*

4. The stroke should begin about 4 inches from your target to give the moving needle a chance to pick up speed. Pretend you're throwing a dart — but don't let go of the syringe. Move your entire forearm and give the wrist a flick at the end of the motion. You shouldn't get hurt. The needle should penetrate the skin for its entire length.
5. As soon as it's in, push the plunger all the way down to inject the fluid. Now promptly remove the needle from the skin.

There's no need to practice injecting oranges, as has been taught in the past. If you're going to practice anything, you might practice "throwing" a syringe with the needle cover on at your skin.

All it takes is enduring one rapid "stick" for you to realize that speed makes it painless. Never has it taken more than a moment for me to get a patient to self-inject. I've had grown men in tears at the prospect of injecting insulin who soon discover that it's easy and painless, and of considerable value in treatment. It doesn't demand much skill, and certainly doesn't require bravery.

HOW TO SELECT AN INSULIN SYRINGE

In recent years, a number of new insulin syringes have appeared on the market in the United States. Although they are all sterile, plastic, and disposable, some are better than others. The important features to consider are described below. Refer to Figure 15-4, which identifies the parts of two typical insulin syringes you might find at your local pharmacy.

The Scale

When selecting a syringe, the scale is the most important feature, because the spacing of the markings determines how accurately you can measure a dose. Think Laws of Small Numbers: accuracy and consistency are both highly important.

Insulin doses, like other injected medications, are measured in "units." One unit of a fast-acting insulin will lower my blood sugar by 40 mg/dl. One unit will lower the blood sugar of a 45-pound child by about 120 mg/dl. Some of my adult patients with mild Type II diabetes find that 1 unit will drop them by 70 mg/dl. Clearly, an error of only ½ unit can make the difference between a normal blood sugar and hypo-

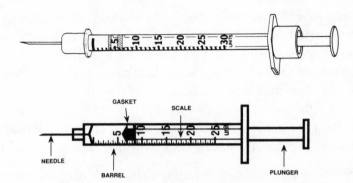

Fig. 15-4. *Typical insulin syringes, neither of which is ideal. Although the one on the bottom has a scale showing half units, I prefer the top syringe because the gasket is flat, making the dosage easier to read. It is also available with a short needle.*

glycemia for many of us. Most of my insulin-using patients rarely inject as much as 8 units in a single dose. It would therefore be ideal to have a long, slender syringe, with a total capacity of 10 units and markings for every ½ unit, spaced far enough apart that ¼ unit can be accurately estimated visually. The numbers on the scale should be easy to read. The lines should be dark, but no thicker than ⅙ unit. Two typical syringes are illustrated above.

The Rubber Gasket

This is the dark-colored piece of synthetic rubber at the end of the plunger nearest the needle. It indicates a given dose by its position along the scale. The best gasket has a surface that's flat and not conical, as some are, so that doses can be read without confusion.

The Needle

The needle should be approximately ⁵⁄₁₆–½ inch long. Longer needles may go too deeply into thin people. Until 1996 all disposable insulin syringes sold in the United States had ½-inch needles. Syringes with shorter (⁵⁄₁₆-inch) needles are now available. With these syringes you usually need not "grab a hunk of flesh" or inject at a 45-degree angle. Just throw it in. Do not, however, use short needles for intramuscular injection as described on page 247.

Needle thickness is specified by gauge number, just like nails and wire. The higher the gauge number, the thinner the needle. With a very thin gauge, even penetrating the skin too slowly may not hurt. With too thin a gauge, the needle might bend or break when puncturing thick skin. The ideal compromise between thinness and strength is probably 30 gauge.

The Point

The needle points of disposable insulin syringes currently sold in the United States are quite sharp. Advertising that claims special sharpness is usually exaggerated.

FILLING THE SYRINGE

This technique for filling a syringe with insulin differs from what is usually taught, but it has the advantage of preventing the retention of air bubbles in the syringe. Although it is not harmful to inject air bubbles into your skin, their presence interferes with accurate measurement of small doses.

General Technique

This step-by-step approach may be followed for all fast-acting (lispro, regular) insulins. If you use longer-acting insulin, be sure to read the section that follows this one before proceeding.

1. Take the cap(s) off your syringe.
2. Draw room air into the syringe by pulling the plunger back until the end of the rubber gasket nearest the needle is set at the dose you intend to inject. If the gasket has a dome or conical shape, the dose should be set at the widest part of the gasket, not at its tip (as indicated by the "gasket" arrow in the lower half of Figure 15-4).
3. Puncture the insulin vial with the needle and inject air into the vial. This seemingly useless step has a purpose. If you were not to inject air to replace the insulin you withdrew, a vacuum would eventually develop in the vial, which would make filling syringes difficult.
4. Invert the syringe and vial and hold them vertically, as shown in Figure 15-5, then rapidly pull back on the plunger until the barrel is filled with insulin well beyond your dose.
5. Slowly push the plunger in, still holding vertically, until the appropriate part of the rubber gasket reaches the desired dose.

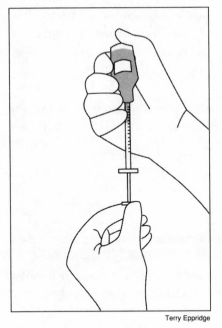

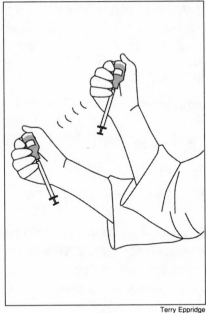

Terry Eppridge   Terry Eppridge

Fig. 15-5. *Filling the syringe, holding*   Fig. 15-6. *Shaking a vial of cloudy*
vial and syringe vertically.   *insulin before drawing out the dose.*

6. Continue to hold syringe and vial vertically as you remove the
   filled syringe and needle from the vial.

Filling a Syringe with Long-Acting Insulin

Most longer-acting insulins (lente, ultralente) are sold today in vials that
contain a clear liquid and a gray precipitate. The gray particles tend to
settle rapidly from the liquid when the vial is left undisturbed. They
must be resuspended uniformly in the liquid immediately prior to every
use. Failure to do this will result in inconsistent effects upon blood sugars from one shot to another. The way to secure a uniform suspension is
to shake the vial. Many years ago, some vaccines in use were of a syrupy
consistency and tended to form a permanent foam when shaken. This is
not the case with today's insulins. Yet most textbooks still tell nurses and
doctors to roll the vial between the hands and not to shake it. This mis-
information is unfortunate, because we don't get consistent results
when vials are rolled.

When filling a syringe with a long-acting (cloudy) insulin, observe the following procedure to ensure an even suspension.*

1–3. Remove cap(s) from syringe, draw air into it, and inject the air into the vial as described in steps 1–3 on page 203.

4. *Before* drawing out any insulin, while still holding the vial and syringe in one hand, vigorously shake them back and forth 6–10 times as shown in Figure 15-6. Holding the inverted syringe and vial vertically, draw back the plunger *immediately* after shaking to fill the syringe with insulin well beyond your dose. Do not delay, as the gray particles will settle very rapidly.

5–6. Still holding vertically, push plunger in until desired dose is reached, then remove needle and filled syringe from vial (see steps 5–6, pages 203–204).

ON THE REUSE OF DISPOSABLE INSULIN SYRINGES

The annual cost of sterile disposable insulin syringes can be considerable, especially if you take multiple daily injections. You may become tempted to reuse your syringes, especially if your medical insurance doesn't reimburse you for the cost. (Most medical insurance policies in the United States do cover this expense.) Although I don't know of any infection caused by reusing syringes, I have encountered the problem of contamination of insulin.

Many of my patients pass through a stage when they routinely reuse their syringes several times, to save money or to enable them to travel with only a small supply. These patients never use the same syringe for two different types of insulin, so we can't say that one insulin is contaminating another. Inevitably, I get a telephone call with the message, "My blood sugars are high and I can't get them down." I ask, "Bring your clear [fast-acting] insulin to the phone. Is it crystal clear, like water?" Inevitably the reply is, "No, it's slightly hazy." Insulin that is hazy has been partially deactivated and will not adequately control blood sugars. This

---

* Long-acting insulins that are not cloudy will probably be marketed within a few years of this writing. They will not require shaking.

is rarely found by people who do not reuse their syringes.* Of course, I advise my patient to replace all insulin vials, whether long- or short-acting, that have been used to fill reused syringes. Replacement of the vials always cures the problem.

What if you encounter a situation where you only have one syringe to last for a week, and have no way of getting new ones? Flush the syringe with air several times after each use to clear out any remaining insulin. When filling the syringe, do not inject air into the insulin vial (step 3), and don't inject the excess insulin back into the vial (step 5). Just draw the needle from the vial and squirt the excess into the air. This way, you won't contaminate your vial with the minute amount of old insulin that may remain in the needle or syringe. If you have a second unused syringe, you can use it just to inject air into your vials, making certain the needle does not come into contact with the insulin in the vials.

If for financial reasons you really must reuse your syringes, the following procedure should help minimize contamination. You will, at the minimum, need three syringes, but four would be better:

- Use one syringe for rapid-acting (clear) insulin and another for long-acting (cloudy) insulin. Put a piece of adhesive tape on the "cloudy" syringe to identify it (but not so much than you can't read the scale).
- Use your insulin vials for a week without injecting air into them. Squirt any excess insulin from each filling into a sink or wastebasket, not back into the vial.
- At the end of a week, remove the plunger from an unused syringe (here it would be best to have two unused syringes, one each for clear and cloudy insulin; again the "cloudy" syringe should be marked with adhesive tape). Stand the vial right side up on a flat surface and push the needle of the unused syringe into the stopper of the vial. Within seconds, the vacuum in the vial will suck in enough air through the needle to displace the vacuum. (If you only have three syringes, use one of them only for replacing air in the vials. When you insert the needle into the stopper, make certain

---

* The reason for this is that the minute amount of insulin remaining in a used needle will become polymerized (inactivated) within a few hours. If it is injected back into the vial, it will eventually cause the polymerization of much of the insulin in the vial.

that it does not touch the insulin. It can then be used for either type of insulin vial.)

- Reinsert the plunger and recap the "air" syringe for use the next week.

MUST YOUR SKIN BE WIPED WITH ALCOHOL?

Most textbooks and instruction sheets that teach insulin injection or finger sticking advise that the skin should be "sterilized" with alcohol before puncturing with a needle. Alcohol will not "sterilize" your skin. At best it will clean off dirt. My patients and I have given hundreds of thousands of injections and finger sticks without using alcohol. None of us has become infected as a result. Certainly it's a sensible idea to clean off visible dirt first, but you can do this with simple soap and water on the rare occasions that it may be necessary. I often inject myself right through my shirt or slacks.

REMOVING BLOODSTAINS FROM CLOTHING

Nowadays, most of us will inject through thin clothing (shirts, stockings, trousers) when it is inconvenient to undress. This can cause a problem on the rare occasion that the needle encounters a small blood vessel. A drop of blood can appear at the puncture site and stain your clothing. Finger punctures sometimes bleed more freely than you expect, so that upon squeezing you may get a squirt in the eye, or blood on your tie, if you're not careful.

The answer to bloodstains on clothing is hydrogen peroxide solution. Hydrogen peroxide is very inexpensive and is sold in all pharmacies. Purchase several small bottles. Keep a bottle of peroxide handy at every location where you measure blood sugars. Carry a small bottle in your luggage when you travel. Once a bottle has been opened, the solution remains stable for perhaps six months, so you might want to have a backup bottle available.

You can make bloodstains disappear very simply without bleaching the dyes in your clothing. It's best if you treat the stain while the blood is still wet, as dried blood bleaches very slowly. Pour some peroxide on a handkerchief and rub it into the stain. The peroxide will foam when it contacts blood. Keep rubbing until the stain has vanished.

SPECIAL DEVICES FOR "PAINLESS" INJECTIONS

Many devices have been advertised with the claim that they inject insulin "without pain." Since most diabetics have not been taught the high-speed painless injection technique described in this chapter, many of these special devices are sold every year. If your injections are already painless, it makes little sense to use them. On the other hand, you may be one of those people taught the old way of injecting who just cannot break the habit. Or perhaps no one is available to help you to learn proper injection technique. If so, read on.

One device gives the entire injection, including the delivery of insulin. It is called the Autojector. To use it, you pull the handle, which cocks a spring. Next you insert a prefilled disposable syringe and hold the tip of the device against your skin. You push a button, and almost instantaneously the entire injection is complete. The Autojector (Owen-Mumford Ltd.) is sold by many diabetes supply dealers in the United States and the United Kingdom. The cost in the United States is about $45.

Other "painless" devices called jet injectors use very precise construction to inject a high-pressure jet of insulin, penetrating the skin without a needle. These injectors do not require a separate syringe since they must be loaded directly with insulin, using special adapters that plug into the insulin vial. Although the concept is very enticing, spray injectors pose some problems. First, they're very expensive, costing from $300 to $600 in the United States. Although this is a substantial initial investment, the cost can be recovered over the course of a year or two if you're giving yourself lots of injections with disposable syringes. Your insurance plan will likely not pay for one but will pay for disposable syringes.

They're not as convenient as disposable syringes because they must be taken apart and sterilized in boiling, deionized water every one to two weeks. Also, the adapters for the insulin vials sometimes leak when the vials are carried in a purse or bag.

You will require considerable training and experimentation with pressure settings in order to give yourself a proper jet injection, which can lead to extra difficulty in getting your blood sugars normalized. You may also experience slightly more pain sometimes than you would with a speedily injected shot from a conventional syringe, and there's a high incidence of black and blue marks on the skin and minor bleeding at the puncture sites.

Despite these drawbacks, jet injectors do have two unique advantages, aside from reducing the number of syringes you must dispose of. First is that you will require about one-third less insulin, since the shots are better absorbed. Second, if you use fast-acting insulin to lower elevated blood sugars, it will work even faster.

I usually experiment with all new injection devices and syringes that are sold in the United States. Since developments in this field advance so rapidly, you may want to drop me a note before purchasing a "painless" injector in order to find out what we currently recommend for our patients. Just write to me at the Diabetes Center, 1160 Greacen Point Road, Mamaroneck, NY 10543.

INSULIN PENS

Several manufacturers are advertising "insulin pens." These are syringes into which small cartridges of insulin can be loaded. They are intended to relieve you of the burden of carrying a vial of insulin if you have to inject away from home. None of those marketed as of this writing can be set at half- or quarter-unit increments, and therefore they cannot give the fine-tuning of blood sugars that our regimens require. Stay away from them.

INHALED INSULIN

Considerable progress has been made in the development of a device that turns insulin into a finely aerosolized "smoke" that can be inhaled by mouth, and clinical trials are now underway. Although absorption of inhaled insulin has been demonstrated, there is still the unanswered question of how accurately blood levels of insulin can be reproduced from one dose to another. My guess is that the precision required for true blood sugar predictability will not be possible for many years, if ever. I hope I will be proven wrong.

16

Important Information About Various Insulins

I f you start using insulin, you ought to understand how its effects can be controlled. It can do some remarkable things, but it must be handled with respect and knowledge. Much of the information in this chapter is based upon my experience with my own insulin needs and with those of many patients. As in many areas of this book, you will likely note that some statements contradict traditional teachings.

AVOID INSULINS THAT CONTAIN PROTAMINE

There are a confusing number of brands and types of insulins being marketed today — and even more are on the way. Insulins may be categorized by how long they continue to affect blood sugars after injection. There are rapid-acting, intermediate-acting, and long-acting insulins. Currently the rapid-acting insulins appear clear, like water, and the other insulins appear cloudy. The cloudiness is caused by an additive that combines with the insulin to form particles that slowly dissolve under the skin. Some of the long- and intermediate-acting insulins contain zinc as the additive. Other insulins are modified with an animal protein called protamine. The zinc is relatively innocuous and does not appear to cause problems. Insulins that contain protamine may stimulate the immune system to make antibodies to the insulin. These antibodies can temporarily bind to some of the insulin, rendering it inactive. Then, unpredictably, they can release the insulin at a time when it's not necessarily needed. This effect, although small, does not facilitate the meticulous control of blood sugars that we seek. Protamine can present another more serious problem if you ever require coronary angiography for the study of arteries that feed your heart (a common procedure nowadays). Just before such a study, you would be given an injection of the anti-coagulant heparin to prevent the formation of blood clots. When the procedure is over, protamine is injected into a vein to "turn off" the heparin. This injection can cause severe allergic reactions, and even death, in a small percentage of people who have previously been treated with insulin containing protamine. Thus, even if an insulin is marketed as a "human" insulin, its effects upon antibody production may be significant if it contains the animal protein protamine.

Table 16-1 lists the long- and intermediate-acting "human" insulins currently sold in the United States together with the additives used to prolong their action. For reasons that should now be obvious, I only recommend lente and ultralente when intermediate- or long-acting insulins are desired. In a few years, some long-acting clear insulins that do not contain additives may become available.

Recently, mixtures of NPH insulin and "regular" (rapid-acting) insulin, designated 70/30 and 50/50 have appeared on the market. Since these contain protamine, I would avoid them.

STRENGTHS OF INSULIN

The biological activity of insulin is measured in units. Two units of insulin should lower blood sugar exactly twice as much as 1 unit. An insulin syringe is therefore graduated in units. If you use the upper syringe illustrated in Figure 15-4 on page 202, each graduation corresponds to

TABLE 16-1

LONG- AND INTERMEDIATE-ACTING INSULINS

Generic Name of Insulin	Action	Principal Additive
NPH (isophane)	Intermediate	Protamine
70/30	Intermediate	Protamine
50/50	Intermediate	Protamine
Lente	Intermediate	Zinc
Ultralente	Long	Zinc

1 unit. The lines are far enough apart so that ½ and even ¼ unit can be reasonably estimated. If you use the lower syringe illustrated in Figure 15-4, each short line on the scale will correspond to ½ unit. Since we know from the packaging that the syringe can dispense up to ¼ cc (cubic centimeter) of fluid, and the scale goes up to 25 units, it is clear that this syringe was designed for an insulin concentration of 100 units per cc. (The top syringe is also designed for a concentration of 100 units per cc, and can dispense up to ³⁄₁₀ cc, or 30 units.) Its strength is designated U-100, meaning "100 units per cc." *In the United States and Canada, this is the only insulin concentration sold,* so you need not specify the strength when you purchase. Other insulin strengths, such as U-40 and U-80, are sold in other countries, and the scales on the syringes are designed for these other strengths. Special strengths such as U-40, U-80, and U-500 are available to your physician in the United States, upon request from the manufacturers, for special applications. The syringes for these alternate strengths are not sold in the United States.

If you travel overseas and happen to lose or misplace your insulin, you may be unable to secure the U-100 strength locally. You can make the best of this by purchasing U-40 or U-80 insulin, together with U-40 or U-80 syringes. You should draw your usual doses in units into the new syringes with the new insulin.

CARING FOR YOUR INSULIN

Insulin is stable for eighteen months at room temperature and thirty-six months if refrigerated. A slight loss of potency may occur if insulin is stored at room temperature longer than 30 days. Insulin can become deactivated with or without a change in its appearance, leading to unexpectedly elevated blood sugars. When I receive a distress call from a patient who has had higher than usual blood sugars for several days, I ask a number of questions in order to determine the source of the blood sugar elevation. Has there been a dietary indiscretion? Is there a possible infection? Or might the insulin be deactivated? Cloudiness of a clear, rapid-acting insulin is a certain sign of deactivation. So is the appearance of visible clumps within, or a gray precipitate on the wall of, a vial of lente or ultralente insulin that will not disappear when it's shaken. Deactivation of insulin, however, may not be possible to distinguish simply by looking. If diet or infection seems unlikely to be the source of the blood sugar elevation, I therefore advise my patient to discard all insulin currently in use, and to utilize fresh vials, even if the insulin *looks* okay.

Here are some simple rules for routine care of your insulin:

- Keep unused insulin in a refrigerator until you are ready to use it for the first time. Vials in current use may be kept at room temperature.
- Never allow insulin to freeze. Even after it thaws out, it may no longer possess its full strength. If you suspect it may have frozen, discard it.
- If your home reaches temperatures above 85°F (29°C), refrigerate all your insulin. If your insulin has been exposed to room temperatures in excess of 99°F (37°C) for more than 1 day, discard it.
- Do not reuse your insulin syringes (page 205).
- Do not put insulin in prolonged sunlight, closed motor vehicles, glove compartments, or car trunks. These areas can become overheated on a sunny day, even in winter. If you inadvertently leave insulin in a hot vehicle, discard it.
- Do not routinely keep insulin close to your body, as in shirt pockets.
- If you keep your currently used insulin out of the refrigerator, mark the date of first use on every vial. Discard all vials whenever three months have elapsed after the marked date.
- When you invert your insulin vial to fill your syringe, observe the level of insulin. When the level drops below the lower edge of the label on the inverted vial, discard the vial. This is especially necessary with longer-acting (cloudy) insulins because the concentration of active particles may change as you use it up.

HOW INSULIN AFFECTS YOUR BLOOD SUGARS OVER TIME

It's important for you to know when your insulin will begin to affect your blood sugar and when it will finish working. This information is printed in the package insert with the insulin. The published information, however, may be inaccurate for patients on our regimen. The reason for this is that we use very small doses of insulin, while most published data are based upon much larger doses. As a rule, larger doses tend to start working sooner and finish working later than smaller doses. Furthermore, the action time of an insulin will vary somewhat from one person to another. Nevertheless, Table 16-2 is a reasonable guide to the approximate starting and finishing times of the insulins we recommend. Your response may not follow a typical pattern, but at least this table can serve as a starting point.

Note when reading Table 16-2 that the apparent action times of lente

TABLE 16-2
APPROXIMATE ACTION TIMES OF PREFERRED INSULINS*

| Generic Name of Insulin | Brand Name | Designation | Action Time After Injection | |
			Action Starts	Action Ends
Regular or Crystalline (R)	Humulin R Novolin R	Rapid-acting	40 minutes	5–6 hours
Lispro (H)	Humalog	Very rapid-acting	15 minutes	4–5 hours
Lente (L)	Humulin L Novolin L	Intermediate-acting	2–3 hours	12 hours if injected in the morning; 8 hours if injected at bedtime†
Ultralente (UL)	Humulin U	Long-acting	Slowly over 4 hours	18 hours if injected in the morning; 9–10 hours if injected at bedtime (apparent)

* Doses exceeding 8 units will usually start sooner and last longer.

† Doses of lente insulin that exceed 8 units may have a peak of action at about 8 hours after injection.

and ultralente insulins are briefer if they are injected at bedtime than if injected in the morning. This bizarre happenstance is probably caused by the dawn phenomenon, described in Chapter 6.

Insulin action will be speeded considerably if you exercise the region of your body into which you injected. As a consequence, it may be, for example, unwise to inject long-acting insulin into your thigh on a day that you run or do lower body exercise, or into your arm on a day that you lift weights, or into your abdomen on a day that you do sit-ups.

ABBREVIATED DESIGNATIONS FOR THE VARIOUS INSULINS

When you're filling in the information on your GLUCOGRAF data sheets, it will be more convenient for you and your doctor if you use the abbreviated designations shown in the first column of Table 16-2 — R, H, L, or UL — instead of the full names. Since it's implied, you also needn't write out the word "units" when noting insulin doses. Seven units of lente insulin would abbreviate as "7L," and so on.

WHY DO WE USE THE LONGER-ACTING INSULINS?

Lente and ultralente, the cloudy, longer-acting insulins, serve a purpose different from that of the rapid-acting, clear insulins. Indeed, for our regimens they have but one principal task — to keep blood sugar from rising *while fasting* (see the discussions of gluconeogenesis and the dawn phenomenon, pages 83–84). They're not intended to prevent the blood sugar rise *after eating*. Furthermore, lente and ultralente are not used to lower a blood sugar that is too high — they work too slowly for this. A secondary purpose of longer-acting insulins in mild Type II diabetes is to help delay or prevent beta cell burnout. As you'll see later, we may use a rapid-acting insulin to cover meals, whether or not the longer-acting insulins are used to cover the fasting state. Which insulin to use, and when, depends upon blood sugar profiles.

Now why do we use both lente and ultralente? Won't just one or the other suffice? Which one to use depends upon blood sugar profiles. If your blood sugar typically rises between noon and bedtime on days that you skip all your meals, you'll need ultralente on arising in the morning. We use ultralente and not lente in the daytime because ultralente lasts longer and will usually carry over until a bit past bedtime. On the other hand, we may use one or the other, or in rare cases, both, at bedtime, to cover the overnight fasting state. When ultralente or lente is needed at bedtime, we usually try the ultralente first. Ultralente is especially valuable if the dawn phenomenon is prolonged or if you sleep longer than 8 hours. If our initial dose of ultralente is not adequate, we may increase it. Sooner or later, however, we may find that late-morning blood sugars are going too low, due to the higher doses of ultralente. We might then switch over to lente at bedtime, to concentrate action during the sleep period. One must be careful, however, not to give too much lente at bedtime, because large doses may cause blood sugars to drop in the middle of the night.

WHEN DO WE USE RAPID-ACTING INSULIN?

If you're a Type I diabetic — or a Type II diabetic who is following our diet and using OHAs and still experiencing blood sugar increases after one or more meals — injecting regular (R) or lispro (H) insulin prior to these meals is indicated. By sheer coincidence, the 5-hour action time of regular corresponds approximately to the time most of us require to digest fully a mixed meal of protein and carbohydrate, and to experience the final effect of the meal upon blood sugars. Regular insulin should usually be injected 40 minutes before a meal, so that it starts to work just as you start to eat.

The beta cells of some Type II's, however, enjoy enough of a rest from one or two small doses of ultralente that they can produce enough insulin to cover meals. Since everyone is different, your insulin regimen must be custom-tailored to normalize your personal glucose profile. All this takes more effort on the part of your physician than just the prescription of one or two daily shots of a long-acting insulin.

Because of its very rapid action, lispro is also the insulin that we use to lower a high blood sugar. Since elevated blood sugars are the cause of the long-term complications of diabetes, we naturally want to see them come down to normal as fast as possible. In Chapter 18, we will teach you how to rapidly get high blood sugars down precisely to your target, using lispro insulin. If your doctor finds that your blood sugars are rarely elevated or appear to rapidly drop down on their own, then it will not be necessary to use lispro for this purpose.

DILUTING INSULIN

Many Type II diabetics, mild Type I diabetics, and small children with Type I diabetes require such small doses of injected insulin that dosage cannot be measured accurately enough with any of the syringes currently on the market. For such people, 1 unit might lower blood sugar by 120 mg/dl. A measurement error of ¼ unit would therefore be equivalent to 30 mg/dl. To solve this problem we dilute the insulin. This is very easy. Your physician or pharmacist can secure, at no charge, empty sterile insulin vials from the insulin makers. The manufacturers will also provide, at no cost, the appropriate diluting fluids for the insulins you use. If your druggist is unwilling to perform the dilution, either find another pharmacist or do it yourself, as follows:

1. Have clear instructions from your physician as to how much insulin and how much diluting fluid should be put into a vial. If your doctor writes "dilute 2:1" (say "two to one"), this means 2 parts of diluent, or diluting fluid, for every 1 of insulin, and so on. He may want to give you a few sterile 3 cc syringes* for this purpose, since they will contain about ten times as much as the 25- or 30-unit syringe you use for injections. Using the larger syringe will speed up the preparation of your vials.
2. Each vial can hold only 10 cc of fluid. You should write down how many cc's of diluting fluid and insulin you will need, remembering that the sum of the two cannot exceed 10. Thus, if your doctor tells you to dilute your insulin 3:1, you might use 6 cc of diluent and 2 cc of insulin.
3. All diluting fluids should be crystal clear, like water. Make sure that the label of the diluting fluid you are using specifies that it is for the insulin you want to dilute. The diluting fluid for ultralente is the same as the diluting fluid for lente.

---

* They should be supplied with relatively wide-bore (about 23 gauge) needles.

4. Pierce the empty vial with the needle of your 3 cc syringe. Draw out air to the dose you wish to transfer (1, 2, or 3 cc).

5. Move the needle and syringe to the diluting fluid vial and inject the air. Invert syringe and vial and hold vertically while you withdraw the predetermined amount of fluid.

6. Inject the diluent into the empty vial from which you took the air, and withdraw more air if you will be delivering more fluid.

7. Repeat steps 4, 5, and 6 until the amount of diluent that you had written down is in the originally empty vial.

8. Draw another 1, 2, or 3 cc of air (depending upon how much insulin you will be transferring) from the vial you've been filling with diluent, but this time inject the air into the insulin vial. Invert syringe and vial and, holding vertically, draw out the predetermined amount of insulin. (If you are working with slow-acting [cloudy] insulins, remember to shake the insulin vial vigorously 6–10 times immediately before withdrawing the dose; see page 204.)

9. Inject the insulin into the vial to which diluent had been added.

10. Repeat steps 8 and 9 until the designated amount of insulin has been added to the diluent.

11. Label the newly diluted insulin vial with the date, the type of insulin (R, L, UL, or H), and the ratio of diluent to insulin used (2:1, 3:2, 4:1, or whatever it happens to be).

12. Put the vial of diluted insulin in the refrigerator for storage until its first use.

I've seen many people, including doctors, nurses, and pharmacists, become confused about how much diluted insulin to inject. With that in mind, we will run through a couple of examples to show you how simply this can be computed.

Example 1. Your doctor wants you to inject 2¼ units of an insulin that has been diluted 1:1. For every 2 parts of liquid in the syringe, only 1 part, or ½, is insulin. To get 2¼ real units of insulin, you will have to inject twice as many diluted units (2 x 2¼ = 4½) as they're measured on the scale of the syringe — which is much simpler to estimate.

Example 2. Your doctor wants you to inject 2¼ units of an insulin that has been diluted 4:1. This time, for every 5 parts of liquid only 1 part is insulin, so we must multiply real units by 5 to set our dose: 5 x 2¼ = 10¾ = 11¼ units on the syringe.

I don't really expect my patients to compute the diluted units they must take. In the case of the second example above, I would ask you to take 11¼ diluted units. If this were ultralente insulin, I'd write "11¼ D UL" on our data sheets, the "D" indicating that the ultralente has been diluted.

LISPRO: A NEW ULTRA-RAPID INSULIN

Lispro was developed to overcome regular insulin's inability to rapidly cover fast-acting dietary carbohydrates. It cannot, however, circumvent the Laws of Small Numbers relating to large amounts of dietary carbohydrate. Since fast-acting carbohydrate foods (bread, pasta, fruit, et cetera) usually contain large amounts of carbohydrate, the hazards of using such foods will still exist.

There are some applications of lispro that the manufacturer may not have considered. For instance, if it is inconvenient to take regular insulin 40 minutes before a meal, you can take a mixture of regular and lispro insulins 15 minutes before the meal. The regular is slow enough to cover digestion of dietary protein, and the lispro should be fast enough to cover slow-acting carbohydrate without the 40-minute delay. This can be very valuable when you eat out, as you will learn in Chapter 18. Also, some insulin users who previously used regular insulin to lower an elevated blood sugar will benefit by using lispro. It will get blood sugar down more rapidly. This, too, will be discussed in Chapter 18.

17

Simple Insulin Regimens

This chapter and the next describe a number of specific insulin regimens. The particular regimen that suits you will depend to a considerable degree upon your blood sugar profiles. Your physician must decide whether you need long-acting insulin to cover the fasting state, short-acting insulin to cover meals, or both. In either event, he or she will require blood sugar profiles and related data, covering at least one week, prior to *every* office visit or telephone call for fine-tuning of doses. Remember that "related data" includes the times of meals, whether you overate or underate, the times of exercise (including seemingly inconsequential activity such as shopping), infections or illnesses you may have had, when and how many glucose tablets were taken to correct low blood sugar — in short, anything that might have affected your blood sugar. Bedtime blood sugar readings are especially important information, because an increase or decrease overnight should most certainly affect your bedtime dosage of longer-acting insulin.

To give you an example of how we might use insulin to bring your blood sugar levels into target range, let's consider several possible blood sugar profile scenarios.

SCENARIO ONE: FASTING BLOOD SUGARS ARE HIGHER THAN BEDTIME BLOOD SUGARS

Let's say you're taking the highest useful dosage of metformin and/or troglitazone at bedtime. Your fasting (i.e., before-breakfast) blood sugars are still consistently higher than your bedtime blood sugars. Because of this, you probably require long-acting (ultralente) or intermediate-acting (lente) insulin at bedtime. Before we'd start you on insulin, however, we'd examine your data sheet carefully in order to make certain that you finished your last meal of each day at least 4 hours prior to your bedtime blood sugar measurement. No one should be given a long-acting insulin to cover an overnight blood sugar increase *caused by a meal* unless gastroparesis (Chapter 21) is present.

For people who customarily sleep 8 hours or longer, we usually start with ultralente; we start with lente for people who sleep 7 hours or less. If you like to sleep more than 8 hours on weekends, it's wise to use ultralente rather than lente *every* night, instead of trying to switch between one and the other.

Estimating the Dose

Your physician may want to use this simple method for estimating your starting bedtime insulin dose. Generally, 1 unit of insulin lowers blood sugar 40 mg/dl for a 140-pound, nonpregnant adult whose pancreas produces no insulin. Since your beta cells may still be producing some insulin, we'd abide by the Laws of Small Numbers and cautiously assume that 1 unit of any insulin would lower you 60 mg/dl, just so we wouldn't bring you dangerously low and risk overnight hypoglycemia.

We would then proceed as follows:

First, we'd look at your blood sugar profiles. The first number we want is the minimum overnight blood sugar increase over the past week. We'd subtract your bedtime blood sugars from your fasting blood sugars and take the number from the night with the lowest rise.

The second number we want is the maximum amount that we'd expect 1 unit of ultralente (or lente) to lower your overnight blood sugar. To get this number, we'd take the maximum anticipated blood sugar drop from 1 unit ultralente. Since our conservative rule of thumb is that 1 unit of ultralente will lower a 140-pound Type II's blood sugar by 60 mg/dl, we would divide 140 by your weight in pounds and then multiply the result by 60 mg/dl. If your weight is 200 pounds, the equation would look like this: (140 ÷ 200) x 60 = 42. So your estimated blood sugar drop will be 42 mg/dl from 1 unit of ultralente.

Let us assume, for example, that your lowest overnight blood sugar rise in the past week was 73 mg/dl. We'd take 73 mg/dl and divide it by the number you derived from the above equation, or 42. Your trial bedtime dose of ultralente (or lente) would be $73 \div 42 = 1.7$ units. This is your starting bedtime dose. Rounding off the dose to the nearest ¼ unit gives you 1¾ units, which you can abbreviate on your data sheet as 2^- (two minus) UL (or L), or just under 2 units.

Fine-Tuning the Dose

That was pretty easy, but it was only a starting point. Most probably this dose won't be perfect — likely a little too low or possibly even a little too high. To fine-tune the bedtime insulin, you merely record bedtime and fasting blood sugars for the first few days after starting the insulin. If the minimum overnight blood sugar rise was less than 10 mg/dl, you've hit the proper dose on the first try. If the rise was greater, your physician may want you to increase the bedtime dose by ½ unit every third night, until the minimum overnight rise is less than 10 mg/dl.

Even one overnight hypoglycemic episode can be quite frightening, especially if you live alone. Such an event can easily turn you off to insulin therapy, so it's wise to take some simple precautions to ensure it doesn't happen. On the night that you take your first shot (and on the first night of any increase in dosage), set your alarm clock to ring 6 hours after your bedtime injection. When the alarm sounds, measure your blood sugar, and correct it to your target value if it's too low (see Chapter 19). Even *one* low blood sugar event suggests that the bedtime dose should be reduced, or that if you're taking lente you should possibly be switched to the slower-acting ultralente.

All but growing children, people with gastroparesis, or the obese usually require less than 8 units of ultralente or lente at bedtime. As the dose of lente is increased above 7 units, its action tends to peak 6–8 hours after the bedtime injection. This may be a great advantage, because it offsets the dawn phenomenon, or it may cause the problem just mentioned — hypoglycemia several hours before arising.

Ultralente in doses greater than 7 units, instead of peaking, tends to last longer. This may be responsible for blood sugars that are too low in the late morning, or even in the afternoon. There are at least two ways to prevent this. First, you can split the ultralente into two approximately equal doses. Both should be injected at bedtime, but into two different sites. If your required dose is 9 units, you might inject 4 units into your arm and the other 5 into your abdomen. You may recall that large doses are not absorbed with consistent timing or total action, so two smaller injections may have the further advantage of making the absorption of both doses more predictable. The same syringe you used for the first shot can be used for the second.

If this method doesn't do the trick for you, your physician may still ask you to inject two separate doses: one lente and the other ultralente. He would customize the relative proportions experimentally. Again, there is no reason not to use the same syringe for both shots — there's no harm in "contaminating" ultralente with lente, or lente with ultra-lente.

SCENARIO TWO: BLOOD SUGAR RISES DURING THE DAY, EVEN IF MEALS ARE SKIPPED

If your blood sugar rises during the day even though you're taking max-imal doses of one or more OHAs before meals, it's time for you and your physician to perform another experiment.

This time you want to determine if meals have caused your increase or if blood sugar increased independently. It's very unusual, by the way, for fasting blood sugars to rise during the day if you don't require in-sulin at bedtime. This is because the dawn phenomenon increases the likelihood that blood sugars will go up overnight, and only overnight. In order to determine when and how much your blood sugar is rising dur-ing the day:

- Start your day with a blood sugar measurement.
- If you're taking an OHA in the morning, continue with your pres-ent dose.
- Do not eat breakfast or lunch, but plan on a late supper — at least 12 hours after your morning blood sugar measurement.
- During the day, check blood sugars approximately every 4 hours, and certainly 12 hours after the first test.
- If, even with a maximal dose of your OHA, your blood sugar rises more than 10 mg/dl during the 12-hour period — without any drops along the way — you probably should be taking ultralente when you arise in the morning. We rarely use lente in the morning, since it probably won't last until bedtime.

This dose of ultralente is calculated the same way we calculated the bedtime dose in the first scenario. Because fasting twice in one week is unpleasant, we may try to wait another week before performing this experiment again to see if our dose of ultralente is adequate. Further experiments in subsequent weeks may be necessary for fine-tuning of the insulin dose.

MONITORING YOUR INSULIN REGIMEN

Once you take insulin, it is essential that you and your family be familiar with the prevention of hypoglycemia (low blood sugar). To this end, you and those who live or work with you should read Chapter 19.

It should not be necessary to measure blood sugar every day if you are taking *only* longer-acting insulin (lente or ultralente) as described in this chapter and you are strictly following our dietary guidelines. Nevertheless, it's wise to assign one day every week for measuring blood sugar on arising, 2 hours after meals, and at bedtime, just to make sure that your insulin requirements are not increasing or decreasing. If any of your blood sugars are consistently 15 mg/dl above or below your target, advise your physician.

It's essential that you also measure blood sugar before and after exercising. If, in your experience, your blood sugar continues to drop one or more hours after finishing your exercise, blood sugar should also be checked then.

As you shall read in Chapter 20, it is important to secure daily blood sugar profiles and report them to your physician whenever you suffer an infectious illness.

Many patients and physicians routinely increase the morning ultralente dose if before-breakfast blood sugars are repeatedly elevated. This is the wrong dose to change. It's the *bedtime* dose that controls fasting blood sugar, and therefore, that dose should be adjusted accordingly. After fine-tuning of bedtime and, if necessary, morning doses of long-acting insulin, your pancreatic beta cells may recover enough function to prevent a blood sugar rise after meals. This frequently turns out to be the case. If, however, you still routinely experience a blood sugar rise of more than 20 mg/dl 1 or 2 hours after any meal, or more than 15 mg/dl 4 hours after any meal, you'll probably require premeal injections of regular insulin, as described in the next chapter.

OTHER CONSIDERATIONS

Weather-Related Changes in Insulin Requirements

Some people experience a sudden decline in their insulin requirements when a long period of cool weather (e.g., winter) is abruptly interrupted by significantly warmer weather. This phenomenon can be recognized by blood sugar well below target when the weather suddenly becomes warmer. In such individuals, insulin requirements will rise as winter occurs and drop in the summer. The reason for this effect is speculative. Whatever the cause, keep careful track of your blood sugar whenever the weather warms suddenly, since potentially severe hypoglycemia can result if insulin dosages are not adjusted.

Air Travel Across Time Zones

Long-distance travel that requires you to shift your clock by 2 hours or less shouldn't have a major effect upon your dosing of OHAs or ultralente or lente insulins covering the fasting state. It should certainly have no effect upon the use of fast-acting insulin or OHAs before meals. A problem does arise when travel shifts the time frame by 3 or more hours. If you're taking different doses of long-acting medication in the morning and at bedtime, the situation becomes particularly complex if you travel halfway around the world, so that day and night are reversed.

When the time shift amounts to 2 hours or less, you need only take your morning medication upon arising in the morning and your bedtime medication at bedtime. One solution to handling larger time shifts is to effect a gradual transition, using 2-hour intervals over a period of days. To do this, you must keep track of the time "back home." If, for example, you're traveling east, so that the time back home is earlier, you would take both of your doses on the first day away 2 hours later on the "back home" clock. On the second day, you would take them 4 hours later, and so on. Thus, if your new location to the east of home is in a time zone 6 hours later than it was at home, it would take you 3 days to achieve a full transition. You would do just the opposite when traveling west. This procedure can be inconvenient because it requires that you set an alarm clock for ungodly hours just to take an insulin shot or a pill — and then, you hope, go back to sleep.

Several of my patients routinely save themselves this kind of annoyance when they travel. At their destinations, they continue to take their morning dose when they arise in the morning and their bedtime dose when they go to bed. They check their blood sugars frequently and lower them, if too high, using the method described in Chapter 18. If their blood sugars drop too low, they raise them using the method described in Chapter 19. Frankly, this is the approach I use myself. Neither I nor my patients have gotten into trouble this way. This carefree approach can cause problems if the bedtime dose is considerably different from the morning dose. If this is the case, the gradual transition of 2 hours per day is certainly safer.

Splitting Larger Doses of Insulin

My patients and I have observed that as larger doses of insulin are injected, the effects upon blood sugar become less predictable. This is due in part to day-to-day variations in absorption of large injections. After some trial and error, I arrived at a cutoff point of 7 units as the largest single injection I would want an adult to take (less for children). Therefore, if an insulin-resistant patient requires 20 units of ultralente at bedtime, I ask him to take 3 separate injections in 3 separate sites of 7 units, 7 units, and 6 units, all using the same syringe.

18

Intensive Insulin Regimens

All Type I diabetics but the mildest should be treated with rapid-acting insulin before each meal, as well as long-acting insulin in the morning and at bedtime to cover the fasting state.

If you are a Type II and preprandial (before-meal) use of OHAs does not prevent your blood sugars from routinely increasing by more than 15 mg/dl 4 hours after eating, or by more than 20 mg/dl 1 or 2 hours after eating, it's probably time for you to use a rapid-acting insulin — lispro (H) or regular (R) — before meals.

Much of this chapter consists of guidelines for computing insulin doses in various situations. They are essentially pretty simple calculations, and your physician or health care provider can and indeed should make them for you. I have rendered them here for several reasons. First, you should understand the information that goes into customizing a dose of insulin, so that you know there's no mystery involved. Second, if you understand how these calculations work, you can also more clearly see what *incorrect* insulin doses look like, and, we hope, avoid them. Finally, despite the dramatic findings of the Diabetes Control and Complication Trial, many physicians and health care professionals are still under the false impression that normalized blood sugars are dangerous or impractical or impossible. My hope is that by providing these calculations, I can help you help your health care provider provide you with better health care.

If you're not the "math type," you can certainly skip the calculations, but do not skip the entire chapter. Herein lies important information about adjusting your insulin dosages or timing to accommodate common variations on your daily routine, such as eating out, and how to adjust your insulin if you skip a meal or have a snack.

DO YOU REQUIRE RAPID-ACTING INSULIN BEFORE EVERY MEAL?

The use of regular or lispro insulin prior to every meal or snack may help to preserve the function of any beta cells that you may still have. Nevertheless, you might not feel terribly enthusiastic about multiple daily injections. It's possible, however, that you may only require insulin before some meals and not others. Several of my patients, for example, maintain normal blood sugars by injecting rapid-acting insulin before breakfast and supper and taking an OHA before lunch. One patient injects before breakfast and supper, and has no medication before the lunch she eats prior to her workout at the gym. The ultimate determinant of when you require preprandial rapid-acting insulin is your glucose profile. If blood sugar remains constant before and after every meal except supper, then you should use rapid-acting insulin only before supper.

You may recall, from our discussion of the dawn phenomenon in Chapter 6, that both your own and injected insulins appear to be less effective when you wake up in the morning. This is why virtually all the people I've seen who require premeal regular insulin must at least have a dose before breakfast.

THE RAPID-ACTING INSULINS: LISPRO (H) VERSUS REGULAR (R) FOR COVERING MEALS

Please reread the section entitled "Lispro: A New Ultra-Rapid Insulin," on page 219.

Clearly, when compared to regular insulin, lispro has both advantages and disadvantages. Figure 18-1 illustrates the reason for a minor dilemma. As you can see, Humalog, or lispro, has a very high early peak level in the blood, and then after 2 hours its level drops below that of regular. Attempting to match this peak with the action of carbohydrate upon blood sugar is very difficult for several reasons. I won't go into them all, but consider the following:

- The timing and shape of the peak will vary from one injection to the next.
- They will also vary with the dose.
- The appearance of carbohydrate in the blood will vary over time from meal to meal.
- The flatter peak of regular insulin is easier to match with slow-acting carbohydrate than is the sharp peak of lispro with either slow- or fast-acting carbohydrate.

On the other hand, regular must be injected about 40 minutes prior to a meal in order to start working as the meal starts. Lispro will start working 15 minutes after injection. This short time interval makes for great convenience if you don't know precisely when your meal will be served, as when dining out (see below). With this in mind, I usually recommend that patients cover meals with regular when time permits, but take a mixture or separate injections of regular and lispro when time is tight. I will usually, therefore, refer to regular as the premeal insulin. This does not rule out the use of lispro or lispro plus regular for situations to be discussed in a few pages.

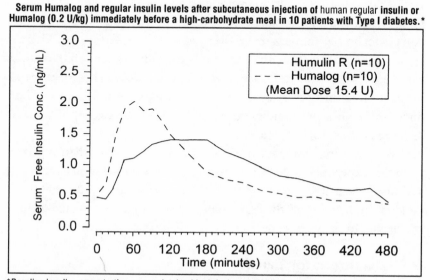

Serum Humalog and regular insulin levels after subcutaneous injection of human regular insulin or Humalog (0.2 U/kg) immediately before a high-carbohydrate meal in 10 patients with Type I diabetes.*

*Baseline insulin concentration was maintained by infusion of 0.2 mU/min/kg human insulin.

Fig. 18-1. *Action times of rapid-acting insulins: regular versus Humalog (lispro).*

HOW MANY MINUTES BEFORE A MEAL SHOULD REGULAR INSULIN BE INJECTED?

Our goal is to minimize or totally prevent any blood sugar increase during or after meals. To achieve this, you must take your shot far enough in advance so that the insulin begins to lower blood sugar as your food starts to increase blood sugar. Yet you should not take it so far ahead of the meal that blood sugar drops faster than digestion can keep up with it. The best injection time for most of us is about 40 minutes before eating. The most common exception would occur if you have gastroparesis, or delayed stomach-emptying. Our approaches to the diagnosis of this condition and to appropriate timing of preprandial insulin if you have it are described in Chapter 21.

Determining When to Inject

The following experiment should be useful in determining how long before a meal you should inject your regular insulin. This test can be conclusive only if your starting blood sugar is near normal—perhaps below 140 mg/dl.

First, inject regular insulin 40 minutes before your planned mealtime. Now, measure blood sugars 25, 30, 35, and 40 minutes after the shot.

The point in time when your blood sugar has dropped 5 mg/dl determines when you should start eating. If this point occurs at 25 minutes, don't even bother to measure further, just start to eat. If no drop is seen at 40 minutes, then delay the meal and continue checking blood sugar every 5 minutes until you see at least a 5 mg/dl drop. Then begin your meal. It shouldn't be necessary to repeat this experiment more than once, unless your preprandial dose of regular is increased by 50 percent or more at some future date.

If your starting blood sugar is higher than 140 mg/dl when you perform this experiment, the lack of precision in blood sugar measurement and insulin sensitivity may be greater than the 5 mg/dl drop that we're looking for. Just put off the experiment until your blood sugar is nearer to normal. In the meantime, assume the 40-minute guideline.

Is There Room for Error?

Suppose after performing the above experiment you find that your regular insulin should be injected 40 minutes before eating — which is the case for most of us. How far off can you be without getting into trouble?

Eating 5 minutes early or late makes no significant difference. If you eat 10 minutes too soon, your blood sugar may rise during the meal, but it probably will return to its starting point by the time the regular finishes acting, about 5 hours after injecting. This is not serious, especially if it occurs only occasionally. If blood sugars go up significantly with *every* meal over many years, you would probably be at risk for long-term complications of diabetes. If you eat 15 or 20 minutes too soon, your blood sugar may go so high (say 180 mg/dl) that you become slightly resistant to the injected insulin. If this occurs, your blood sugar will not drop all the way to the premeal level when the regular finishes its action. If it happens often, your risk for developing the long-term complications of diabetes will increase.

What if you delay your meal by 10 or 15 minutes beyond the proper time after your shot? Now you're asking for trouble! Regular starts to work slowly, but its effect on blood sugar accelerates over the first 2 hours or so. Even a delay of 10 minutes can send your blood sugar dropping more rapidly than your food can raise it. This, of course, can be hazardous.

USING RAPID-ACTING INSULIN WHEN DINING OUT

Part of the pleasure of eating out is having someone else serve you something you couldn't make at home — but the difficulty for the insulin-taking diabetic is that you're served on their schedule, not yours. Hostesses, restaurants, and airlines — as well intentioned as they may be — rarely serve you at the time they promise. For nondiabetics, waiting may be annoying. For those of us who are diabetic, annoyance is compounded with danger. When planning your premeal insulin shot, you cannot afford to rely on the word of your hostess, waiter, or airline staff. I've been taking premeal regular insulin for nearly thirty years and I've been "burned" more times than I care to count. Now that we have lispro, I inject a dose when I see the waiter approaching my table with the first course. If I suspect that the main course will be delayed, I'll split my dose in half and take the second half when the waiter arrives with the main course. You should do the same. A transient blood sugar elevation is a small price to pay for the assurance that you will not experience severe hypoglycemia because the meal was delayed.

On airplanes, you can "jump the gun" slightly by taking your injection when the food wagon (not the beverage wagon) starts serving. Even seated at the far end of the aisle, you will be served within 40 minutes unless sudden heavy weather is encountered. It is also a good idea to look over the actual airline meal before taking your shot. Just walk over to the galley and ask a member of the flight crew to show you a meal. You may find that the portions are too small to cover your insulin dose. Or you may find that there is nothing on the tray that fits your dietary guidelines. This is especially true of breakfasts, which may consist only of juice, cereal, and sweet rolls. If I find that the protein or salad or vegetable portion of my meal is too small to match my usual dose of regular, I may explain that I'm a diabetic and ask for two portions before I take my shot. Alternately, I may inject only half my usual dose of regular and eat only half the amount of carbohydrate and half the amount of protein that my meal plan calls for.

By the way, never order "diabetic" meals when traveling by air. As of this writing, airlines are still serving as "diabetic" meals a high-carbohydrate diet loaded with simple sugars. The salads in these meals may even contain fruit. My trick is to preorder "seafood" meals when I reserve my flight. This ensures that I get reasonable portions of protein. Unfortunately, many airlines do not serve seafood for breakfast. On the newer, no-frills discount airlines that serve nothing but drinks and a bag of peanuts, you may actually be better off. You can pack your own brown bag breakfast or lunch, stick to your diet, and time exactly when you're going to take your shot and eat your food.

OTHER MEALTIME CONSIDERATIONS

Must Meals Be Eaten at the Same Time Every Day?

Ever since the introduction of long-acting insulin in the late 1930s, diabetics have been advised that they must have meals and snacks at the same times every day. This very inconvenient rule still appears in current litereature describing the treatment of diabetes. Prior to our use of low doses of long-acting insulins to cover the fasting state, most physicians prescribed 1 or 2 large daily doses of long-acting insulin to cover both the fasting state and meals. (Many still do.) Such regimens *never* succeed in controlling blood sugars, and hypoglycemia is an ever-present threat. Patients are told to eat meals and several snacks at exactly the right times, to offset the continuous blood sugar drop caused by the long-acting insulin.

But if, as outlined in this chapter, we now cover our meals with rapid-acting insulin, we're free to eat whenever we want, provided we take our shot beforehand. We can also skip a meal if we skip the shot. When I was in medical training and worked 40-hour shifts, I sometimes skipped breakfast and ate lunch at 3 A.M. On some days I did not eat at all. This worked out fine because I followed a flexible insulin regimen.

What If You Forget to Take Your Regular 40 Minutes Before Eating?

If it's now *less* than 15 minutes before a fixed mealtime (e.g., your lunch break at work), take lispro instead of regular.

If you still have 15 minutes before you'll be eating, take half of your dose of insulin for this meal as regular and half as lispro. Ideally they should be taken as separate shots. If you want to take them together as one injection, be careful not to contaminate the lispro vial with regular or the regular vial with lispro. If you ate your meal after forgetting your regular insulin, take lispro instead — immediately.

HOW TO ESTIMATE PREPRANDIAL DOSES OF REGULAR INSULIN

We know that for Type I diabetics who make no insulin at all, 1 unit of regular insulin usually lowers blood sugar 40 mg/dl in a 140-pound adult. We also know that 1 gram of carbohydrate raises blood sugar 5 mg/dl. Thus 1 unit regular usually covers 8 grams of carbohydrate. We also know that 1 unit of regular insulin covers approximately 1½ ounces of protein.

There are variables, however. These figures apply *only* to people who produce none of their own insulin and who are not insulin-resistant. Doses must be tailored to the individual, so if you're obese, pregnant, or a growing child, you may require more insulin than these guidelines suggest. On the other hand, if your beta cells are still producing some insulin, you may need considerably less insulin than indicated here. I have patients who require only one-third of these amounts of insulin.

Another variable in figuring a proper dose of regular is our old friend the dawn phenomenon. The regular insulin you inject before eating will be perhaps 20 percent less effective at breakfast than at other meals, even though it comes from the same vial.

The biggest factor is, of course, what you eat. Since we cannot know exactly how regular insulin will affect you until you begin to use it, your initial trial doses before meals must be based upon your precisely formulated meal plan. With that, we can make a safe estimate of how much insulin you're likely to need.

It's not easy for your physician to balance out all these variables and come up with just the right doses of regular insulin on the first try. Because of this, we try, for safety's sake, to underestimate your insulin needs initially, and then gradually to increase your preprandial doses after checking subsequent blood sugar profiles. This is yet another example of the Laws of Small Numbers in action. Because of the complexity of this task, let us examine how your physician might proceed with two very different scenarios.

Scenario One

You're a Type I diabetic and are switching to our regimen from an outdated regimen of 1 or 2 large daily doses of long-acting insulin. Remember that many Type II diabetics eventually lose all beta cell function and then, in effect, have Type I diabetes. So this scenario would apply to these people too.

Assume that the meal plan you negotiated with your physician is the following:

> Breakfast: 6 grams carbohydrate, 3 ounces protein
> Lunch: 12 grams carbohydrate, 4½ ounces protein
> Supper: 12 grams carbohydrate, 6 ounces protein

Because we want to play it safe and stay with the lowest possible insulin doses, we will for the moment ignore any effect of the dawn phenomenon upon your breakfast dose, as well as the possibility of insulin resistance due to obesity. Our calculations, based on the numbers mentioned above, are as follows:

> To cover carbohydrate: number of grams ÷ 8 = units of regular insulin

To cover protein: number of ounces ÷ 1½ = units of regular insulin

Breakfast

- 6 grams of carbohydrate ÷ 8 = ¾ unit of regular insulin (which you'd note on your data sheet as 1⁻ [1 minus] R)
- 3 ounces of protein ÷ 1½ = 2 units of regular (2 R)
- Total trial dose for breakfast will be 2¾ units of regular (3⁻ R)

Lunch

- 12 grams of carbohydrate ÷ 8 = 1½ units of regular (1½ R)
- 4½ ounces of protein ÷ 1½ = 3 units of regular (3 R)
- Total trial dose = 4½ units of regular (4½ R)

Supper

- 12 grams of carbohydrate ÷ 8 = 1½ units of regular (1½ R)
- 6 ounces protein ÷ 1½ = 4 units of regular (4 R)
- Total trial dose = 5½ units of regular (5½ R)

Your physician will probably want to lower these doses if your pancreas is making any insulin (as shown by the C-peptide test, page 50).

It's virtually a certainty that your trial doses will be a bit too high or too low. In other words, your blood sugars may either rise or drop after some or all of these meals. It is most unlikely, however, that your postprandial blood sugars will be dangerously low, unless you have gastroparesis. If you're insulin-resistant, you will likely need more insulin on the second try.

Both you and your physician will want to get your blood sugars into line as rapidly as possible. So you'll probably be asked to fax, phone, or bring in your blood sugar profiles during the second day (and perhaps subsequent days) of this intensive insulin regimen for fine-tuning of doses. Remember that the important blood sugar measurements for fine-tuning your doses of regular are 5 hours after each dose of regular (4–5 hours for lispro), as it takes this long for the insulin to finish working. Let's assume that on the first day your blood sugar profile looked like this:

5 hours after breakfast: increased 70 mg/dl
5 hours after lunch: decreased 20 mg/dl
5 hours after supper: increased 20 mg/dl

Clearly, our initial insulin doses were a bit off and require adjustment to prevent further increases or decreases of more than 15 mg/dl. These changes are easy, if you remember that for 140-pound adults who make no insulin (Type I diabetics), 1 unit of regular lowers blood sugar by 40 mg/dl. If you weigh 100 pounds, 1 unit of regular will lower you about 56 mg/dl, or (140 ÷ 100) x 40 mg/dl. If you weigh 180 pounds, 1 unit of regular will lower you about 30 mg/dl, or (140 ÷ 180) x 40 mg/dl. We will assume, for this exercise, that your weight is close enough to 140 pounds to use the 40 mg/dl drop from 1 unit of regular. Type II diabetics might do better by using Table 18-1, on page 243.

Now let's look again at the hypothetical blood sugar profiles and work out the changes in preprandial regular that will be necessary:

Meal	Blood Sugar Change	Change ÷ 40 mg/dl	Change in Dose Rounded Off to Nearest 1/4 Unit
Breakfast	+ 70 mg/dl	+ 1.75	+ 1¾ R
Lunch	− 20 mg/dl	− 0.5	− ½ R
Supper	+ 25 mg/dl	+ 0.625	+ ½ R

We now fine-tune our premeal regular insulin by making the above changes to the original trial doses.

Meal	Trial Dose	Change	New Dose
Breakfast	2¾ R	+ 1¾	4½ R
Lunch	4½ R	− ½	4 R
Supper	5½ R	+ ½	6 R

That was pretty easy. Remember, however, that the content of your meals, in terms of grams of carbohydrate and ounces of protein, must be kept constant from one day to the next, because your insulin doses will not be changing every day. If you're consistently hungry after a particular meal, you can increase the amount of protein at that meal, but you must then have the extra protein every day. When you raise the protein portion of your meal, you look at your blood sugar profiles (or your physician does) to see how much your blood sugar goes up, and increase your dose of regular insulin for that meal accordingly. Do not increase your carbohydrates — the Laws of Small Numbers dictate that such a rise will cause real problems with your blood sugar normalization attempts.

Scenario Two

You have Type II diabetes and are following our diet. You've been taking an OHA in the morning and/or at bedtime. Your blood sugars are fine when you skip meals, but they go up after meals, even with the maximal doses of your OHA.

Since you're not a Type I diabetic and are making some insulin of your own, we cannot use the simple rules that apply to those who make no insulin. We have to assume that your beta cells still make a portion of the insulin needed to cover your meals, yet we do not know the magnitude of that portion. So we see how much a meal will raise your blood sugars without premeal regular insulin. We then use this blood sugar increase as a guide for the doses you will be needing. We do not use this method with Type I's because their blood sugars might go so high without insulin as to cause the dangerous condition known as ketoacidosis.

Further fine-tuning of preprandial regular insulin might be performed by reviewing your blood sugar profiles over a week. If you've been taking a premeal OHA, as assumed in this scenario, you probably have already collected blood sugar profiles that show how much your blood sugar increases after each meal. If these profiles cover only 1 day, okay. If they cover a week, better. We want to start you with the lowest reasonable insulin doses, so we pick the smallest blood sugar increases for each meal that we can find for that meal, and then adjust your preprandial insulin accordingly. To find the increase before you begin taking regular, subtract the preprandial blood sugar from the 3-hour postprandial blood sugar measurement (we wait 3 hours to allow the OHA to finish working).

On pages 221–222, we showed you how to compute a starting dose of ultralente to cover overnight blood sugar rises. We can use the same simple formula to calculate doses of regular insulin to cover meals. But, for safety's sake, and to obey the Laws of Small Numbers, we're deliberately going to keep the trial doses on the low side. We'll use, as a guide, the blood sugar data you collected while you were taking your OHA, even though we will likely discontinue the OHA when you start using premeal regular insulin.

To finish this example, let us assume that your 3-hour postprandial increases in blood sugar over the past week can be summarized as follows:

> Smallest increase after breakfast: 105 mg/dl
> Smallest increase after lunch: 17 mg/dl
> Smallest increase after supper: 85 mg/dl

Now, we must estimate the premeal doses of regular insulin that would approximately offset these increases. You may remember that our formula in estimating trial doses of ultralente insulin is that 1 unit of insulin will lower a 140-pound, insulin-requiring Type II diabetic's blood sugar by 60 mg/dl. Your physician may want to be even more conservative and assume that 1 unit will lower your blood sugar by 70 mg/dl. We now only need to divide the above postprandial blood sugar increases by 70 to get the trial doses of premeal regular insulin, as in the following table:

Meal	Blood Sugar Increase	Increase ÷ 70 mg/dl	Round Off to Nearest 1/4 Unit for Trial Dose of R
Breakfast	105 mg/dl	1.5	1½ R
Lunch	17 mg/dl	0.24	¼ R
Supper	85 mg/dl	1.2	1¼ R

As in the previous scenario, you will need to take periodic blood sugar measurements to monitor the effect of the insulin. If, after one day on the trial doses of premeal regular insulin, your postprandial blood sugars still go up by more than 10 mg/dl at 5 hours, your physician may ask you to increase the appropriate preprandial doses by ¼ unit. (Note that we now look at 5-hour blood sugars instead of 3-hour values, because injected regular insulin requires 5 hours to finish working.) If your postprandial blood sugar elevations hardly respond to the ¼-unit increase, he may choose 1-unit increases. We rarely increase a prepran-dial dose in steps greater than 1 unit because of the danger of hypo-glycemia.

The above trial-and-error procedure should be repeated until your 5-hour postprandial blood sugars do not consistently change from the preprandial values by more than 10mg/dl up or down. This all assumes that the carbohydrate and protein contents of your meals remains con-stant.

WHAT ABOUT SNACKS?

If you've ever been on one of the conventional regimens that utilizes 1 or 2 large daily doses of longer-acting insulin, you're probably familiar with mandatory snacks. These were required, usually midway between meals and at bedtime, in the hopes of offsetting the continuous blood sugar–lowering effect of large amounts of insulin, thereby preventing daily episodes of hypoglycemia.

Our regimen, as you know, uses such low doses of lente and ultralente insulins that blood sugars hold level during the fasting state. With our regimen, there is no need for mandatory snacks! This does not mean that you must wait until the next meal before eating if you're hungry. *Theoretically,* you can eat a snack almost anytime, provided that you cover it with regular insulin, just as you would a meal. There are, how-ever, some guidelines to remember.

Snacking Guidelines

Try to avoid snacks during the initial fine-tuning stage of your insulin doses. This is especially true of bedtime snacks. Snacks and their doses of regular insulin can confuse the issue of what caused what change in blood sugar. If, for example, you wake up with a high or low fasting blood sugar, was it your bedtime dose of ultralente or lente, or was it the dose of regular that you took for the snack, that was wrong?

Anytime you snack, try to wait until your prior meal has been fully digested, and the dose of regular insulin for that meal has run its course, about 5 hours after the preprandial regular. This is especially important if you are measuring blood sugars every day, which, as explained later in this chapter, is not mandatory for everyone. Suppose you were to eat a snack 2 hours after a meal and then check your blood sugar 5 hours after the regular you took to cover the snack; you would have no way of telling whether it was the meal or the snack, and the respective doses of regular insulin, that was responsible for any increase or decrease in your blood sugar.

If you snack, don't eat "snack food." Try to snack on a food — such as a single serving of sugar-free Jell-O gelatin or three sheets of toasted nori — that will not affect your blood sugar and will not have to be covered with insulin. Most snacks other than these muddy the waters when you're trying to analyze data. If you really make no insulin you shouldn't snack, because your blood sugar depends entirely on what you eat and inject, so that snacking interferes with meticulous blood sugar control. Full Type I's who do snack will have to refrain from correcting high blood sugars until 5 hours after the presnack injection of regular (4 hours if the snack is covered with lispro). If you make some insulin and your routine injected doses have been fine-tuned, blood sugar *corrections* after a snack may not be needed, as you may be able to make enough insulin to cover high blood sugars (or "turn off" insulin production if blood sugars are heading too low). But you will still need to inject the correct dosage prior to the snack to cover it, and to check your blood sugar levels 4 or 5 hours later to make sure they have returned to your target.

For these reasons, most of my patients do not snack on foods that will affect blood sugars. If you do snack, the same carbohydrate limit that applies to meals should also be applied to snacks. If you consume 12 grams of carbohydrate for lunch and for dinner, 12 grams of carbohydrate would be the upper limit for carbohydrate for any single snack. Lesser amounts of carbohydrate for a snack — as the Laws of Small Numbers would indicate — will naturally pose lesser problems.

If you're hungry several hours after a meal, check your blood sugar before snacking. Hunger may reflect hypoglycemia, reflecting in turn too much insulin, and should be treated with glucose tablets as indicated in Chapter 19 and a possible reduction of insulin dosage the next day.

Estimating the Dose of Regular Insulin for a Snack

There are several different approaches to this problem.

The simplest is to decide in advance that you will eat for your snack exactly half the amount of carbohydrate *and* protein that you eat for lunch or supper. Remember that fat has no direct effect on blood sugar, so you need only consider the carbohydrate and protein. Cover the snack with exactly half the dose of regular that you take for lunch or supper. If your snack is one-third or one-quarter of your lunch or supper amounts, then you'd naturally take one-third or one-quarter your usual dose of regular for those meals — rounded off to the nearest ¼ unit. You should inject the regular insulin as far in advance of the snack as you would for a meal. In a pinch, you can take lispro instead of regular and wait 15 minutes instead of, say, 40 minutes before snacking.

If you select a snack containing carbohydrate and/or protein that is not in the same proportion as one of your meals, use the computational method outlined on pages 234–239 for regular meals. To test the validity of your computations, skip lunch and lunch insulin and take the snack and snack insulin instead. Check your blood sugar before taking the snack insulin, and then check it again 5 hours afterward. This will help you determine the dosage correction to make when you next decide to do the same experiment (perhaps a few days later, as you may not enjoy skipping lunch 2 days in a row). You may have to try this several times before you get the dose exactly right. Thereafter, you won't have to skip lunch in order to have a snack.

If you've decided that your snacks will consist only of protein, you can take your regular insulin 15 minutes before eating instead of 40 minutes before. This is because protein is converted to glucose much more slowly than is carbohydrate. Be sure to keep the protein and/or carbohydrate content of your snack(s) the same from one day to the next, as you probably won't want to do more experiments to determine doses of regular.

Last but not least, blood sugars will be easier for you to control if you don't snack at all, or if you make your snack a small amount of sugar-free Jell-O instead of real food.

RAPID CORRECTION OF ELEVATED BLOOD SUGARS: CALCULATING THE DOSE

Sooner or later a dietary indiscretion, an infection, emotional stress, or even errors in estimating meal portions may cause your blood sugar to rise substantially over your target value. If your beta cells are still capable of producing moderate amounts of insulin, your blood sugar may drop back to target within a matter of hours. On the other hand, you may be like me and make little or no insulin, or you may be very resistant to your own insulin. If any of these is the case, your physician may want you to inject lispro (H) whenever your blood sugar goes too high. Because lispro works faster than regular insulin, it is much preferred for this purpose. (If you are presently covering elevated blood sugars with regular insulin, use care when switching to lispro — see "Some Final Considerations Regarding Lispro Insulin," page 251.) To do this properly, you must first know how much ½ or 1 or 5 units of lispro insulin will lower your blood sugar.

This requires yet another experiment.

Wait until you have a blood sugar that is at least 20 mg/dl above your target (but this should not be an elevated measurement taken on arising — the dawn phenomenon can make the experiment useless). To make sure that your prior mealtime dose of regular has finished working, this blood sugar should be measured at least 5 hours after your last dose. Be sure that you have taken your morning dose of ultralente or lente.

Now refer to Table 18-1, which suggests the amount that 1 unit of lispro (H) might lower your blood sugar, *for the purpose of this trial only*. The left-hand column represents the total daily dose of ultralente or lente (or both) that you are taking just to keep your *fasting* blood sugars level. The middle column shows the amount that 1 unit of lispro will probably lower your blood sugar. The right-hand column shows the amount that 1 unit, as read on a syringe, would lower blood sugar using a dilution of 3:1. Again, *this table is only approximate*. Its only purpose is to suggest how much lispro (H) you might try for this experiment. The column for diluted insulin is for those few individuals who find a little goes a long way.

After recording your elevated blood sugar, determine the amount of lispro insulin suggested by the table to bring your blood sugar down to your current target. Let's assume that the sum of the morning and bedtime doses of lente and ultralente that will just keep your blood sugars level (if no meals) is 9 units. Then, by interpolating between lines in the table, 1 unit of lispro (H) will probably lower your blood sugar about 45 mg/dl. Let's assume that your blood sugar is 175 mg/dl and that your

TABLE 18-1

APPROXIMATE EFFECT OF 1 UNIT LISPRO (H) IN LOWERING BLOOD SUGAR

Total Daily Dose of Ultralente and Lente	1 Unit H (Full Strength) Might Lower Blood Sugar		1 Unit H (3:1 Dilution) Might Lower Blood Sugar	
2 units	200 mg/dl	11.1 mmol/l*	50 mg/dl	2.8 mmol/l
3	150	8.3	38	2.1
4	100	5.6	25	1.4
5	80	4.4	20	1.1
6	67	3.7	17	0.94
7	57	3.2	14	0.8
8	50	2.8	12	0.7
10	40	2.2	10	0.6
13	31	1.7	8	0.4
16	25	1.4	6	0.3
20	20	1.1	5	0.3
25	16	0.9	4	0.2

* Reminder: Mmol/l, or millimoles per liter, is the standard international measure of blood glucose level (1 mmol/l = 18 mg/dl).

target is 100 mg/dl. You therefore would like to lower your blood sugar 75 mg/dl. One and a half units of H should lower you about 1.5 x 45 = 68 mg/dl. This is certainly close enough, so you would inject 1½ units.

Check and record your blood sugar again 4, 5, and 6 hours after the shot.[†] The lowest value will not only tell you how much your blood sugar dropped but also how long it took. For most of us, the lispro finishes working in about 5 hours. If your lowest value occurs at or after 6 hours, you should wait at least this long in the future before checking your blood sugars to see if an extra shot of lispro really brought you down to target. Let's say that the 1½ units of lispro in the above example

---

[†] Note that this experiment requires that you refrain from eating for 5 hours after your last shot of regular and another 6 hours after the lispro, for a total of 11 hours. Hopefully, you'll have to do this only once in your life.

brought your blood sugar from 175 down to 91 mg/dl after 5 hours, and it did not drop further at 6 hours. Now you've learned that 1½ units H will lower your blood sugar by 84 mg/dl (or 175 − 91). Divide 84 mg/dl by 1.5 (units of lispro) to find that 1 unit H will lower your blood sugar 56 mg/dl. Whatever this value turns out to be, write it down on your GLUCOGRAF data sheet in the box 1 UNIT H WILL LOWER BG. In this case, we have learned that our initial estimate that 1 unit would lower you 45 mg/dl was off by about 25 percent. This can happen, and this is precisely why we do this experiment.

If at any point during this experiment your blood sugar drops 15 mg/dl or more below your target, immediately correct to target with glucose tablets, as detailed in the next chapter. This will offset the hazard of hypoglycemia. On your data sheet, record the number of glucose tablets that you used. When you read the next chapter, you will see how you can use the number of tablets in completing the above calculation without terminating the experiment.

As stated at the beginning of this chapter, it shouldn't be necessary for you to perform any of the above calculations on your own. This is the job of your health care professional, who can use our table and should have much more experience than you. He or she might want to try a simple option. For example, your doctor might instruct you to measure your 5-hour, postlunch blood sugar and, if it's over 180 mg/dl, to inject 1 unit of lispro (H) and see how far your blood sugar drops in another 5 hours. This will tell you how much 1 unit will lower your blood sugar.

WHEN TO COVER HIGH BLOOD SUGARS

Once you know how much 1 unit of lispro will lower blood sugar, you're in a position to bring down your blood sugar rapidly if it goes much above your target. All you need to do is to inject the proper dose. Within hours, your blood sugar will probably return to target, unless for you small doses of lispro work more slowly, or unless you have a very high blood sugar and take more than 7 units. These extra doses are what is known as coverage. Once your insulin doses have been fine-tuned it should rarely be necessary for you to cover with more than 2 units of lispro, unless you are very insulin-resistant, overeat, or suffer from gastroparesis.

Never cover an elevated blood sugar with lispro if you have not waited for the last dose of regular or lispro to finish working. After all, if two doses are working at the same time, your blood sugar can drop too low. This is one reason you should know how long it takes for a dose of regular or lispro to complete its action.

Suppose target blood sugar is 90 mg/dl, and you wake up in the morning and find that your fasting blood sugar is 110, an elevation of 20 mg/dl. If 1 unit of lispro lowers you 40, you'd immediately inject ½ unit as coverage. If you plan on having breakfast in 40 minutes, just add this ½ unit to your usual breakfast dose of regular.

Another time you may find that 5 hours after your lunchtime regular was injected, your blood sugar is 60mg/dl above your target. If 1 unit of lispro lowers you 40 mg/dl, take 1½ units of lispro right away.

At first, after you cover with lispro, you may want to check your blood sugar when the insulin has finished working to make sure that the numbers from your original experiment were correct. After a few times, however, you will become confident that your calibration is proper. If I find my blood sugar to be slightly elevated 4½ hours after lunch, I take the necessary coverage and forget it. I don't have to bother to recheck my blood sugar before dinner, because I know the coverage will work.

IF RESULTS DON'T MATCH EXPECTATIONS

Under certain circumstances, lispro insulin will not lower your blood sugar as much as you would expect based upon your calibration. Let's take a look at some factors that can cause this.

Your lispro is cloudy. If your blood sugar does not drop as much as you expect, hold the insulin vial to the light to make sure that it's not cloudy. Compare it with a fresh vial to be sure. Lispro insulin should be crystal clear; if it is cloudy it has been deactivated and should be discarded. Also discard the vial if it has been frozen or kept in a hot place, since temperature extremes will also affect its potency.

Your fasting blood sugar was high on arising in the morning. The dawn phenomenon causes more insulin resistance in the morning for some people than for others. If you start the day with an elevated blood sugar, you may require more coverage for that period than you would 4 or more hours later in the day. If you find that early-morning coverage is not very effective, review your blood sugar profiles with your physician. You'll probably be told that you should increase your coverage by one-third, one-half, or some other proportion during the first few hours after you wake up. By late morning, this increased coverage should no longer be necessary.

Your blood sugar was higher than 200 or 300 mg/dl. At such high blood sugars we become more resistant to the effects of injected insulin. This increased resistance may become very significant as blood sugar rises above 250 mg/dl. But the point at which resistance develops is not precise, and its magnitude is difficult to determine. We rarely encounter such high blood sugars once insulin doses and diet are appropriate. If you do measure a very high blood sugar, cover it with your usual calibration for lispro and wait the usual 5 hours or so. Then check your blood sugar again. If it has not come all the way down to your target, take another coverage dose based on the new lower blood sugar. This time the coverage will probably be fully effective.

Infections. If your lispro coverage or any other insulin dose is less effective than usual, you may have an infection. We once discovered that a patient had an intestinal inflammation called diverticulitis, only because he was wise enough to telephone me when his blood sugars were a little less responsive to insulin than he had been accustomed to. *It's important that you notify your physician whenever you find that your insulin is losing its efficacy.*

INTRAMUSCULAR SHOTS WILL GET YOUR BLOOD SUGAR DOWN FASTER

Intramuscular shots of insulin can be quite useful for bringing down elevated blood sugar more rapidly than our usual subcutaneous shots. You should not ordinarily use them for your usual meal doses of regular insulin, and you should never inject lente or ultralente into a muscle — it makes no sense to speed up the action of a long-acting insulin.

Typically, an intramuscular shot of lispro will begin to lower an elevated blood sugar within about 5 minutes. It will finish acting about 1 hour sooner than your usual subcutaneous injection, and it will have your blood sugar close to your target within about 2 hours.

Problems to Consider

With intramuscular shots, you may encounter several problems that you do not encounter with subcutaneous shots. Because of this, I give my patients the option of using or not using this method of self-injection, and fully appreciate the feelings of those few who turn it down. Here are some obstacles you may confront:

Fat arms. If you have fat arms, don't even try intramuscular shots. If you have a lot of fat over the muscle on your upper arm, the needle on your insulin syringe will be too short to penetrate the underlying muscle.

Missing the muscle. Even moderately slim people sometimes "miss" the muscle because the needle may not penetrate deeply enough. Since we cannot always tell whether or not the needle hit the muscle, all of us must wait as long before rechecking our blood sugars as we would for a subcutaneous shot.

Hitting a blood vessel. You are much more likely to hit a blood vessel than with subcutaneous injections. This can be briefly painful. You can also get blood on your shirt, if you shoot right through the sleeve as I do. I estimate that I hit a blood vessel once in every thirty intramuscular injections.

Pain. If, for whatever reason, you're unable to throw the needle in rapidly like a dart, all your intramuscular shots may be briefly painful — if so, do not even bother to attempt them.

Intramuscular Injection Technique

Please refer to Figure 18-2 as you read the following step-by-step instructions. Do not use a syringe with the new short needles. I keep on hand a supply of syringes with ½- or ⅝-inch needles just for intramuscular shots.

1. Locate your deltoid muscle, illustrated in Figure 18-2. It begins at the shoulder and ends about one-third of the way down your upper arm. It's wide at the shoulder and tapers to a V shape farther down. You may be able to feel the V with your fingers if you lift your arm to the side until it is parallel to the floor. This will tighten the muscle and make it feel thicker. We usually use the deltoid muscle because it is easy to find, is relatively large and thick, and is less likely to be covered with a deep pad of fat than most other muscles.

2. Now, allow your nondominant arm (left if you're right-handed) to dangle loosely at your side. This will relax the muscle, so that the needle can penetrate easily.

3. The site for injection will be near the upper (wider) end of the deltoid, about 1½ inches below your shoulder (at about the position of the arrow in Figure 18-2). We use the wide end of the muscle because you are less likely to miss it with the needle, and because you would not want to pierce the axillary nerve, which is located near the tip of the V, at the lower end.

4. As your nondominant, target arm dangles loosely at your side, pick up the syringe with your dominant hand and "throw" the needle straight into the injection site as you would a dart — but, of course, don't let go of the syringe. Do not grab any flesh, as you do for subcutaneous shots. Do not inject at an angle, but go in per-

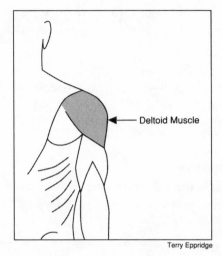

Terry Eppridge

Fig. 18-2. *The deltoid muscle (arrow indicates preferred site for intramuscular injection).*

pendicular to the skin. Be fast, as a slow intramuscular shot can hurt. Push in the plunger to inject your insulin. Now pull out the needle. Touch the injection site with your finger, to make sure you have not bled.

5. If the shot hurts, you probably hit a small blood vessel, so be prepared for some blood. In such a case, press the injection site firmly with a finger. Hold it there for about a minute. This will prevent or stop any bleeding. If you do not press, you will develop a slightly painful lump where the blood accumulates under the skin. The lump will turn yellow or black and blue after a number of hours. If you get blood on your shirt or blouse, apply hydrogen peroxide, as described on pages 207–208.

Once you have given a number of intramuscualr shots using your dominant hand to operate the syringe, try switching hands and arms. This may seem cumbersome at first, but with practice you will be able to inject into either arm.

"MIXED" THERAPY — INSULIN PLUS OHAS

As indicated previously, you may be able to take troglitazone or metformin instead of regular insulin before certain meals. This will depend upon your postprandial blood sugar profile. There is no therapeutic advantage to such a substitution, but it may prove more convenient. Remember, however, that you will probably have to wait about 90 minutes to 2 hours after taking metformin or 60–90 minutes after troglitazone before starting your meal. It is usually more convenient to take a shot of regular insulin, since the waiting time after injecting is generally only 40 minutes.

A more important use for an OHA in combination with insulin occurs if you are overweight and your bedtime dose of lente or ultralente is more than 8–10 units. This suggests that you may have insulin resistance, which may respond to metformin or troglitazone. Recall that these two OHAs increase your sensitivity to insulin. Large doses of insulin help build fat, of course, and can also cause further down-regulation, or desensitization, of insulin receptors. If you're obese, the less insulin you have swimming around in your system storing away fat while you're asleep, the better. So there may be some advantage in reducing your bed-time insulin dose.

If your physician decides to add one of these OHAs to your bedtime regimen, he or she will want you to build up the dose of the OHA grad-ually while simultaneously reducing your dose of lente or ultralente. If your bedtime insulin requirements are not reduced while taking 2,500 mg of metformin or 600 mg of troglitazone before sleeping, then the bedtime OHA is serving no purpose and should be discontinued.

IS IT NECESSARY TO RECORD DAILY BLOOD GLUCOSE PROFILES AFTER INSULIN DOSES HAVE BEEN FINE-TUNED?

Type I diabetics, and those Type II's whose beta cells are producing little or no insulin, both tend to show significant blood sugar changes follow-ing relatively small changes in what they eat, their activity level, and so on. If your blood sugars commonly show changes of more than 30 mg/dl in the course of a day, you probably should measure blood sugar profiles daily for the rest of your life. Such frequent monitoring is nec-essary so that you can correct high blood sugars with lispro or low blood sugars with glucose tablets (see next chapter).

I've seen many individuals on our regimen whose blood sugars are quite stable even though they require the 5 daily shots typical of inten-sive insulin therapy. These people usually require small doses of insulin, typically under 8 units daily for all doses combined. If you fit into this category, your beta cells are probably still producing some insulin. This enables your system automatically to smooth out the peaks and valleys that your blood glucose profile would otherwise show. With such stable blood sugars (varying less than 30 mg/dl daily), there's no reason to bother taking daily blood sugar profiles. You would, instead, prepare a full blood glucose profile (four or five tests) for 1 day every week. If you spotted a change in your blood sugar ranges, you'd check the next few days to see if it continued. If it did, you would contact your physician, who might want to explore the possible reasons for such changes. If you become ill, or if, say, you have a school-age child who brings home a cold, you might want to check your blood sugars if you suspect an infection.

SOME FINAL CONSIDERATIONS REGARDING LISPRO INSULIN

Perhaps as a result of reading one of my prior books, you may already be covering elevated blood sugars with regular insulin. If this is the case, be very careful when using lispro for this purpose. I and many of my patients have found it to be more effective than regular — that is, a given dose of lispro is likely to lower blood sugar more than the same dose of regular. For example, I find that while 1 unit R will lower my blood sugar 40 mg/dl, 1 unit H will lower it 55 mg/dl. I advise, therefore, that you initially take half as much lispro (H) as your prior regular (R) for this purpose. Based upon the initial effect on your blood sugar, you can then adjust subsequent doses of lispro. The same consideration applies if you eat out and use H to cover a meal.

We have also observed that when lispro is used to cover meals, blood sugars are less predictable than with regular. This result was not mentioned in reports of clinical trials of lispro — probably because the trial population followed a high-carbohydrate diet and had such wide blood sugar fluctuation that this effect was not apparent.

In spite of these considerations, I believe that lispro will be of considerable benefit to those who use it properly. I am most grateful for its availability!

INSULIN PUMPS

Much effort and expense are being devoted to promote and market insulin pumps. These devices were designed to make multiple daily injections easier. They also do away with the need for long-acting insulins.

The instruments consist of three basic elements:

- A pump unit about the size of a small pocket calculator that you can hang from a belt, keep in a pocket, or pin to your clothing.
- A very large bore needle that stays in your skin, typically above your waist. The needle usually should be changed every 2–3 days.
- Flexible plastic tubing that connects the pump to the needle.

The pump unit can be loaded with a supply of regular (R) insulin that lasts a number of days. It delivers a basal flow of insulin all day long, giving an effect similar to that of 2 daily injections of long-acting insulin. This basal rate can be preset by the user and can even be set to change automatically at various times of the day. Premeal or corrective doses of R are readily produced by setting the dose and then pushing a button.

Insulin pumps offer the following advantages over multiple daily injections:

- There is no need to carry insulin vials and syringes when away from home.
- Corrective injections are elegantly simple.
- Pumps can be set to automatically increase the delivery rate shortly before arising in the morning, thereby circumventing problems associated with the dawn phenomenon. They thus render it unnecessary for you to arise early on weekends to take your long-acting insulin.

On the other hand, insulin pumps can pose some problems:

- Pump failure, insulin coagulation, tubing blockage, or kinking can occur in spite of sophisticated alarms and safeguards. As a result, ketoacidosis has occurred overnight in Type I users.
- Many people are turned off by the idea of constantly having a large-bore needle sticking in their abdomens.
- There is a moderate incidence of infections at needle sites. These have formed abscesses requiring surgical drainage.
- Severe hypoglycemia is more common among pump users, possibly because of mechanical problems.
- Insulin pumps cannot be used to give intramuscular injections for more rapid lowering of elevated blood sugars.

In our experience, insulin pumps do not provide better blood sugar control than multiple injections. Contrary to a common misconception, they do not measure what your blood sugar is and correct it automatically.

19

How to Prevent and Correct Low Blood Sugars

When using medications such as insulin or OHAs that lower blood sugar, you're exposed to the ever-present possibility that your blood sugars may drop below your target value.* Because your brain requires glucose in order to function properly, a deficit of glucose — or hypoglycemia — can lead to some occasionally bizarre mental symptoms. In extreme cases, it can result in death. Although severe hypoglycemia can be dangerous, it is preventable, and treatable. I encourage you to have your family or workmates read this chapter so they will be able to assist you in the event you have a hypoglycemic episode and cannot correct it alone.

HYPOGLYCEMIA: SIGNS AND SYMPTOMS

For our purposes in this chapter, we will use the term "hypoglycemia" to designate any blood sugar that's more than 10 mg/dl below target. "Mild" hypoglycemia is any blood sugar that's 10–20 mg/dl below target. As it drops lower, it's progressively more "severe," and can, if left uncorrected, become the condition known as neuroglycopenia, which means "too little glucose in the brain."

Glucose diffuses in and out of your brain slowly, whereas blood sugar

---

* It has been claimed that the OHA metforim (Glucophage) cannot cause abnormally low blood sugars. This is not so. As we discussed in Chapter 14, I've seen it happen — in a very mild diabetic who was using it to facilitate weight loss. Nevertheless, this is a rare occurrence and will be similarly rare for troglitazone.

in the rest of your body can rapidly drop to zero in half an hour from an intramuscular overdose of lispro insulin. If your blood sugar drops rapidly, you may notice the physical symptoms, and because of the slow diffusion of glucose out of the brain, you may still be able to think clearly enough to measure blood sugar and correct it. If, on the other hand, your blood sugar drops slowly, you may not be able to think clearly enough to realize that it's low as the symptoms progress.

Progression of Symptoms

Below is a list of signs of hypoglycemia, ranging from mild (early) to severe (late), which together make up neuroglycopenia:

- Delayed reaction time — e.g., failure to slow down fast enough when driving a car.
- Irritable, stubborn behavior and lack of awareness of the physical symptoms of hypoglycemia (see box, pages 256–257).
- Confusion, clumsiness, difficulty speaking, weakness.
- Somnolence (sleepiness) or nonresponsiveness.
- Loss of consciousness (very rare if you do not take insulin).
- Convulsions (extremely rare if you do not take insulin).
- Death (extremely rare if you do not take insulin).

Some Common Causes of Hypoglycemia

In various chapters, particularly those covering insulin, we've discussed a number of different potential causes of low blood sugar. Below is a list of some common causes. As we will discuss later in the chapter, certain aspects of hypoglycemia may make you resistant to the idea that you could be having an episode.

- Too much delay before eating a meal after taking regular or lispro insulin or certain OHAs.
- Delayed stomach-emptying (see Chapter 21).
- Reduced activity of counterregulatory hormones during certain phases of the menstrual cycle.
- Sudden termination of insulin resistance after abatement of illness or stress that required higher than usual doses of OHAs or insulin.
- Injecting from a fresh vial of insulin after having used progressively higher doses of insulin that slowly lost its activity over a period of months.

- Eating less than the planned amount of carbohydrate or protein for a meal or snack.
- Taking too much insulin or OHA.
- Engaging in unplanned physical activity or failing to cover physical activity with appropriate carbohydrates.
- Drinking too much alcohol, especially prior to or during a meal.
- Failure to shake vials of lente or ultralente insulins vigorously before using.
- Inadvertently injecting long-acting or premeal regular insulin into a muscle.
- Injecting near a muscle that will be strenuously exercised.
- Taking aspirin in large doses, or anticoagulants, barbiturates, antihistamines, or certain other pharmaceuticals that may lower blood sugar or inhibit glucose production by the liver (see Appendix C).

Very Common Early Signs and Symptoms

Hunger. This is the most common early symptom. A truly well-controlled, well-nourished diabetic should not be unduly hungry — unless he's hypoglycemic. This symptom, although frequently ignored, should not be. On the other hand, hunger is also very often a sign of tension or anxiety. One cannot assume that it automatically signals hypoglycemia. Perhaps half of so-called insulin reactions may merely reflect hunger pangs provoked by mealtime, emotional factors, or even *high* blood sugars. When blood sugars are high, the cells of the body are actually being deprived of glucose, and you may feel hungry. Thus, hunger is very common in poorly controlled diabetics. *If you feel hungry, measure your blood sugar.*

Elevated pulse rate. Always carry a watch with a sweep second hand. Know your maximum resting pulse rate. When possible symptoms of hypoglycemia appear and you have no handy means of testing your blood sugar, measure your resting pulse. Many people find it more convenient to measure the temporal pulse (at the temple, on the side of the head between eyebrow and hairline) or carotid pulse (on the side of the neck near lower edge of jaw about 1–2 inches forward of the ear) than the radial, or wrist, pulse. If resting pulse exceeds your *maximum* resting value by more than one-third, assume hypoglycemia. This measure-

Symptoms of Hypoglycemia

Many diabetics develop physical symptoms or signals that enable them to recognize a hypoglycemic episode. Some are listed here. You may not notice these signals, however, if neuroglycopenia is present. Severely deprived of glucose, the brain is less capable of comprehending these things. "Hypoglycemia unawareness" (reduced or absent ability to experience early signs of hypoglycemia) is also common in individuals who have recently had frequent hypoglycemic episodes, because of a phenomenon called down-regulation of adrenergic receptors (see page 271). It can also be caused by a class of cardiac drugs (beta blockers) that slow the heart and lower blood pressure. Signs and symptoms of hypoglycemia include the following:

- Confusion (e.g., inability to read the time or to find things)
- Blurred or double vision
- Headache
- Hand tremors
- Tingling sensation in fingers or tongue
- Buzzing in ears
- Elevated pulse rate
- Great hunger
- Tight feeling in throat or near rear of tongue
- Numbness or strange sensations in lips or tongue
- Clumsiness
- Impaired ability to detect sweet tastes
- Stubbornness
- Irritability
- Nastiness

ment may be normally elevated if you've been walking about during the prior 10 minutes. Your health care professional can help you learn how to measure your pulse.

Nystagmus. This symptom may be demonstrated by slowly moving your eyes from side to side while keeping your head immobile. If another person is asked to watch your eyes, she will notice — when your blood sugar is low — that they may jerk briefly in the reverse direction, or "ratchet," instead of moving smoothly. You can observe the effect of this by looking at the sweep second hand of your watch. If it seems occasionally to jump ahead, you are experiencing nystagmus (actually, as

- Anxiety
- Pounding hands on tables and walls
- Miscellaneous visual impairments, such as blurred or double vision, seeing spots, visual hallucinations (e.g., letters or numbers seem to be printed in Chinese)
- Poor physical coordination (e.g., bumping into walls and dropping things)
- Tiredness
- Weakness
- Sudden awakening from sleep
- Shouting while asleep
- Rapid shallow breathing
- Nervousness
- Light-headedness
- Faintness
- Hot feeling
- Cold or clammy skin
- Restlessness
- Insomnia
- Nightmares
- Pale complexion
- Nausea
- Slurred speech
- Nystagmus

Several of these symptoms may occur at the same time. One symptom alone may be the only indicator. In some cases, there may be no clearly apparent early symptoms at all.

your eyes jumped to the side for brief instants, you missed seeing bits of motion of the second hand).

Absence of erections. For a man, a fairly reliable sign of early-morning hypoglycemia is awakening without an erection, assuming that he ordinarily experiences morning erections.

Denial. As hypoglycemia becomes more severe, or if blood sugar has been dropping slowly, many patients will insist that their blood sugars are fine. An observer suspecting hypoglycemia should insist on a blood sugar measurement before accepting the diabetic's denial.

TREATING MILD TO MODERATE HYPOGLYCEMIA, WITHOUT BLOOD SUGAR OVERSHOOT

Historically, the advice for correction of low blood sugar has been to consume moderately sweet foods or fluids, such as candy bars, fruits, cookies, hard candies, peanut butter crackers, orange juice, milk, and soda pop. Such treatment has never worked properly, for reasons you can probably guess, knowing what you now know about various foods and how they affect your blood sugar.

These moderately sweet foods contain mixtures of slow- and rapid-acting carbohydrates. If, for example, you eat or drink enough that the rapid-acting carbohydrate raises your blood sugar 40–90 mg/dl over the course of half an hour, you may have simultaneously consumed so much slow-acting carbohydrate that your blood sugar will go up to 300 mg/dl several hours later.

In the old days, before I learned to maintain my blood sugar in normal ranges, my physicians insisted that very high blood sugars after hypoglycemic episodes were due to an "inevitable" hypothetical effect they called rebound, or the Somogyi phenomenon. Once I learned to avoid the usual foods for treating low blood sugar, I never experienced blood sugar rebound. Nevertheless, the scientific literature does describe occasional mild insulin resistance that lasts up to 8 hours following an episode of very low blood sugar. This is not the dramatic rebound caused by eating the wrong thing to bring up blood sugar.*

Hypoglycemia can be hazardous, as the list of its progression on page 254 demonstrates. We therefore want to correct it as rapidly as possible. Complex carbohydrate, fructose, lactose (in milk), and even sucrose, which is used in most candies — all must be digested or processed by the liver before they will fully affect blood sugar. This delay makes these types of carbohydrate a poor choice for treating hypoglycemia. Furthermore, you need to know *exactly* how much your blood sugar will rise after eating or drinking something to raise it — and it's relatively easy if you know how. With most of the traditional treatments you must continually check your blood sugar many hours later to gauge the unpredictable effect.

---

* If your physician still believes what he learned in medical school about this fictional phenomenon, ask him to read "The Somogyi Phenomenon — Sacred Cow or Bull?," *Arch Intern Med* 1984; 144: 781–787.

Raising Blood Sugars Predictably

What, then, can we use to raise blood sugars rapidly with a predictable outcome? The answer, of course, is glucose.

Glucose, the sugar of blood sugar, does not have to be digested or converted by the liver into anything else. Unlike other sweets, it's absorbed into the blood directly through the mucous membranes of the mouth, stomach, and gut. Furthermore, as we discussed in Chapter 13, "Using Exercise to Enhance Insulin Sensitivity," we can compute precisely how much a fixed amount of glucose will raise our blood sugar. If you have Type II diabetes and weigh about 140 pounds, 1 gram of pure glucose will raise your blood sugar about 5 mg/dl — provided that your blood sugar is below the point at which your pancreas starts to make insulin to bring it down. If you weigh 140 pounds and have Type I diabetes, 1 gram of glucose will raise your blood sugar about 5 mg/dl no matter what your blood sugar may be, because you cannot produce any insulin to offset the glucose. If you weigh twice that, or 280 pounds, 1 gram will raise your blood sugar only half as much. A 70-pound diabetic child, on the other hand, will experience double the blood sugar increase, or 10 mg/dl per gram of glucose consumed. Thus, the effect of ingested glucose on blood sugar is inversely related to your weight. Table 19-1 gives you the approximate effect of 1 gram glucose upon low blood sugar for various body weights.

TABLE 19-1

EFFECT OF 1 GRAM GLUCOSE UPON LOW BLOOD SUGAR

Body Weight		1 Gram Glucose Will Raise Low Blood Sugar	
35 pounds	16 kilograms	20 mg/dl	1.11 mmol/l
70	32	10	0.56
105	48	7	0.39
140	64	5	0.28
175	80	4	0.22
210	95	3.3	0.18
245	111	3	0.17
280	128	2.5	0.14
315	143	2.2	0.12

Many countries have available as candies or confections products that contain virtually all of their nutritive ingredients as glucose. These glucose tablets are usually sold in pharmacies. Some countries even have glucose tablets marketed specifically for the treatment of hypoglycemia in diabetics. Table 19-2 lists a few of the products with which we are familiar.

TABLE 19-2

GLUCOSE TABLETS USED FOR TREATMENT OF HYPOGLYCEMIA BY DIABETICS

Country of Manufacture	Name of Product	Grams of Glucose Per Tablet	1 Tablet Will Raise Blood Sugar of 140-Pound Person with Low Blood Sugar Approximately	
USA	Dextrotabs	1.6	8 mg/dl	0.44 mmol/l
USA	Sweetarts or Wacky Wafers	2*	10	0. 56
USA	B-D Glucose Tablets	5	25	1.40
USA	Dex 4	4	20	1.10
UK	Dextrosol	3	15	0.83
FRG	Dextro-Energen	4	20	1.10

* Tablet size may vary.

Of the glucose tablets listed, I personally prefer Dextrotabs because they're very easy to chew, raise blood sugar quite rapidly, taste good, are conveniently packaged, and are inexpensive. They are also small enough that they usually need not be broken in halves or quarters to make small blood sugar adjustments (except for children). Each jar of 100 Dextrotabs[†] comes with a small plastic envelope that holds 12 tablets. This envelope fits easily into your pocket or purse and can be refilled as often as needed. Dextrotabs begin to raise blood sugar in about 3 minutes and finish after about 40 minutes (if you don't have gastroparesis — see Chapter 21).

[†] Available from Harrison Chemists, (800) 829-1493.

With this background in mind, how should you proceed when you encounter a low blood sugar?

Using Glucose Tablets

If you experience any of the symptoms of hypoglycemia detailed earlier — especially *hunger* — measure blood sugar. If blood sugar is 10 mg/dl or more below target, chew enough glucose tablets to bring blood sugar back to your target. If you have no symptoms but discover a low blood sugar upon routine testing, again, take enough glucose tablets to bring blood sugar back to your target. If you weigh about 140 pounds and your blood sugar is 60 mg/dl but your target is 90 mg/dl, then you might eat 4 Dextrotabs. This would raise your blood sugar, according to Table 19-2, by 32 mg/dl, bringing you to 92 mg/dl. If you are using Dextro-Energen, you'd take 1½ tablets. With B-D tablets, you'd take 1. Simple.

If your low blood sugar resulted from taking too much insulin or OHA, it may continue to drop after taking glucose tablets if the insulin or OHA hasn't finished working. You should, therefore, recheck your blood sugar about 45 minutes after taking the tablets, to rule out this possibility and see if you're back where you belong. If blood sugar is still low, take additional tablets. If you have delayed stomach-emptying, you may have to wait as much as 2 or more hours for full effect.*

What if you're out of your home or office and don't have your blood sugar meter? (A minor crime, as noted earlier.) If you think you're hypoglycemic, play it safe and take enough tablets to raise your blood sugar about 60 mg/dl (7 Dextrotabs, for example, or 2 B-D tablets). You may worry that this will bring you too high. If you take insulin, this poses no problem. Simply check your blood sugar when you get back to your meter. If it's above your target, take enough lispro to bring you back to target. If you don't take insulin, your blood sugar should eventually come back on its own, because your pancreas is still making some insulin. It may take several hours, or even a day, depending upon how rapidly you can produce insulin. In any event, you may have saved yourself an embarrassing or even disastrous situation.

---

* This time frame can be reduced by drinking special glucose solutions (see page 298).

WHAT IF YOUR SYMPTOMS PERSIST AFTER YOU HAVE CORRECTED THE HYPOGLYCEMIA?

Many of the symptoms of hypoglycemia are actually effects of the hormone epinephrine (which you may know as adrenaline). If you do not have the problems listed on page 272, your adrenal glands will respond to hypoglycemia by producing epinephrine. Epinephrine, like glucagon, signals the liver to convert stored glycogen to glucose. It is epinephrine that brings about such symptoms as rapid heart rate, tremors, pallor, and so on. (Beta blockers can interfere with the ability of epinephrine to cause these symptoms.) Epinephrine has a half-life in the blood of about 1 hour. This means that an hour after your blood sugar comes back to target, about half the epinephrine you made is still in the bloodstream. This can cause a persistence of symptoms, even if your blood sugar is normal. Thus, if you took some glucose tablets an hour ago, and still feel symptomatic, check your blood sugar again. If it's on target, try to control the temptation to eat more. If your blood sugar is still low, more tablets are warranted.

COPING WITH THE SEVERE HUNGER OFTEN CAUSED BY HYPOGLYCEMIA

Mild to moderate hypoglycemia can cause severe hunger and an associated panic. The drive to eat or drink large amounts of sweet foods can be almost uncontrollable. New patients have told me stories of eating an entire pie, a jar of peanut butter, a quart of ice cream, or drinking a quart of orange juice in response to hypoglycemia. Before I stumbled onto blood sugar self-monitoring and learned how to use glucose tablets, I did much the same. The eventual outcome, of course, was extremely high blood sugar several hours later.

Since the effects of glucose tablets are so predictable, the panic element has vanished for me and for most of my patients.

Unfortunately, rapid correction of blood sugar does not always correct the hunger. This may be somehow related to the long half-life of epinephrine and the persistence of symptoms even after restoration of normal blood sugars. My patients and I have successfully coped with this problem in a very simple fashion. You can try the same trick that we use.

First, consume the appropriate number of glucose tablets.

If overwhelming hunger persists, consider what might satisfy it. Typical options include a full meal (such as another breakfast, lunch, or supper), half a meal, or a quarter of a meal. A full meal means exactly the amount of carbohydrates plus protein that you would ordinarily eat at that meal. Half a meal means exactly half.

Even if your blood sugar has not yet come back to target, since you know you have consumed the proper amount of glucose to eventually bring it back, you can confidently inject the amount of insulin or swallow the dose of the OHA that you normally use to cover that meal. For half a meal, take half the dose.

Don't frustrate yourself by waiting the usual 40 minutes or so after injecting regular insulin or the 60–120 minutes after taking an OHA. Just eat. An extra meal now and then won't make you fatter or cause harm. Since you're eating within the controlled boundaries of your meal plan and not gorging on sugars or unlimited amounts of food, you're still abiding by the Laws of Small Numbers.

Instead of a meal, if you know how much insulin or OHA you usually take to cover a certain snack, you might have the snack instead of the meal.

HOW FAMILY AND FRIENDS CAN HELP YOU CATCH A HYPOGLYCEMIC EPISODE WITHOUT MUTUAL ANTAGONISM

Two of the most common effects of hypoglycemia can make the job of helping you difficult and unpleasant. These effects are irritable, nasty behavior and failure to recognize symptoms. At my first interview with many new patients and their families, instances of violence during hypoglycemic episodes are commonly reported. The most common scenario I hear goes like this: "Whenever I see that he's low, I hand him a glass of orange juice and tell him to drink it, but he throws the juice at me. Sometimes he throws the glass, too." Such stories come as no surprise to me, because as a child I used to throw orange juice at my mother, and when I was first married, I did the same to my wife. Why does this happen, and how can we prevent such situations?

First, it's important to try to understand what's going on in the minds of you and the family member during a bout with hypoglycemia. The cognitive difficulties that hypoglycemia can cause can make the slightest frustration or irritation overwhelming. Your low blood sugar may cause you to act bizarrely, as if intoxicated — and in a sense, you are intoxicated. Because your thinking is impaired, you may be totally unaware that your blood sugar is low. The similarity to drunkenness is not a coincidence, since the higher cognitive centers of the brain, which control rational behavior, are impaired in both cases.

You probably have been taught that high blood sugars are to be avoided, and at some level, you remember this, perhaps even cling to it, despite your hypoglycemia. If someone tries to cajole you into eating something sweet, you may decide that it's the *other* person who's irrational. This is especially true if the other person has done the same thing in the past, when blood sugars were actually normal or even high. In "self-protection" against the supposed irrational attempt to get you to eat something sweet, you instinctively may become violent. Most commonly, this occurs if an attempt is made to put food or drink in your mouth. You might view this as an "attack." In less rational moments, you may even decide, since you know that high blood sugars are harmful, that your spouse or relative is trying to kill you.

The helping relative, usually a spouse or parent, may be terrified to see such strange behavior. If your loved one has been through many such encounters, he or she may, for self-protection, keep candies or other sweets around the house in the hopes that you will eat them, and thus avoid such situations. The fear can be exacerbated if your loved one has seen you unconscious from hypoglycemia, or is merely aware that hypoglycemia can cause dire consequences. On other occasions, when your blood sugar wasn't really low, your loved one may have erroneously asked you to eat something sweet. Such diagnoses are especially common during family squabbles. The spouse or parent may feel that "his blood sugar is low, and that's why he's yelling at me." Your loved one would rather play it safe and give you something sweet, even if your blood sugar isn't low.

There is a solution to this apparent dilemma. First of all, both parties must recognize that, as a rule, about half the time that the relative suspects hypoglycemia, you do *not* have a low blood sugar; the other half of the time, blood sugar is indeed low.

No one has ever contradicted me when I make this point.

Encouraging a diabetic to eat sweets when hypoglycemia is suspected, despite conventional teaching, does as much harm as it does good. A better approach would be for the loved one to say, "I'm worried that your blood sugar may be low. Please check it and let me know the result so that I'll feel less anxious." As a patient, you should realize that living with a diabetic can often be as much or more of a strain than having diabetes. You, the diabetic, owe some consideration to the needs of your loved ones. Try to look upon the request to check your blood sugar not as an intrusion but as your obligation to relieve someone else's fear. With this obligation in mind, you should automatically check your blood sugar if asked, just to make the other person feel better. It doesn't matter whether your blood sugar is low or normal. If your blood sugar is low, you can correct it and find out why. If it's normal, then you probably will have diffused the tension of the situation, and now you'll be able to get back to whatever you were doing, unworried that blood sugar is off target. When you look at blood sugar as something like a clock that you can set — and reset — you take some of the mystery out of it, and can diminish the emotion involved.

If you're without your meter, take enough glucose tablets to raise your blood sugar about 60 mg/dl — again to make the other person feel better. This is the least you can do for someone who may worry about you every day.

Believe it or not, this simple approach has worked for me and for many of my patients. As I've said previously, I went through this with my parents and have gone through it with my wife. Spouses report that it relieves them of a great burden. Some have even cried when expressing their gratitude.

HOW FAMILY AND FRIENDS CAN HELP WHEN YOU ARE CONSCIOUS BUT UNABLE TO HELP YOURSELF

This more serious hypoglycemic state is often characterized by extreme tiredness and inability to communicate. You may be sitting and banging your hand on a table, walking around in a daze, or merely failing to respond to questions. It's important that those who live or work with you learn that this is probably a fairly severe stage of hypoglycemia. The likelihood that it's hypoglycemia is so great that valuable time may be wasted if treatment is delayed while someone fumbles about trying to measure your blood sugar. It's quite possible that if you're given glucose tablets you will not chew them, and may even spit them out.

The treatment at this stage is glucose gel by mouth.

Glucose prepared as a syrupy gel is sold in the United States under several brand names. At least one of these products is not pure glucose (dextrose), but contains a mixture of long- and short-acting sugars, and therefore will not exert its full effect as rapidly as we'd like. At present, I ask my patients to purchase a product called Glutose 15 (Paddock Laboratories, Minneapolis, MN 55427). Glutose 15 is packaged in a plastic tube (like toothpaste), with a twist-off cap. Each tube contains 15 grams of glucose. From Table 19-1 (page 259), we see that this amount will raise the blood sugar of a 140-pound person by 75 mg/dl (15 x 5). An appropriate dose for most adults in this condition would be 1½ tubes. These would typically raise one's blood sugar by 100 mg/dl.

Some of the tubes of decorative icing used to write on birthday cakes contain almost pure glucose (dextrose), so you might save money by purchasing those. Look in the baking section of most supermarkets, but make sure of the contents and weight. To convert ounces to grams, multiply by 30. Make sure that the major ingredient is glucose, as some brands are mostly sucrose.

We recommend that two tubes of Glutose, secured together with a rubber band, be placed at strategic locations about the house and place of work, as well as in luggage when you travel with a companion. To administer, someone should insert the tip of an open tube into the corner of your mouth, in between your lower gum and your cheek, and squeeze slowly. You will probably swallow the small amount present in your mouth. After you swallow, more of the gel should be gently squeezed from the tube. Within 5 minutes of ingesting, you should be able to answer questions.

Although glucose gels may not be available in many countries, most industrialized nations have pharmacies and surgical dealers that sell flavored glucose drinks to physicians for performing oral glucose-tolerance tests. These are usually bottled in 10-ounce (330 ml) screw-top bottles and usually contain 100 grams of glucose. A dose of 2 fluid ounces (60 ml) will provide about 20 grams of glucose, enough to raise the blood sugar of a 140-pound person by 100 mg/dl. This can be administered with the help of a plastic squeeze bottle. Whoever feeds you the liquid or gel must exercise caution, as the possibility exists that you could breathe in some of it, causing you to choke.

TREATING HYPOGLYCEMIA IF YOU ARE UNCONSCIOUS

Hypoglycemia is not the only cause of loss of consciousness. Stroke, heart attack, a sudden drop in blood pressure, and even a bump on the head can render you unconscious. In fact, very high blood sugar (above 400 mg/dl) over several days, especially in a dehydrated individual, can also cause loss of consciousness. We will assume, however, that if you are carefully observing the treatment guidelines of this book, you will not allow such prolonged blood sugar elevation to occur.

If you're found unconscious by someone who knows how to check your blood sugar, a measurement should be made. Treatment should not be delayed, however, while people are scampering about trying to find your testing supplies.

The treatment under these conditions is injection of glucagon, a hormone that rapidly raises blood sugar. For this reason, it is imperative that those who live with you know how to give an injection. If you use insulin, you can give them some practice by teaching them how to give you insulin injections. Glucagon is sold in pharmacies in the United States and Canada as the Glucagon Emergency Kit. This consists of a small plastic box containing a syringe filled with an inert waterlike solution and a little vial of white powder (glucagon). The kit also contains an illustrated instruction sheet that your family should read before an emergency develops. The user injects the water into the vial, shakes the vial to dissolve the powder in the water, and draws the solution back into the syringe. The entire contents of the syringe should be injected, either intramuscularly or subcutaneously. Any of the sites shown in Figure 15-1 on page 199 can be used, as can the deltoid muscle (page 248), or even the calf muscle. Your potential benefactors should be warned that if they choose the buttocks, injection should go into the upper outer quadrant, so as not to injure the sciatic nerve. An injection may be given through clothing provided it is not too thick (for example, through a shirtsleeve or trouser leg, but not through a coat or jacket).

Under no circumstances should anything be administered by

mouth while you are unconscious. Since you will not be able to swallow, oral glucose could asphyxiate you. If your glucagon cannot be found, your companions should dial 911 and get the emergency medical squad, or you should be taken to the emergency room of a hospital.

When an individual has lost consciousness from hypoglycemia, he may experience convulsions. Signs of this include tooth-grinding and tongue-biting. This can cause permanent damage in the mouth and should be prevented. A simple protective measure is to roll up a handkerchief and insert it between the rear teeth on one side of the mouth. The handkerchief should not protrude so far into the mouth that it will block the airway. It is a good idea to attach a folded handkerchief, by rubber band, to each of your Glucagon Emergency Kits. If you start to convulse before a handkerchief is in place, this exercise should not be attempted, as you might bite off someone's fingers.

You should begin to show signs of recovery within 5 minutes of a glucagon injection. You should fully regain consciousness and be able to talk sensibly within 20 minutes at most. If prompt recovery does not occur, the only recourse is the emergency squad or hospital. The emergency squad should be asked to inject 40 cc of a 50 percent dextrose (glucose) solution into a vein. Individuals weighing under 100 pounds (45 kilograms) should receive half this amount.

Glucagon can cause retching or vomiting in some people. Your head should therefore be turned to the side so that if you do vomit, you won't breathe the vomitus. Keep a 4-ounce (120 ml) bottle of Reglan syrup (metoclopramide), also attached with a rubber band to the Glucagon Emergency Kit. One gulp of Reglan, taken after you are sitting up and speaking, should almost immediately stop the feeling of nausea. Do not consume more than one gulp, as large doses can cause unpleasant side effects (see page 293). In most of the United States, Reglan is available only upon prescription by a physician.

One dose of glucagon can raise your blood sugar by as much as 250 mg/dl, depending upon how much glycogen was stored in your liver at the time of the injection and subsequently converted to glucose. After you've fully recovered your senses, you should check your blood sugar. If at least 5 hours have elapsed since your last dose of regular insulin, or at least 4 hours since your last dose of lispro, take enough intramuscular (or subcutaneous) lispro insulin to bring your blood sugar back down to your target. This is important, because if your blood sugar is kept normal for about 24 hours, your liver will rebuild its supply of glycogen. This glycogen reserve is of great value for protection from possible subsequent hypoglycemic events.

By the way, if we tried to give glucagon to someone twice in the same day, the second shot might not raise blood sugar. This is possible because liver glycogen reserves may have been totally depleted by the first injection. Thus, monitoring and correction of blood sugar every 5 hours for 1 full day is mandatory after the use of glucagon. Additional blood sugar measurements should be taken every 2½ hours to make sure that you're not again hypoglycemic (but do *not* correct for *high* blood sugars every 2½ hours).

Although reading about possible loss of consciousness may be frightening, remember that this is an extremely rare event, and usually results when a Type I diabetic makes a major mistake, such as those included in the list on pages 254–255. I know of no case where a Type II diabetic experienced severe hypoglycemia when using OHAs that we recommend.

KNOW WHY YOU WERE HYPOGLYCEMIC

Review your Glucograf data sheet after all hypoglycemic episodes, even mild ones. It's important that you reconstruct the events leading up to any episode of low blood sugar, even if it caused no notable symptoms. This is one of the reasons why we recommend (page 68) that most insulin-taking diabetics keep faithful records of data pertinent to their blood sugar levels and why we went into so much detail in Chapter 5 teaching you how to record the information. Since severe hypoglycemia can lead to amnesia for events of the prior hour or so, habitual recording of relevant data can be most valuable for this scenario. It is certainly helpful to record times of insulin shots, glucose tablets, meals, and exercise, as well as to note if you overate or underate, and so on. Merely recording blood sugar data will not help you to figure out what caused a problem. If you experience a severe hypoglycemic episode or several mild episodes and cannot figure out how to prevent recurrences, read or show your Glucograf data sheet to your physician. Your doctor may be able to think of reasons that did not occur to you.

BE PREPARED

Keeping Hypoglycemia Supplies

Glucose tablets, glucose gel (Glutose 15), and glucagon can each potentially save your life. They won't help if they're not around or are allowed
to deteriorate. Here are some basic rules:

- Place supplies in convenient locations around your house and
  workplace.
- Show others where your supplies are kept.
- Keep glucose tablets in your car, pocket, or purse.
- When traveling, keep a full set of supplies in your hand luggage,
  and also in your checked luggage — just in case a piece of luggage
  is lost or stolen.
- Replace glucagon before the expiration date on the vial. Usually
  glucagon dating is two to three years after purchase. Check new
  vials for possible short-dating and return the kit if dating is less
  than two years.
- Always replace supplies when some have been used. Never allow
  your stock to become depleted. Keep plenty of extras on hand.

Your Hypoglycemia Tool Kit

To make sure you are not caught unprepared by low blood sugars, you
should always keep the following supplies on hand at both your home
and your workplace:

If You Take OHAs
- 1–3 bottles (100 tablets each) Dextrotabs or other glucose
  tablets; always carry glucose tablets with you

If You Take Insulin, You Also Need
- 2 or more tubes Glutose 15 or 1–2 ten-ounce bottles glucose-
  tolerance test beverage
- Glucagon Emergency Kit
- 4-ounce bottle Reglan syrup

Emergency Identification Tags

If you use insulin or OHAs, you should wear an identification tag that displays a recognizable medical emblem, such as a red serpent encircling a red staff. The tag, which may be worn as a bracelet or necklace, should be engraved with a message that relates to the treatment of hypoglycemia. My own bracelet is engraved with the following message: *"Diabetic. If conscious — give candy or sweet drink. If unconscious — to hospital."*

Most pharmacies and jewelers sell medical ID tags. Prices begin at $5 for stainless steel and go into hundreds of dollars for solid gold. The Medic Alert Foundation, Turlock, CA 95381, will keep a record of your medical history, and will send you a stainless steel ID bracelet or necklace, with their emblem, for $35. Sterling silver or gold-plated IDs cost slightly more. Beautiful 14-carat gold IDs are available at considerably higher cost. They will also engrave the tag for the same cost. All tags are stamped with your special ID number and with their "call collect" 24-hour telephone number. By phoning this number, a hospital can secure your name and address, those of your next of kin and physician, a list of all your medical conditions, and the doses of medications that you take. You can obtain an application form by writing to the above address or by phoning (800) ID-ALERT.

Emergency Alarm Service

If you live alone, you may want to consider using an emergency alarm system. These can automatically phone a friend, relative, or emergency squad when you push a button on a necklace. The system can also be activated if you do not "check in" at predetermined time intervals. The least expensive system that I have encountered is supplied by the Medic Alert Foundation (see prior section). Their "failure to check in" alert unfortunately can only be activated at 24-hour intervals, so you can be unconscious for 24 hours before someone is notified.

"HYPOGLYCEMIA UNAWARENESS"

Some diabetics have absent or diminished ability to experience the warning signs of hypoglycemia. This occurs under five circumstances that have been documented in the scientific literature:

- Severe autonomic neuropathy (injury, by chronically high blood sugars, to the nerves that control involuntary bodily functions).
- Adrenal medullary fibrosis (destruction, by chronically high blood sugars, of the cells in the adrenal glands that produce epinephrine). This is especially common in long-standing poorly controlled diabetes.
- Blood sugars that are chronically low.
- The use of beta-blocking medication for treatment of hypertension or cardiac chest pain.
- The use of large (nonphysiologic) doses of insulin, as is common for individuals on high-carbohydrate diets.

All of these situations result in lowered production of, or sensitivity to, epinephrine, the hormone that produces tremor, pallor, rapid pulse, and other signs that we identify with hypoglycemia. It is ironic that epinephrine production or sensitivity is most commonly diminished in those whose blood sugars have been chronically either very high *or* very low.

Injury to the autonomic nervous system by elevated blood sugar has been discussed on pages 54–55. Individuals whose heart rate variation on the R-R interval study is severely diminished may be especially susceptible to this problem.

People who have frequent episodes of hypoglycemia or chronically low blood sugar tend to adapt to this condition. They appear to be less sensitive to the effects of epinephrine. This condition cannot be predicted by R-R studies. It is, however, readily detectable if you measure your own blood sugar frequently. If caused by chronically low blood sugar, this condition can be reversed by taking measures to ensure that blood sugar is maintained at normal levels.

Hypoglycemia unawareness can deprive one of potentially lifesaving warning signals. To compensate for this disability, blood sugar should be checked more frequently. For rare individuals who take insulin, it may be necessary, for example, to measure blood sugar every hour for 4½ hours after meals, instead of only once after each meal. Fortunately, we now have the tools to circumvent this problem; we need only to use them diligently.

POSTURAL HYPOTENSION —
THE GREAT DECEIVER

Syncope, or fainting, is fairly common as people get older. It is especially common among diabetics. Even more common is near-syncope. This is merely the feeling that you will pass out unless you lie down right away. Simultaneously, your surroundings may look gray or your vision may fade. There are many causes of syncope and near-syncope. These include cardiac and neurological problems, certain medications, and dehydration. These causes are not nearly as common in diabetics as are sudden drops of blood pressure caused by autonomic neuropathy or by inappropriate use of antihypertensive medications — especially diuretics ("water pills") and alpha-1 antagonists, such as prazosin and terazosin.

When most of us stand from a seated, supine, or squatting position, the brain sends a message to the blood vessels in our legs to constrict reflexively and instantly. This prevents blood from pooling in the legs, which would deprive the brain of blood and oxygen. If you've had high blood sugars for many years, the nerves that signal the vessels in the legs may conduct the message poorly (a sign of autonomic neuropathy). A drop in blood pressure upon standing is called postural, or orthostatic, hypotension.

Alternately, if you eat a big meal, blood may concentrate in your digestive system, also depriving the brain. The normal mechanisms that protect the brain from this shunting of blood may be deficient if you have autonomic neuropathy. It is in part to gauge potential for these reactions that I measure supine and standing blood pressures, and perform R-R interval studies on all diabetic patients. A recent study of medical (mostly nondiabetic) outpatients in the United States suggests that 20 percent of individuals over the age of 65 and 30 percent of those over age 70 have documentable postural hypotension. For diabetics the incidence is probably much greater.

A common scenario for syncope or near-syncope involves the diabetic who gets up in the middle of the night to urinate and keels over on the way to the bathroom. A simple way to avoid this is to sit at the edge of the bed with feet dangling for a few minutes before standing.

Another syncope scenario involves the person who goes to the toilet and passes out while trying to produce a bowel movement or urinate.

Again, the reflexes that prevent shunting of blood away from the brain are blunted by autonomic neuropathy.

If syncope is caused by transient low blood pressure as a result of autonomic neuropathy, one should lay the victim out flat and elevate his feet high above his head. He should return to consciousness almost immediately.

The symptoms of syncope are similar to those of moderate to severe hypoglycemia. In both cases, the brain is being deprived of a basic nutrient — oxygen in the case of syncope, glucose in the case of hypoglycemia. Furthermore, postural hypotension can also occur as a *result* of hypoglycemia. Some symptoms of near-syncope include faintness, visual changes, and disorientation.

Whatever the cause of fainting or near-syncope, blood sugar must be checked to rule out hypoglycemia. If blood sugar is normal, no amount of glucose will cure the problem.

TWO FINAL NOTES

If you've heard horror stories about the frequency and severity of severe hypoglycemia in Type I diabetes, the people you've been hearing about are probably taking industrial doses of insulin to cover large amounts of dietary carboyhdrate. On our regimen, this hazard is virtually nil. Someone would have to make a major mistake, such as taking an insulin dose twice, for life-threatening episodes to occur. Many Type I diabetics seek me out because of their frequent hypoglycemic episodes and not necessarily because of their high blood sugars. Our regimen takes care of both.

Please don't neglect to ask others to read this chapter. When you are most in need of help for treating hypoglycemia, you may be incapable of rendering it yourself. So show this chapter to your close relatives, friends, and coworkers and ask them to read it. It should increase their own confidence in coping with such situations, and the potential payoff to you may be considerable.

20

How to Cope
with Dehydrating Illness

When you experience vomiting, nausea, fever, or diarrhea, you should immediately contact your physician.

We all get sick from time to time, but if you're on our diet and treatment plan, and if you're reasonably healthy, you shouldn't get sick any more frequently than the average person. For diabetics, however, illness can pose special problems.

As you know, sickness or infection can cause your blood sugar to increase, and injected insulin — even if you don't normally take insulin — can help preserve beta cell function during illness (as well as help keep your blood sugar under control). One of the most pressing concerns for diabetics during illness is dehydration, which can lead to life-threatening consequences if not handled effectively and rapidly.

DIABETES AND DEHYDRATION:
A DANGEROUS COMBINATION

Common causes of dehydration include multiple episodes of diarrhea or vomiting; fever and resulting perspiration; failure to drink adequate fluids, especially during hot weather or prolonged exercise; and very high blood sugars.

Dehydration causes transitory insulin resistance, and consequently during periods of dehydration, blood sugar will tend to rise. This blood sugar rise comes in addition to the blood sugar elevation caused by the viral or bacterial infection that led to your vomiting, fever, or diarrhea.

High blood sugar, as you know, also leads to insulin resistance. If all that isn't bad enough, high blood sugar causes *further* dehydration as your kidneys attempt to unload glucose by producing large amounts of urine. The increased dehydration causes higher blood sugars, which in turn cause further dehydration — a classic vicious circle.

The good news is, however, that simple interventions can halt this spiraling of blood sugars and fluid loss. It's the purpose of this chapter to give you the knowledge to prevent what can be grave consequences.

KETOACIDOSIS AND HYPEROSMOLAR COMA

There are two acute conditions that can develop from the combination of high blood sugars and dehydration. The first is called diabetic ketoacidosis, or DKA. It occurs in people who make no insulin on their own (either Type I diabetics or Type II diabetics who eventually lose all beta cell activity). Very low serum insulin levels, combined with the insulin resistance caused by high blood sugars and dehydration, result in the virtual absence of insulin-mediated glucose transport to the tissues of the body. In the absence of adequate insulin, the body metabolizes stored fats to produce the energy that tissues require to remain alive. A by-product of fat metabolism is the production of substances called ketones and ketoacids. One of the ketones, acetone, is familiar as the major component of nail polish remover. Acetone may be detected in the urine by using a dipstick such as Ketostix (see Chapter 3, "Your Diabetic Tool Kit"). Acetone may also be detected on the breath as a fruity aroma, which is why unconscious diabetics are often mistaken for passed-out drunks.

Since ketones and ketoacids are poisonous in large amounts, they can be toxic. More important, your kidneys will try to eliminate them with even more urine, thereby causing further dehydration. Some of the hallmarks of severe ketoacidosis are large amounts of ketones in the urine, extreme thirst, dry mouth, nausea, frequent urination, deep labored breathing, and high blood sugar (usually over 350 mg/dl).

The other acute complication of high blood sugar and dehydration, hyperosmolar coma, is a potentially more severe condition, and occurs in people whose beta cells still make some insulin. ("Hyperosmolar" refers to high concentrations of glucose, sodium, and chloride in the blood due to inadequate water to dilute them.) Diabetics who develop this condition usually have some residual beta cell activity, making enough insulin to suppress the metabolism of fats, but not enough to prevent very high blood sugars. As a result, ketones may not appear in the urine or on the breath. Because this condition most commonly occurs in elderly people, who do not become very thirsty when dehydrated, the degree of fluid loss is usually greater than in ketoacidosis. Early symptoms of a hyperosmolar state include somnolence and confusion. Extremely high blood sugars (as great as 1,500 mg/dl) have been reported in cases of hyperosmolar coma. Fluid deficit may become so severe that the brain becomes dehydrated. Loss of consciousness and death can occur in both the hyperosmolar state and severe DKA.

The treatment for DKA and hyperosmolar coma includes fluid replacement and insulin. Fluid replacement alone can have a great effect upon blood sugar because it both dilutes the glucose level in the blood and permits the kidneys to eliminate it. Fluid also helps the kidneys eliminate ketones in DKA. Our interest here, though, is not in treating these conditions — this must be done by a physician or in a hospital — but in *preventing* them.

VOMITING OR NAUSEA

Vomiting or nausea are most commonly caused by bacterial or viral infections sometimes associated with flulike illness. An essential part of treatment is to stop eating. Since you can certainly survive a day or two without eating, this should pose no problem. But if you're not eating, it makes sense to ask what dose of insulin or OHA you should take.

Adjusting Your Diabetes Medication
If you're on one of the medication regimens described in this book, the answer is simple: you take the amount and type of medication that you'd normally take to cover the basal, or fasting, state and *skip* any doses that are intended to cover meals. If, for example, you ordinarily take ultralente or lente insulin upon arising and at bedtime, and regular or lispro insulin before meals, you'd continue the ultralente or lente and skip the preprandial regular or lispro for those meals you won't be eating. Similarly, if you take metformin or troglitazone on arising and/or at

bedtime for the fasting state, and again to cover meals, you skip the doses for those meals that you do not plan to eat.

In both of the above cases, *it's essential that the medications used for the fasting state continue at their full doses.* This is in direct contradiction to traditional "sick day" treatment, but it's a major reason why patients who carefully follow our regimens do not develop DKA or hyperosmolar coma when they are ill.

Remember, because infection and dehydration may each cause blood sugar to increase, you may need additional coverage for any blood sugar elevation. Such additional coverage should usually take the form of lispro insulin. This is one of the reasons that we advocate the training of all diabetics in the techniques of insulin injection — even those who, when not sick, can be controlled by just diet and OHAs. Using insulin when you're sick may be especially important for you, because it helps to relieve the added burden on beta cells that leads to burnout. This is but one of the reasons it's mandatory that you contact your physician *immediately* when you feel ill. He or she should be able to tell you how much coverage with lispro will be necessary, and when to take it. The protocol for such coverage is discussed on pages 241–244, but because of its importance, it bears repeating again briefly:

- Measure blood sugars on arising and every 4 hours thereafter.
- Inject enough lispro at these times to bring your blood sugars down to your target value. Intramuscular shots are preferred (see pages 246–247) because of their rapid effect, but subcutaneous injection is also acceptable. It is prudent to continue blood sugar measurements and insulin coverage, even during the night, for as long as blood sugars continue to rise.

If you're so ill that you cannot check your own blood sugars and inject your own insulin, someone else must do this for you, or you should be hospitalized. The potential consequences are so serious that you have no other options.

Controlling the Vomiting

The other mainstay of treatment is fluid replacement, but if you've been vomiting, you'll probably be unable to hold anything down, including fluids. Ordinary vomiting can be suppressed with Tigan (trimethobenzamide hydrochloride) suppositories, administered rectally about every 5 hours if vomiting persists. These should be stored in your refrigerator, as they tend to melt in hot weather. When you experience vomiting, nausea, fever, or diarrhea, you should immediately contact your physician. If vomiting or nausea continues for more than 4 hours, or if it cannot be halted by Tigan within 1 hour, he or she may want you to try a second dose or to visit a hospital emergency room to receive intravenous fluid (saline) and to have the cause established. Some surgical emergencies such as intestinal obstruction can lead to vomiting, as can poisoning, gastroparesis (Chapter 21), DKA, and so on. Vomiting is a serious problem for people with diabetes, and should not be treated casually.

Large doses of Tigan can cause bizarre neurological side effects, especially in children and in slim, elderly people. It should not be administered more often than every 4 hours, or in doses greater than that prescribed by your physician. I usually recommend 100 mg suppositories for children and people older than 65 years; 200 mg suppositories, for all others.

Fluid Replacement

Once vomiting has been controlled, you should immediately begin to drink fluids. Two questions naturally arise at this point: What fluid? And how much? There are three factors that must be considered in preparing the fluid to be used.

First, it must be palatable. Second, it should contain no carbohydrate (therefore *no* Gatorade or other sports drinks), but artificial sweeteners are okay. This guideline also contradicts conventional treatment, which usually calls for sweetened beverages to offset the excessive amounts of insulin that many diabetics use. Finally, the fluids should replace the electrolytes — sodium, potassium, and chloride — that are lost from the body when we lose fluids. Beverages commonly used by my patients include diet soda, diluted iced tea, seltzer, water, and carbohydrate-free bouillon or clear soup. To these fluids, we add electrolytes.

> *To each quart of liquid, add:*
> 1 level teaspoon table salt (½ teaspoon if it tastes too salty) (provides sodium and chloride)
> ¼ teaspoon salt substitute (see list, page 60)(provides potassium and chloride)

In anticipation of these rare "sick days," you should always have on hand several 2-quart bottles of diet soda, or two empty 2-quart plastic iced tea pitchers. The pitchers can be used to store whatever concoction you may prefer instead of diet soda. When the need arises, one pitcher of fluid can be kept by your bedside, while the second is kept cool in the refrigerator.

The volume of fluid you will require each day, when not eating, depends upon your size, since large people utilize more fluid than small people. If your blood sugars are elevated or if your urine is dipstick-positive for ketones, you will need much more fluid than otherwise. The ongoing fluid requirement for most adults without these problems comes to about 2–3 quarts daily while fasting. In addition, within the first 24 hours you should replace the estimated fluid loss caused by vomiting, fever, or diarrhea. This may come to another few quarts, so clearly you will have to do a lot of drinking. Your physician should be consulted for instructions regarding your fluid intake while ill. If for any reason you cannot consume or keep down the amount of liquid that she or he recommends, you may have to be hospitalized to receive intravenous fluids.

Diarrhea

Here again we are faced with three basic problems: blood sugar control; control of the diarrhea to prevent further water and electrolyte loss; and fluid and electrolyte replacement.

The guidelines for blood sugar control are the same as if you have been vomiting (see prior section). Fluid and electrolyte replacement should be the same as for vomiting, except that 1 level teaspoon of sodium bicarbonate (baking soda) should be added to each quart of the electrolyte-replacement mixture. The primary treatment for diarrhea, as for vomiting, is to stop eating. Medications to relieve diarrhea, if any, should be specified by your physician. Some forms of diarrhea caused by bacteria, such as "traveler's diarrhea," may warrant the use of antibiotics. I sometimes avoid medications that slow the motility of the gut (e.g., Imodium, or loperamide), because bacterial infections frequently produce toxins that irritate the gut, and diarrhea is the body's way of diminishing them naturally. A benign way to treat diarrhea is with emulsified pectin and kaolin (clay), commonly sold in the United States under the brand name Kaopectate. Kaopectate increases stool bulk and coats the walls of the gut, offering protection from inflammatory toxins. It must be used in large amounts (6 tablespoons after each loose stool) to be truly effective. Since it contains a small quantity of sucrose, you may experience a slight blood sugar increase, which can be corrected with insulin after you check your blood sugar. If Kaopectate fails to control the diarrhea, the aforementioned agents should be tried.

If, in spite of using antidiarrheal medications, frequent loose or watery stools persist, you'll have to be treated in a hospital with intravenous fluid administration. Bring plenty to read because you may be kept in the emergency room for 8 hours or more.

FEVER

No doubt you've heard the advice, "Drink plenty of fluids," for a fever. This is because fever causes considerable fluid loss through the skin as perspiration. Your loss of fluid can be difficult to estimate, so your physician may want to assume that you'd require 1–2 more quarts of fluid daily than you'd normally need. Ordinarily, a mild fever helps to destroy the infectious agent (virus or bacteria) that caused the fever. The tendency to sleep out fever may also be beneficial. For a diabetic, however, the somnolence that you experience with fever may discourage you from checking your blood sugar, covering with insulin, drinking adequate fluid, and calling your physician. It is therefore appropriate to use aspirin or acetaminophen, in accordance with your doctor's instructions, to help fight the fever. Beware, however, that aspirin can cause false positive readings on tests for urinary ketones. *Never use aspirin for fever in children.*

If you have fever, the guidelines for blood sugar control and replacement of fluid are almost the same as indicated previously for vomiting. There is one difference, however. Since there is very little electrolyte loss in perspiration, it's not necessary to add salts to the fluid you consume if you're not vomiting or experiencing diarrhea. Certainly there is no reason not to eat if you feel hungry.

ADDITIONAL SUGGESTIONS

Like hypoglycemia, dehydrating illness can be life-threatening to a diabetic. Encourage the people you live with to read this chapter carefully. The supplies mentioned should be kept in locations known to all. Phone your physician at the first sign of fever, diarrhea, or vomiting. The chances are that he/she would much rather be contacted early, when dehydration and loss of blood sugar control can be prevented. Emergency situations make treatment more difficult, so you can make your physician's life a bit easier (and look out for your own well-being) by phoning *before* major problems occur.

Your physician will probably ask you whether your urine shows ketones, so use the Ketostix before you call. Also, let your doctor know if you have taken any aspirin in the prior 24 hours, as this can cause a false positive Ketostix reading. Similarly, the antihypertensive ACE inhibitor drug Captopril can also cause false positive Ketostix tests. In both cases, a simple solution is to put urine on Acetest tablets, which change color without giving false positive results.

One last point about aspirin. Large doses can cause prolonged severe hypoglycemia in people who take insulin. Adults should therefore limit themselves to no more than 12 standard tablets in a day.

21

Delayed Stomach-Emptying: Gastroparesis

A number of times throughout this book, you've come across the term "delayed stomach-emptying" or "gastroparesis." As I explained in Chapter 2, elevated blood sugars for prolonged periods can impair the ability of nerves to do what they're supposed to. It's very common that the nerves that stimulate the muscular activity, enzyme secretion, and hormone production essential to digestion function poorly in long-standing diabetes. These changes affect the stomach, the gut, or both. Dr. Richard McCullum, a noted authority on digestion, has said that if a diabetic has any other form of neuropathy (dry feet, reduced feeling in the toes, diminished reflexes, et cetera), he or she will also experience delayed digestion.

What happens when digestion is delayed, and why should it affect blood sugar control? Slowed digestion can be fraught with unpleasant symptoms (rarely), or it may only be detectable when we review blood sugar profiles or perform certain diagnostic tests (commonly). The picture is different for each of us. For more than twenty-five years, I suffered from many unpleasant symptoms myself. I eventually saw them taper off and vanish after thirteen years of essentially normal blood sugars. Some of the physical complaints possible (usually after meals) include burning along the midline of the chest ("heartburn"), belching, feeling full after a small meal (early satiety), bloating, nausea, vomiting, constipation, constipation alternating with diarrhea, cramps a few inches above the belly button, and an acid taste in the mouth.

GASTROPARESIS: CAUSES AND EFFECTS

Most of these symptoms, as well as effects upon blood sugar, relate to delayed stomach-emptying. This condition is called gastroparesis diabeticorum, which translates from the Latin as "weak stomach of diabetics." It is believed that the major cause of this condition is neuropathy (nerve impairment) of the vagus nerve. This nerve mediates many of the autonomic or regulatory functions of the body, including heart rate and digestion. In men, neuropathy of the vagus nerve can also lead to problems in having penile erections. To understand the effects of gastroparesis, refer to Figure 21-1.

On the left, is a representation of a normal stomach after a meal. The contents are emptying into the intestines, through the pylorus. The pyloric valve is wide open (relaxed). The lower esophageal sphincter (LES) is tightly closed, to prevent regurgitation of stomach contents. Not shown is

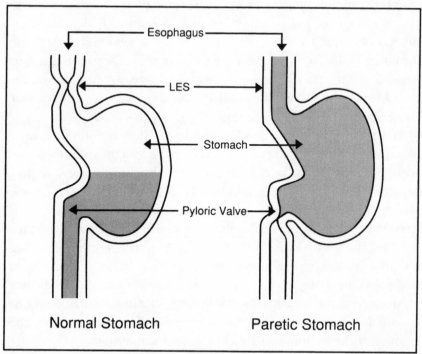

Terry Eppridge

Fig. 21-1. *Normal and paretic stomachs.*

the grinding and churning activity of the muscular walls of the stomach.

On the right is pictured a stomach with gastroparesis. The normal rhythmic motions of the stomach walls are absent. The pyloric valve is tightly closed, preventing the unloading of stomach contents. A tiny opening about the size of a pencil point may permit a small amount of fluid to dribble out. When the pyloric valve is in tight spasm, some of us can feel a sharp cramp above the belly button. Since the lower esophageal sphincter is relaxed or open, acidic stomach contents can back up into the esophagus (the tube that connects the throat to the stomach). This can cause a burning sensation along the midline of the chest, especially while lying down. I have seen patients whose teeth were actually dissolved by regurgitated stomach acid.

Because the stomach does not empty readily, one may feel full even after a small meal. In extreme cases, several meals accumulate and cause severe bloating. More commonly, however, you may have gastroparesis and not be aware of it. In mild cases, emptying may be slowed somewhat, but not enough to make you feel any different. Nevertheless, this can cause problems with blood sugar control. Certain medications, such as tricyclic antidepressants, can further slow stomach-emptying and other digestive processes.

Some years ago, I received a letter from my friend Bob Anderson. His diabetic wife Trish, who has since passed away, had been experiencing frequent loss of consciousness from severe hypoglycemia, caused by delayed digestion. His description of an endoscopic exam, when he was allowed to look through a flexible tube into Trish's stomach and gut, paints a graphic picture:

> **All this brings me to today's endoscopy exam. I watched through the scope and for the first time, I now understand what you have been saying about diabetic gastroparesis. Not until I viewed the inside of the duodenum did I understand the catastrophic effect of 33 years of diabetes upon the internal organs. There was almost no muscle action apparent to move food out of the stomach. It appeared as a very relaxed smooth-sided tube instead of having muscular ridges ringing the passage. I suppose a picture is worth a thousand words. Diabetic neuropathy is more than a manifestation of a tilting gait, blindness, and other easily observable presentations; it wrecks the whole system. This you well know. I am learning.**

HOW DOES GASTROPARESIS AFFECT BLOOD SUGAR CONTROL?

Consider the individual who has very little phase I insulin release and must take fast-acting insulin or one of the older (sulfonylurea) OHAs before each meal. If he were to take his medication and then skip the meal, his blood sugar would plummet. When the stomach empties too slowly, it can have the same effect as skipping a meal. If we knew when the stomach would empty, we could delay the insulin shot or add some lente insulin to the regular to slow down its action. The big problem with gastroparesis, however, is its unpredictability. We never know when, or how fast, the stomach will empty. If the pyloric valve is not in spasm, the stomach contents may empty within minutes. On another occasion, when the valve is tightly closed, the stomach may remain loaded for days. Thus, blood sugar may plummet 1–2 hours after eating, and then rise very high, say 12 hours later, after emptying eventually occurs. It is this unpredictability that can make blood sugar control impossible if significant gastroparesis is ignored in people who take insulin or certain OHAs before meals.

For most Type II diabetics, fortunately, even symptomatic gastro-paresis may not grossly impede blood sugar control, because they may still produce some phase I and phase II insulin. They therefore may not require substantial amounts of injected insulin to cover their meals. Much of their insulin is produced in response to blood sugar elevation. Thus, if the stomach does not empty, only the low basal (fasting) levels of insulin are released, and hypoglycemia does not occur. Of course, the sulfonylurea OHAs (which I don't recommend) can cause hypoglycemia under such circumstances. If the stomach empties continually but very slowly, the beta cells of most Type II's will produce insulin concurrently. Sometimes the stomach may empty suddenly, as the pyloric valve re-laxes. This will produce a rapid blood sugar rise, caused by the sudden absorption of carbohydrate following the entrance of stomach contents into the small intestine. Most Type II beta cells then cannot counter rapidly enough. Eventually, however, insulin release catches up and blood sugar drops to normal, if a reasonable regimen is followed. This latter effect may explain the occasional elevation of fasting blood glu-cose that many Type II's experience the morning after a large supper, followed by a normal blood sugar at bedtime.

In any event, if you do not require insulin or use a sulfonylurea before meals, there is no hazard of hypoglycemia due to delayed stomach-emptying. This assumes that any long-acting insulin or sulfonylurea is administered in doses that cover only the fasting state, as discussed in prior chapters. The traditional use of large doses of these medications, meant to cover both the fasting and fed states, brings with it the hazard of postprandial hypoglycemia when gastroparesis is present.

DIAGNOSING GASTROPARESIS

Efforts at diagnosis are usually unnecessary if there is no reason to suspect the presence of gastroparesis. So first we must have an index of suspicion. If at the initial history-taking interview with your physician you mention symptoms like those described earlier in this chapter, he should have a high index of suspicion. If your R-R interval study (Chapter 2) at the initial physical exam is grossly abnormal, he can be quite certain of gastroparesis. Remember that this study checks the ability of the vagus nerve to regulate heart rate. If the nerve fibers going to the heart are impaired, the branches that activate the stomach are probably also impaired. In my experience, the correlation of grossly abnormal R-R studies with demonstrable gastroparesis is very real.

Diagnostic Tests

Given the physical symptoms or the abnormal R-R study, your physician may want to consider further tests to evaluate your condition. The most sophisticated of these studies is the gamma-ray technetium scan. This test is performed at major medical centers, and is quite costly. It works this way: You eat some scrambled eggs to which a minute amount of radioactive technetium has been added. A gamma-ray camera trained on your abdomen measures (from outside your body) the low levels of radiation the technetium emits as the eggs pass from your stomach into your small intestine. If the gamma radiation drops off rapidly, the study is considered normal.

A less precise study can be performed at much lower cost by any radiologist. This is called the barium hamburger test. In this test, you eat a 1/4-pound hamburger and then drink a liquid that contains the heavy element barium. Every half hour or so, an X-ray photo is taken of your stomach. Since the barium shows up in these photos, the radiologist can estimate what percent of the barium remains in your stomach at the end of each time period. Total emptying within 3 hours or less is usually considered normal.

Despite their theoretical usefulness, neither of these studies is any-where near 100 percent sensitive, because of the unpredictable nature of the paretic stomach. One day it may empty normally, another day it may be a bit slow, and on yet another day its emptying may be severely de-layed. Because of this unpredictability factor, the study may have to be repeated a number of times before a diagnosis can be made. The possi-bility exists that you could have several normal studies but still have abnormal stomach-emptying.

Telltale Blood Sugar Patterns

Having medical tests is bad enough, but having to repeat them incon-clusively has naturally proven quite annoying to many of my patients. Worse than annoyance, the studies are not cheap, and most insurance companies will not pay for repeats of the same study unless they're sep-arated by many weeks or months. If you're regularly measuring your blood sugar levels and trying to keep them in the normal range, it's re-ally not difficult to spot gastroparesis that's severe enough to affect blood sugars. For practical purposes, this is just the degree of gastro-paresis that should concern us.

Below are some of the typical blood sugar patterns that I look for. To call these patterns, though, is slightly misleading. The hallmark of gas-troparesis is randomness, unpredictability from one day to the next. These "patterns" come and go in such a fashion that blood sugar profiles are rarely similar on 2 or 3 successive days. The first two patterns to-gether are highly indicative of gastroparesis, while the third by itself is usually adequate for diagnosis.

- Low blood sugar occurring 1–3 hours after meals.
- Elevated blood sugar occurring 5 or more hours after meals with no other apparent explanation.
- Significantly higher fasting blood sugars in the morning than at bedtime, especially if supper was finished at least 5 hours before retiring. If bedtime long-acting insulin or OHA is gradually in-creased in an effort to lower the fasting blood sugars, we may find

that the bedtime dose is much higher than the morning dose. On some days fasting blood sugar may still be high, but on other days it may be normal or even too low. We're thus giving extra bedtime medications to accommodate overnight stomach-emptying — but sometimes the stomach doesn't empty overnight and fasting blood sugars drop too low.

Having seen such patterns of blood sugar, we can then perform a simple experiment to confirm that they really are caused by gastroparesis.

Skip supper and its premeal insulin or OHA one night. When you go to bed, measure your blood sugar, and then measure your fasting blood sugar the next morning on arising. If, without supper, your blood sugar has dropped or remained unchanged overnight, gastroparesis is the most likely cause.

Repeat this experiment several days later, and again a third time, after another few days. If each experiment results in the same effect, delayed stomach-emptying is virtually certain. When you had previously been eating suppers, at least *some* of the following mornings had shown an overnight rise in blood sugars. Since such rises occurred on nights when you had eaten supper, but *not* on the nights when you did *not* eat, the rise must have been caused by food that did not leave your stomach until after you went to bed.

"False Gastroparesis"

I've seen a number of patients whose blood sugar profile or physical symptoms could have been diagnostic of gastroparesis, yet their R-R interval studies were normal or only slightly impaired. These people had impaired stomach-emptying but properly functioning vagus nerves. The conflicting data obliged me to order endoscopic studies for these people. Endoscopy uses a thin, flexible, lighted fiber optic cable to look directly into the stomach or bowel.

The endoscopic tests demonstrated that they all had abnormalities unrelated to their diabetes. Such findings have included gastric or duodenal ulcers, erosive gastritis, irritable gastrointestinal tract, hiatal hernia, and other gastrointestinal disorders. Each of these conditions required treatment distinct from treatment for diabetes. Only in one case, the hiatal hernia, were we unable to alleviate the digestive problem.

The loud and clear message from this is that the R-R interval study should be performed on every diabetic patient whose blood sugar profiles resemble those outlined above.

APPROACHES TO CONTROL OF GASTROPARESIS

It is worth noting at the outset that *gastroparesis can be cured by extended periods of normal blood sugars.* I've seen several relatively mild cases where special treatment was terminated after about 1 year, and blood sugar profiles remained flat thereafter. At the same time, R-R studies normalized. Since my late teens, I experienced severe daily belching and burning in my chest. These symptoms gradually eased off, and eventually disappeared, but only after thirteen years of nearly normal blood sugars. My R-R study is now normal. The "sacrifices" in lifestyle required for treatment of gastroparesis may really pay off months or years later. The vagus nerve doesn't control only stomach-emptying — there are a number of other complications resulting from impaired vagus function that can be reversed by maintaining normal blood sugars. The regained ability to sustain a penile erection is an important one for many of my male patients.

Once gastroparesis has been confirmed as the major cause of high overnight blood sugars and wide random variations in blood sugar profiles, we can begin to attempt to control or minimize its effects. If your blood sugar profiles reflect significant gastroparesis, there is no way to get them under control by only juggling doses of insulin or OHAs. There's just too much danger of either very high or very low blood sugars for such approaches to work. The only chance for effective treatment is to concentrate on improving stomach-emptying.

How do we do this?

We have four basic approaches. First is the use of medications. Second is special exercises after meals. Third is meal plan modification utilizing ordinary foods, and fourth is meal plan modification utilizing semiliquid or liquid meals.

It's unusual for a single approach to normalize blood sugar profiles fully, so most often we try a combination of these four approaches, adapted to the preferences and needs of the individual. As these attempts start to smooth out blood sugars, we must modify our doses of insulin or OHAs accordingly. The guidelines that we use to judge the efficacy of a given approach or combination of approaches are these:

- Reduction or elimination of physical complaints such as early satiety, nausea, regurgitation, bloating, heartburn, belching, and constipation.
- Elimination of random postprandial hypoglycemia.
- Elimination of random, unexpected high fasting blood sugars — probably the most common sign of gastroparesis that we encounter.
- Flattening out of blood sugar profiles.

Remember that the last three of these improvements may not be possible if you're following conventional dietary and medication regimens for "control" of your blood sugar. For example, I know of no way that will truly flatten out blood sugar profiles if you're on a high-carbohydrate diet and the associated large doses of insulin or OHAs.

Medications That Facilitate Stomach-Emptying

There is no medication that will cure gastroparesis. The only "cure" is months or years of normal blood sugars. There are, however, some pharmaceutical preparations that may speed the emptying of your stomach after a meal. This will help smooth your blood sugar profiles after that meal. Most diabetics with gastroparesis will require medication before every meal.

When gastroparesis is very mild, it may be possible to get away with medication only before supper. For some reason — perhaps because most people tend not to be as physically active after supper, and may have their largest meal of the day in the evening — digestion of supper appears to be more impaired than that of other meals.

Medications for gastroparesis may take the form of liquids or pills. The question immediately arises that if pills must dissolve in the stomach to become effective, just how effective are they going to be? My experience is that they're of questionable value. The time required for a pill to dissolve in a paretic stomach is unpredictable, and consequently the medication may take several hours to become effective. I generally prescribe only liquid medications for stimulating gastric (stomach) emptying.

Cisapride suspension (Propulsid, Jansen Pharmaceutical) is usually my first choice. I begin with 1 tablespoon (25 mg), 15–30 minutes before meals for adults. Many people will require 2 tablespoons for maximum effect. Larger doses appear to be of little added value. The manufacturer recommends doses only up to 20 mg (2 teaspoons) for the treatment of esophageal reflux disease. This condition is much more responsive to treatment than diabetic gastroparesis, which, as a rule, requires the larger doses. The package insert also recommends a bedtime dose, which serves no purpose for gastroparesis. In many cases, cisapride alone will not bring about complete stomach-emptying. We may add other medications if blood sugar profiles don't level off.

Cisapride can inhibit or compete for liver enzymes that clear certain medications from the bloodstream. Your physician should therefore review *all* your medications, especially antidepressants, antibiotics, and antifungal agents, before prescribing cisapride.

George's Distilled Aloe Juice is a waterlike liquid sold by the quart or gallon in many health food stores. You can purchase it from Harrison Chemists, (800) 829-1493, if you cannot procure it locally. I recommend this particular brand of aloe juice because most users do not complain of the medicinal taste common to most aloe products. The usual dose of George's is one 8-ounce glass with the cisapride, 15–30 minutes before eating.

Even the combination of cisapride and aloe juice frequently fails to empty the stomach consistently. Gastroparesis is not easily controlled.

Super Papaya Enzyme Plus has been praised by many of my patients for its rapid relief of some of the physical symptoms of gastroparesis — bloating and belching, for example. Some claim that it also helps to level off the blood sugar swings caused by gastroparesis. The product consists of pleasant-tasting chewable tablets that contain a variety of enzymes (papain amylase, proteases, bromelain, lipase, and cellulase) that digest protein, fat, carbohydrate, and fiber while they are still in your stomach. You would normally chew 3–5 tablets during and at the end of each meal. The tablets are available in most health food stores and are marketed by American Health, Bohemia, NY 11716. Some of my kosher patients use a similar product called **Freeda All Natural Parvenzyme** which is distributed by Freeda Vitamins, 36 East Forty-first Street, New York, NY 10017. The small amount of sorbitol and similar sweeteners contained in these products should not have a significant effect on your blood sugar if consumption is limited to the quantities detailed above. Readers of my last book have written to me praising the effects of chewable enzyme tablets.

Domperidone (Motilium, Jansen Pharmaceutical) is currently not available in the United States. It is, however, marketed in Canada and overseas. We usually fax prescriptions to Canadian pharmacies for our patients here, who then phone in their credit card numbers for mail order shipments. Since it is not available as a liquid, we ask patients to chew 2 tablets (10 mg) 1 hour before meals and to swallow with 8 ounces of water or diet soda. I limit dosing to 2 tablets because larger amounts can cause sexual dysfunction in males and absence of menses in women. Since it works by a mechanism different from those of the preceding products, its effects can be additive (that is, useful with other preparations, *not* addictive). We always try the liquid preparations mentioned above first. Jansen may market a liquid form of this product in the United States at some time in the future.

Metoclopramide syrup (Reglan, A. H. Robins) may possibly be the most powerful stimulant of gastric emptying. It works in a fashion similar to domperidone, by inhibiting the effects of dopamine in the stomach. Because it can readily enter the brain, it can cause serious side effects, such as somnolence, depression, and neurologic problems that resemble Parkinsonism. These side effects can appear immediately in some individuals or only after many months of continuous use in others. I use this medication only as a last resort and limit dosing to 1 tablespoon (25 mg), 15–30 minutes before meals.

If you use metoclopramide, you should keep on hand the antidote to its side effects — diphenhydramine elixir (Benadryl syrup). Two tablespoons usually work. If side effects become serious enough to warrant use of the antidote, the metoclopramide should be immediately and permanently discontinued.

Erythromycin ethylsuccinate is an antibiotic that has been used to treat infections for many years. It has a chemical composition that resembles the hormone motolin, which stimulates muscular activity in the stomach. Apparently when stimulation of the stomach by the vagus nerve is depressed, as with autonomic neuropathy, motolin secretion is diminished. Three papers delivered to the 1989 annual meeting of the

American Gastroenterological Association demonstrated that this drug can stimulate gastric emptying in patients with gastroparesis. In people without gastroparesis, erythromycin can cause nausea, unless taken after drinking fluids. I ask my patients to drink two glasses of water or other fluid before each dose. I usually prescribe erythromycin ethylsuccinate oral suspension just before meals. We start with 1 teaspoon of the 400 mg/tsp concentration, and increase to several teaspoons if necessary. As each teaspoon of this suspension contains 3.5 grams of sucrose (table sugar), it will be necessary to increase slightly the doses of insulin or OHA covering meals while this medication is used. If the liquid is kept in a refrigerator, the taste begins to deteriorate after 35 days. At room temperature, taste deteriorates after 14 days. I have seen no side effects from this medication. I insist that patients who use it chronically take 1 acidophilus capsule with each dose. This is to restore natural bacteria to the intestine that can be destroyed by this antibiotic.

Exercises That Facilitate Stomach-Emptying

The paretic stomach may be described as a flaccid bag, deprived of the rhythmic muscular squeezing present in a stomach that is properly "wired" to the vagus nerve. Any activity that rhythmically compresses the stomach can crudely replicate the normal effect. You may perhaps have observed how a brisk walk can relieve that bloated feeling.

A patient of mine learned a trick from her yoga instructor that eliminated the erratic blood sugar swings caused by her moderate gastroparesis. The trick is to pull in your belly as far as you can, then push it out all the way. Repeat this with a regular rhythm as many times as you can, immediately after each meal. Over a period of weeks or months, your abdominal muscles will become stronger and stronger, permitting progressively more repetitions before you tire. Eventually shoot for 100 reps. This should require less than 4 minutes of your time — a small price to pay for an improvement in your blood sugar profiles.

Another patient discovered an exercise that I call the "back flex." Sit or stand while bending backward as far as you can. Then bend forward, about the same amount. Repeat this about 20 times.

Although these exercises may sound excessively simple, even silly, their potential benefit to you if you suffer from gastroparesis can be inestimable.

Chewing Gum Can Make a Big Difference

The act of chewing produces saliva, which not only contains digestive enzymes but also stimulates muscular activity in the stomach and tends to relax the pylorus. Trident "sugarless" gum contains only 1 gram of sugar per piece and so will have very little effect upon your blood sugar. Chewing gum for 1 hour after meals is probably the most effective treatment of gastroparesis outside of major dietary changes.

Meal Plan Modifications, Utilizing Ordinary Foods

More often than not, changes in your meal plan will prove more effective than medication. The problem is that such changes are unacceptable to many patients. We usually proceed from most to least convenient in five stages:

1. Reduction of dietary fiber.
2. Virtual elimination of red meat.
3. Reduction of protein at supper.
4. Introduction of four or more small daily meals, instead of three larger meals.
5. Semiliquid or liquid meals.

In the paretic stomach both soluble fiber (gums) and insoluble fiber can form a plug at the very narrow pyloric valve. This is no problem in the normal stomach, where the pyloric valve is wide open. Many patients with mild gastroparesis have reported better relief of fullness and improved blood sugar profiles after modifying their diets to reduce fiber content. This means, for example, that mashed well-cooked vegetables must be substituted for salads, and high-fiber laxatives such as those containing psyllium (e.g., Metamucil) should be avoided. It also means that you would have to give up a valuable source of slow-acting carbohydrate — bran crackers. On the other hand, *very small amounts* of faster-acting carbohydrate foods such as bread and rice will raise your blood sugar more slowly because of the slowed digestion, and may be more acceptable until your gastroparesis has a chance to clear up.

Most people in the United States like to eat their largest meal in the evening. Furthermore, they usually consume their largest portion of meat or other protein food at this time. These habits make control of fasting blood sugars very difficult for people with gastroparesis. Apparently animal protein, especially red meat, like fiber, tends to plug up your pylorus if it's in spasm. An easy solution is to move most of your animal protein from supper to breakfast and lunch. Many of my patients have observed remarkable improvements when they do this. We usually suggest a limit of 2 ounces of animal protein at supper. This is not very much. Yet people are usually so pleased with the results that they will continue with such a regimen indefinitely (of course, as protein is shifted from one meal to another, doses of insulin or OHA must also be shifted). With a reduction of delayed overnight stomach-emptying, the bedtime dose of longer-acting insulin or OHA must usually be reduced so that fasting blood sugar will not drop too low.

Some people find that by moving protein to earlier meals, they increase the unpredictability of blood sugar after these meals. For such a situation, we suggest four or more smaller meals each day, instead of three larger meals. We try to keep these meals spaced about 4 hours apart, so that digestion and doses of regular insulin or OHA for one meal are less likely to overlap those for the next meal. We also try to continue the timing of the last meal so that it precedes bedtime by 4–5 hours. This enables you to make any bedtime blood sugar correction after the preprandial regular has finished working.

Semiliquid or Liquid Meals

A last resort for gastroparesis is the use of semiliquid or liquid meals. I say "last resort" because such a restriction takes much of the pleasure out of eating, but it may be the only way to assure near-normal blood sugars. With this degree of improvement, the gastroparesis will slowly reverse, as mine did. The restriction can then eventually be removed. In this section I'll try to give you some ideas that you can use to create meal plans using semiliquid foods that still follow our guidelines.

Baby food. Low-carbohydrate vegetables and nearly zero-carbohydrate meat, chicken, and egg yolk protein meals are readily available as baby food. Remember to read the labels. Also remember that for a typical protein food, 6 grams of protein on the label corresponds to about 1 ounce of the food itself by weight. To avoid protein malnutrition, you must consume at least 0.8 grams of protein for every kilogram (2.2 pounds) of ideal body weight. Thus, a slim person weighing 150 pounds should consume at least 54 grams of protein daily. This works out to 9 ounces of protein foods. People who are still growing or who exercise vigorously must consume considerably more than 0.8 grams per kilogram of ideal body weight.

I've already pointed out that when vegetables that only slowly raise blood sugar are ground or mashed, they can raise blood sugar more rapidly. How, therefore, can we justify the use of baby foods? The answer is obvious. We only recommend such foods for people whose stomach already empties very slowly. Thus even with baby food your blood sugar may still have difficulty keeping pace with injected regular insulin. As you will see later in this chapter, we still have some tricks for circumventing this problem.

Below is a brief list of some typical baby foods that can be worked into the meal-planning guidelines set forth in Chapters 10 and 11. Do not exceed those guidelines for carbohydrate, since most of the Laws of Small Numbers still apply, even if you have gastroparesis.

Vegetables	Carbohydrate
Beech Nut Green Beans (4.5-ounce jar)	8 grams
Beech Nut Garden Vegetables (4.5-ounce jar)	11
Heinz Squash (4.5-ounce jar)	8

Meats — Strained	Protein
Beef (3-ounce jar)	2.25 ounces
Chicken (3-ounce jar)	2.25
Ham (3-ounce jar)	2.25
Egg Yolks (3-ounce jar)	1.50 (plus 1 gram carbohydrate)

Unflavored whole-milk yogurt. Some brands of yogurt, such as Erivan, have no added sugars or fruits. As noted previously, Erivan is sold at health food stores throughout the United States. Again, always specify "whole-milk, unflavored." Remember that "low-fat" dairy foods usually contain more carbohydrate than the whole-milk product.

Erivan yogurt contains 11 grams of carbohydrate and 2 ounces protein per 8-ounce container.

Bland foods like plain yogurt can be made quite tasty by adding one of the sources of carbohydrate-free flavorings listed on page 137. The amounts used should suit your taste.

Whole-milk ricotta cheese. While not as liquid as yogurt or baby food, ricotta cheese goes down better than solid foods. It can also be put into a blender with some water or cream to render it more liquid. Each 8-ounce serving of ricotta contains about 8 grams of carbohydrate and 2 ounces protein. To my taste, ricotta is a very bland food, but when flavored with carbohydrate-free flavorings, it can be a real treat.

Liquid meals. When semiliquid meals are not fully successful, the last resort is high-protein, low-carbohydrate liquid meals. These are sold in health food stores for use by bodybuilders. They should be used only under the supervision of your physician.

TREATING LOW BLOOD SUGARS WHEN YOUR STOMACH IS SLOW TO EMPTY

A patient from Indiana with a hiatal hernia once told me, "These Dextrotabs don't raise my blood sugar one bit. What really works is one stick of that sugar-free chewing gum."

Her comment illustrates a major hazard associated with any condition that retards stomach-emptying (gastroparesis, ulcers, and so on): it's nearly impossible to treat hypoglycemia rapidly. Note the qualifier, "nearly." There are some tricks to circumvent the problem.

If your hypoglycemia occurred because your last meal is still sitting in your stomach, you might try some chewing gum to help it empty.

Since chewed glucose tablets can take several hours to leave your stomach, you should try a liquid glucose solution. Such a product is available as glucose-tolerance test beverage under a number of brand names in the United States. These include Glucola, Limeondex, Dexicola, and Sun-Dex. The drinks are bottled by manufacturers of clinical laboratory reagents and are stocked in every hospital lab and private clinical laboratory. If your physician cannot get you a few cases, call Harrison Chemists, (800) 829-1493. Pick a flavor — cola, orange, or lemon-lime. Glucose-tolerance test beverage comes in 10-ounce glass bottles with screw caps. Each ounce contains 10 grams of glucose. One teaspoon will raise the blood sugar of a 150-pound adult about 8 mg/dl and 1 tablespoon by about 25 mg/dl. If you don't have a tablespoon handy and are in a hurry, assume that one swallow from the bottle is equivalent to 1 tablespoon.

If you're traveling and forget to bring along a bottle of your glucose-tolerance test beverage, get some lactose-free milk. This product has been treated with an enzyme that converts the lactose to glucose. In the United States, the most widely marketed brand is Lactaid. Every 4 ounces contains 6 grams of glucose and will raise the blood sugar of a typical 150-pound adult by 30 mg/dl. Remember, however, that Lactaid will spoil after a few days if not refrigerated.

Even if you've used the glucose-tolerance test drink or Lactaid, you can speed up the action by chewing gum or doing the back-flex and stomach exercises described earlier in this chapter.

MODIFICATIONS OF PREPRANDIAL INSULIN OR OHA REGIMENS TO ACCOMMODATE DELAYED STOMACH-EMPTYING

It takes a while for your physician to select and fine-tune a program to improve stomach-emptying. In the meantime, it's possible to reduce the frequency and severity of postprandial hypoglycemia. To do this, you must *slow the action* of preprandial insulin or OHA to match more closely the delay you experience in digesting your meals.

Let's suppose, for example, that you'll be using a preprandial OHA. If you have gastroparesis, your doctor may ask you to take it 10, 30, or 45 minutes before eating, instead of the usual 60–120 minutes. If you'll be getting preprandial shots of regular insulin, your physician may want you to inject immediately before eating, instead of the usual 40 minutes. If regular still works too rapidly for your slow digestion, you may be asked to take it *after* your meal. Alternately, you might substitute 1 or more units of lente for 1 or more units of regular in your syringe, to slow the action. If, for example, you are asked to inject a preprandial mixture containing 4 units of regular and 1 unit of lente, you would draw the 4 units of regular into the syringe in the usual manner (see pages 203–204). Now, insert the needle into the vial of lente and shake the vial and syringe together vigorously a few times, as illustrated in Figure 15-6.

Immediately but carefully draw 1 unit of lente into the syringe. Now remove the needle from the vial and draw in about 3 units of air. The exact amount of air is not important. The air bubble will act a bit like the metal ball in a can of spray paint to help mix the insulins. Invert the syringe a few times to permit the air bubble to move back and forth, thereby mixing the two insulins.

Now you can inject the contents of the syringe, including the air. This tiny amount of air will dissolve in your tissue fluids and cannot do any harm.

If this process confuses you, don't worry. Your physician or diabetes educator should demonstrate it for you and check your technique.

If you use this procedure to slow down your preprandial dose of regular insulin, it'll keep working for an unknown period of time beyond the usual 5 hours. If you routinely correct elevated blood sugars with additional shots of lispro as described on page 241, you now have a real problem — when do you correct an elevated blood sugar?

The answer is actually simple. Under these conditions, you are limited to correcting a high blood sugar only once daily — when you arise in the morning. This will be about 12 hours after your suppertime shot of the regular-lente mixture. Twelve hours is enough time for the mixture to have finished acting.

Do not use lispro to cover meals if you have delayed stomach-emptying. The reasoning here should be self-evident. Feel free, however, to use it to bring down an elevated blood sugar using the methods previously mentioned.

THOUGH "CURABLE," GASTROPARESIS IS SERIOUS BUSINESS

The effects upon blood sugar of even asymptomatic (symptom-free) delayed stomach-emptying from any cause can be dramatic. Don't think that because you have no symptoms you're free from its effects upon blood sugar. If you're uncertain, ask your physician to perform an R-R interval study. If you're following the guidelines of this book and your blood sugars are still unpredictable, suggest that he or she read this book.

22

Routine Follow-up Visits to Your Physician

Taking responsibility for the care of your own diabetes may force you to break habits that have been with you for many years. It also requires the establishment of new habits, such as exercise and blood sugar self-monitoring, that are easier to avoid than to follow.

Once your blood sugars have become controlled, it may only take a few months for you conveniently to forget about the pain you used to have in your toes, or the parent or friend who lost a leg or vision due to complications of diabetes, and so on. As time goes on, you will find that with diabetes, as with life in general, you will gradually tend to do what is easiest or most enjoyable at the moment. This backsliding is quite common. When I haven't seen a patient for six months, I'll usually take a meal history, and find that some of the basic dietary guidelines have been forgotten. Concurrently blood sugar profiles, glycosylated hemoglobin levels, lipid profiles, and even fibrinogen levels have deteriorated. Such deterioration can be short-circuited when I see patients every two months. We all need a little nudge to get back on track, and it seems that a time frame of about two months does the trick for most of us. I was not the first diabetologist to observe this, and your physician may likewise want you to visit him at similar intervals.

Dosage requirements for insulin or OHAs may change over time, whether due to weight changes, to deterioration or improvement of beta cell output, or just to seasonal temperature changes. So there's an ongoing need for readjustment of these medications. Again, two-month intervals are appropriate.

What are some of the things that your physician may want to examine at these follow-up visits?

First of all, your doctor will try to answer any new questions that you may have. These may cover a host of subjects, from something you read in the newspaper to new physical complaints or dissatisfaction with your diet. Write down your questions in advance, so that you won't forget them.

Your physician will, of course, want to review your blood sugar data sheets covering a period of one or two weeks. It makes no sense for your doctor to review prior data, as that is old history. If he or she wants to adjust your medications or meal plan, the changes should be based upon current information. Remember, however, that the data must be complete and honest. This means, for example, that if you spent a few hours shopping or overate, it should be noted on your data sheet. It doesn't make sense, and can be dangerous, for your doctor to change your medications based upon high blood sugars caused by a few unrecorded dietary indiscretions.

Your physician will also want to draw some blood. At each visit your HgbA$_{1C}$ (glycosylated hemoglobin) should be checked. You need not be fasting for this test. At least once annually, a complete lipid profile should be performed, and fibrinogen levels should be checked; also check lipoprotein(a), if you can afford the cost. Kidney function studies should also be made. You'll recall that these require a 24-hour urine collection, which must be completed on the day of the visit (see Chapter 2). Remember that the "normal values" for lipid profiles are based upon fasting determinations. So if your physician has planned a lipid profile, try to book an early-morning appointment, and don't eat breakfast. If you skip breakfast be sure also to skip your preprandial insulin or OHA, if you usually use these medications. Do not omit glucose tablets or Humalog (lispro) needed to correct low or elevated blood sugars. Also remember to take your basal dose of OHA or long-acting insulin, as the purpose of these is merely to hold blood sugar level while fasting. Your physician may also want to perform other blood tests from time to time, such as a blood count and a chemical profile.

A partial physical examination should be performed every two months. Usually the most important element of these visits should be examination of your feet. Such an examination is not merely to look for injuries, blisters, or what have you. Equally important is the discovery of dry skin, athlete's foot, pressure points from ill-fitting shoes, ingrown or fungus-infected toenails, and calluses. Any of these can cause or may indicate problems that could lead to ulcers of the feet and should be corrected. Dry skin is best treated with daily applications of animal or vegetable oils such as vitamin E oil, olive oil, purified mink oil, or emulsified lanolin. The cure for ill-fitting shoes is new shoes (possibly custom-made) with a wide toe box and a deep rise. Calluses frequently require the purchase of custom orthotics that redistribute the pressure on the bottoms of your feet. Grinding off calluses is not the solution, as calluses are a symptom, not a cause, of excess pressure.

Resting blood pressures, repeated every few minutes until the lowest reading is obtained, are mandatory at every visit if your blood pressure is even slightly elevated. If your blood pressure is usually normal, it should be checked every twelve months anyway.

Over the course of a year or two, other aspects of physical examination should be performed. All the tests need not be done at one visit, but may be staggered. These include oscillometric studies of the blood circulation in your legs, an electrocardiogram, tests for sensation in your feet, and a complete eye exam. The eye exam should include pupillary reflexes, visual acuity, intraocular pressure, the Amsler grid test, a test for double vision, and examination of your lenses and retinas through dilated pupils. This last exam must be performed with certain specialized equipment that should include direct and indirect ophthalmoscopes and a slit lamp. If your physician is not so equipped, or if he has previously found vision-threatening changes in your eyes, you should be referred to an ophthalmologist or retinologist.

The best treatment for the complications of diabetes is prevention. The second best treatment is detection in the very early stages, while reversal is still possible. For these reasons, I strongly recommend visits to your physician every two months, or at least every three months.

23

What You Can Expect from Virtually Normal Blood Sugars

I am convinced, from my personal experience, from the experiences of my patients, and from reading the scientific literature, that people with normal blood sugars do not develop the long-term complications of diabetes. I am further convinced that diabetics with slightly elevated blood glucose profiles may eventually develop some of the long-term complications of diabetes, but they will develop more slowly and likely be less severe. In this chapter, I will try to describe some of the changes that I and other physicians have observed when the blood sugars of our patients dramatically improve.

MENTAL CHANGES

Most common, perhaps, is the feeling of being more alert, and no longer chronically tired. Many people who "feel perfectly fine" before their blood sugars are normalized comment later that they had no idea they could feel so much better.

Another common occurrence relates to short-term memory. Very frequently patients or spouses will refer to their "terrible memory." When I first began my medical practice, I would ask patients to phone me at night with their blood sugar data for fine-tuning of medications. My wife, a physician specializing in psychoanalytic medicine, sometimes overheard my end of the conversation and would comment, "That person has a dementia." Weeks later, she would again hear my end of a conversation with the same individual, and would comment on the great improvement of short-term memory. This became so common that I introduced an objective test for short-term memory into the neurologic exam that I perform on all new patients. About half my new patients indeed display this mild form of dementia, which appears to lift after several weeks of improved blood sugar. The improvement is usually quite apparent to spouses.

DIABETIC NEUROPATHIES

Diabetic neuropathies seem to improve in two phases — a rapid partial improvement that may occur within weeks, followed by sustained very slow improvement that goes on for years if blood sugars continue to remain normal. This is most apparent with numbness or pain in the toes. Some people will even comment, "I know right away if my blood sugar is high, because my toes feel numb again." On the other hand, several patients with total numbness of their feet have complained of severe pain after several months of near normal blood sugars. This continues for a number of months and eventually resolves as sensation returns. It is as if nerves generate pain signals while they heal or "sprout." The experience is very frightening and distressing, especially if you haven't been warned that it might occur.

Erectile impotence affects about half of diabetic males, and is the result of years of elevated blood sugars. It may be defined as an inability to maintain a rigid enough penile erection for adequate time to perform intercourse. It usually results from neuropathy, blocked blood vessels, or both. We can perform simple tests to determine which of these causes predominates. When the problem is principally neurologic, I frequently hear the comment, sometimes after only a few weeks of near-normal blood sugar profiles, "Hey, I'm able to have intercourse again!" Unfortunately, this turnaround only appears to occur if the man was able to attain at least partial erections before. If at the original interview, I'm told, "Doc, it's been dead for years," I know recovery is unlikely to occur. If testing shows that the problem was due primarily to blocked blood vessels, I never see improvement. Note, however, that it's normal to be unable to have erections when blood sugars are too low, say below 75 mg/dl.

Another remarkable change relates to autonomic neuropathy and associated gastroparesis. I have documented major improvement of R-R interval studies in many patients, and total normalization in a few. Along with this, we see reduction in symptoms of gastroparesis. Usually such improvement takes place over a period of years. Although it occurs most dramatically in younger people, I've also seen it occur in seventy-year-olds.

VISION IMPROVEMENTS

Diplopia, or double vision, is caused by neuropathy of the nerves that activate the muscles that move the eyes. It is a very common finding on physical examination, but rarely severe enough to be noticed by patients on a day-to-day basis. Here, again, when testing is redone after a few years, we find improvement or even total cures with blood sugar improvement.

Vacuoles are tiny bubbles in the lens of the eye. They are thought to be precursors of cataracts. I have seen a number of these vanish after a year or two of improved blood sugars. I have even seen the disappearance of small spokes on the lens that signify very early cataracts.

I've seen cases of glaucoma cured by normalization of blood sugars.

OTHER IMPROVEMENTS

Improvements in risk factors for heart disease, such as mild hypertension, HDL-cholesterol ratios, triglycerides, and fibrinogen levels, are commonplace. They usually can be observed after about two months.

Similarly, improvements in early changes noted on renal risk profiles are often obtained, usually after one or two years, but sometimes after a few months.

Most dramatic and commonplace is the feeling of satisfaction and control that nearly everyone experiences when they produce normal blood sugar profiles. This is especially true for individuals who had already been taking insulin, but appears also to occur in those who do not take insulin.

Last but not least is the feeling that we are not doomed to share the fate of others we have known, who died prematurely after years of disabling or painful diabetic complications. We come to realize that with the ability to control our blood sugars comes the ability to prevent the consequences of high blood sugars.

I have long maintained that diabetics are entitled to the same blood sugars as nondiabetics. But it is up to us to see that we achieve this goal.

What About the Widely Advocated Dietary Restrictions on Fat, Protein, and Salt, and the Current High-Fiber Fad?

Most of this book is instructional, of the how-to variety. The intent of this appendix is to provide you with a little of the science that surrounds the program described in the rest of the book. I hope that I can cut through some of the myths that cloud diet and the treatment of diabetic complications so that you will have the why that supports the how-to. We've already discussed some of the myths. We'll look at the origins of those myths to try to give you as many of the facts as are available at this writing. If your only interest is in the how-to, feel free to skip this chapter.

Once you've started to follow a restricted-carbohydrate diet, you may find yourself pressured by well-meaning but uninformed friends or family, or even newspaper articles, to cease penalizing yourself and eat more "fun" foods, sweets, and treats. This chapter will provide you with specific scientific information that underpins my philosophy and will perhaps give you some ammunition for responding to this pressure. Even if you skip it now, you may want to come back to it later, or show it to your loved ones to lay their concerns to rest. As I don't expect most readers to be scientists, I've tried to keep all these explanations relatively simple. Some of the explanations may at this moment represent more theory than fact, but they're based on the latest information available to us.

HOW DID THE COMMONLY PRESCRIBED
HIGH-CARBOHYDRATE DIET COME ABOUT?

If, like me, you've had diabetes for a while, you've probably been told to cut way down on your dietary intake of fat, protein, and salt, and to eat lots of complex carbohydrate. You may even have read this advice in publications circulated to diabetic patients.

Why is such advice being promulgated, when the major cause of such diabetic complications as heart disease, kidney disease, high blood pressure, and blindness is high blood sugar?

When I first developed diabetes, in 1947, little was known about why this disease, even when treated, caused early death and such distressing complications. Prior to the availability of insulin, about twenty-five years earlier, people with Type I diabetes usually died within a few months of diagnosis. Their lives could be prolonged somewhat with a diet that was very low in carbohydrate and usually high in fat. Sufferers from the milder Type II diabetes frequently survived on this type of diet, without supplemental medication. When I became diabetic, oral hypo-glycemic agents were not available, and many people were still following very low carbohydrate, high-fat diets. It was at about this time that diets very high in saturated fats, with resultant high serum cholesterol levels, were experimentally shown to correlate with blood vessel and heart disease in animals. It was promptly assumed by many physicians that the complications of diabetes, nearly all of which related to abnormalities of large or small blood vessels, were caused by the high-fat diets. I and many other diabetics were therefore treated with a high-carbohydrate, low-fat diet. This new diet was adopted in the mid-1940s by the ADA, the New York Heart Association, and eventually by the American Heart Association (AHA) and other groups around the world. On the new diet, many of us had even higher serum cholesterol levels, and still developed the grave long-term complications of diabetes. Seemingly unaware of the importance of blood sugar control, the ADA raised the recommended carbohydrate content to 40 percent of calories, and then more recently to 60 percent.

RECENT DEVELOPMENTS REGARDING RISK FACTORS FOR HEART DISEASE

In the past twenty years, research studies have generated considerable new information about heart disease and vascular (blood vessel) disease in general, and their relationship to diabetes in particular. Some of this more recent information is summarized here.

A number of fatty substances have been found in the blood which relate to risk of heart attacks and vascular disease. These include HDL (high-density lipoprotein), LDL (low-density lipoprotein), triglyceride, fibrinogen, and lipoprotein(a). High serum levels of LDL, triglyceride, fibrinogen, and lipoprotein(a) tend to increase cardiovascular risk, while high levels of HDL tend to protect from cardiovascular disease. Cholesterol is a component of both LDL and HDL particles. The fraction of total cholesterol found in LDL particles is an index of risk, while the fraction of cholesterol found in HDL particles is an index of protection. Nowadays, when we want to estimate the effects of *lipids* upon the risk of coronary artery disease, we look at the ratio of total cholesterol to HDL and also at fasting triglyceride levels. Someone with high serum HDL can thus have a high total cholesterol and yet be at low statistical risk for a heart attack. Conversely, a person with low total cholesterol and very low HDL may be at high risk.

Recently a very large multicenter study (the Lipid Research Clinics Trial) investigated the effects of a low-fat, high-carbohydrate diet on middle-aged men. The study followed 1,900 people for seven years. Throughout this period, total cholesterol had dropped 5 percent from baseline in the low-fat group, but serum triglyceride went up about 10 percent! (Serum triglyceride rises very rapidly after a high-carbohydrate meal in nondiabetics, and moves up and down with blood sugar levels in most diabetics.) As with prior studies, no significant correlation was found between serum cholesterol levels and mortality rates.

On average, diabetics with chronically high blood sugars have elevated levels of LDL (the "bad" cholesterol) and depressed levels of HDL (the "good" cholesterol), even though the ADA low-fat diet has now been in use for many years. Of great importance is the recent discovery that the forms of LDL that harm arteries are small, dense LDL, oxidized LDL, and glycosylated LDL. All of these increase as blood sugar increases. In addition, independently of blood sugars, high serum insulin levels caused by high-carbohydrate diets bring about increased production of small, dense LDL particles and enlargement of the cells lining and surrounding arteries.

Under normal conditions, receptors in the liver remove LDL from the bloodstream and signal the liver to reduce its manufacture of LDL when serum levels rise even slightly. Glucose may bind to the surface of the LDL particle and also to liver LDL receptors, so that LDL cannot be recognized by its receptors. In people with high blood sugars, many LDL particles thus become glycosylated, and are therefore not cleared by the liver. They accumulate in the blood, where they can become incorporated into the walls of arteries, forming fatty deposits called atherotic plaques. Since liver LDL production cannot be turned off by the glycosylated LDL (and also the presence of glycosylated LDL receptors), the liver continues to manufacture more LDL, even though serum levels may be elevated.

The proteins in the walls of arteries can also become glycosylated, rendering them sticky. Other proteins in the blood then stick to the arterial walls, causing further buildup of plaque.

Serum proteins also glycosylate in the presence of glucose. White blood cells called macrophages ingest glycosylated proteins and glycosylated LDL. The loaded macrophages swell up, becoming very large. These transformed macrophages, loaded with fatty material, are called foam cells. The foam cells penetrate the sticky arterial walls, causing disruption of the orderly architecture of the artery, and narrow the channel through which blood can flow.

In recent years, the tendency of blood to clot has come into focus as a major cause of heart attacks. People whose blood clots too readily are at very high risk. You may recall that one of the medical names for a heart attack is coronary thrombosis. A thrombus is a clot, and coronary thrombosis refers to the formation of a large clot in one of the arteries that feed the heart. People who have elevated levels of certain clotting precursors or depressed levels of clotting inhibitors in their blood are at high risk of dying from heart attacks. The risk probably far exceeds that caused by high LDL or low HDL. Some of the blood factors that enhance clotting include fibrinogen and factor VII. Another factor, lipoprotein(a) — abbreviated Lp(a) — inhibits the destruction of small thrombi before they become large enough to cause a heart attack. All of these factors have been found to increase in people with chronically high blood sugars. Platelets, or thrombocytes, are particles in the blood that play major roles in the blocking of arteries and the formation of clots. These have been shown to clump together and stick to arterial walls much more aggressively in people with high blood sugars. What is exciting is that all of these factors, including sticky platelets, tend to normalize as long-term blood sugars improve.

Diabetics die from heart failure at a rate far exceeding that of people with normal glucose tolerance. Heart failure involves a weakening of the cardiac muscle so that it cannot pump enough blood. Most long-term, poorly controlled diabetics have a condition called cardiomyopathy. In diabetic cardiomyopathy, the muscle tissue of the heart is slowly replaced by scar tissue over a period of years. This weakens the muscle so that it eventually "fails." There is no evidence linking cardiomyopathy with dietary fat intake or serum lipids.

A fifteen-year study of 7,038 French policemen in Paris reported that "the earliest marker of a higher risk of coronary heart disease mortality is an elevation of serum insulin level." A study of middle-aged nondiabetic women at the University of Pittsburgh showed an increasing risk of heart disease as serum insulin levels increased. Other studies in nondiabetics have shown strong correlations between serum insulin levels and other predictors of cardiac risk such as hypertension, elevated triglyceride, and low HDL. The importance of elevated serum insulin levels (hyperinsulinemia) as a cause of heart disease and hypertension has taken on such importance that a special symposium on this subject was held at the end of the 1990 annual meeting of the ADA. A report in a subsequent issue of the journal *Diabetes Care* quite appropriately points out that "there are few available methods of treating diabetes that do not result in systemic hyperinsulinemia" unless the patient is following a low-carbohydrate diet.

Although the AHA and the ADA have been recommending low-fat, high-carbohydrate diets for diabetics for many decades, no one had compared the effects on the same patients of low- versus high-carbohydrate diets until the late 1980s. Independent studies performed in Texas and California demonstrated lower levels of blood sugar *and* improved blood lipids when patients were put on lower-carbohydrate, high-fat diets. It was also shown that, on average, for every 1 percent increase in $HgbA_{1C}$ (the test for average blood sugar over the prior four months), total serum cholesterol rose 2.2 percent and triglycerides increased 8 percent.

The National Health Examination Follow-Up Survey, which followed 4,710 people, reported in 1990 that "in the instance of total blood cholesterol, we found no evidence in any age-sex group of a risk associated with elevated values." That's right — they found *no risk* associated directly with elevated total cholesterol. On the same page, this study lists diabetes as by far the single most important risk factor affecting mortality. In males aged 55–64, for example, diabetes was associated with 60 percent greater mortality than smoking and double the mortality associated with high blood pressure.

The evidence is now simply overwhelming that elevated blood sugar is the major cause of the high serum lipid levels among diabetics and, more significantly, the major factor in the high rates of various heart and vascular diseases associated with diabetes. Many diabetics were put on low-fat diets for so many years, and yet these problems didn't stop. It is only logical to look elsewhere, to elevated blood sugar and hyperinsulinemia, for the cause of what kills and disables so many of us.

My personal experience with diabetic patients is very simple. When we reduce dietary carbohydrate, blood sugars improve dramatically. After about two months of improved blood sugars, we repeat our studies of lipid profiles and thrombotic risk factors. In the great majority of cases, I see normalization or improvement of abnormalities. This parallels what happened to me nearly thirty years ago when I abandoned the high-carbohydrate, low-fat diet that I had been following since 1947.*

WHY IS PROTEIN RESTRICTION SO COMMON?

About 30 percent of diabetics develop kidney disease (nephropathy). Diabetes is the greatest single cause of kidney failure in the United States. Early kidney changes can be found within two to three years of the onset of high blood sugars. As we discussed briefly in Chapter 9, the common restrictions on protein intake by diabetic patients derive from

---

* If your physician finds all of this hard to believe, he might read the seventy articles and abstracts on this subject contained in the Proceedings of the Fifteenth International Diabetes Foundation Satellite Symposium on "Diabetes and Macrovascular Complications," *Diabetes* 45, Supplement 3, July 1996. Also worth reading is "Effects of Varying Carbohydrate Content of Diet in Patients with Non-Insulin Dependent Diabetes Mellitus," by Garg et al., *Jnl Amer Med Assoc* 1994; 271:1421–1428.

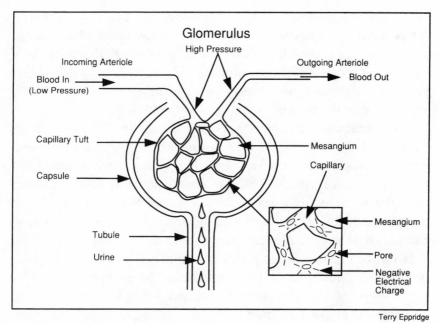

Terry Eppridge

Fig. A-1. *The microscopic filtration*
unit of the kidneys

fear regarding this problem, and ignorance of the actual causes of diabetic kidney disease.

By looking at how the kidney functions, one can better understand the relative roles of glucose and protein in kidney failure of diabetes. The kidney filters wastes, glucose, drugs, and other potentially toxic materials from the blood and deposits them into the urine. It is the urine-making organ. A normal kidney contains about 6 million microscopic blood filters, called glomeruli. Figure A-1 illustrates how blood enters a glomerulus through a tiny artery called the incoming arteriole. The arteriole feeds a bundle of tiny vessels called capillaries. The capillaries contain tiny holes or pores that carry a negative electrical charge. The downstream ends of the capillaries merge into an outgoing arteriole, which is narrower than the incoming arteriole. This narrowing results in high fluid pressure when blood flows through the capillary tuft. The high pressure forces some of the water in the blood through the pores of the capillaries. This water dribbles into the capsule surrounding the capillary tuft. The capsule, acting like a funnel, empties the water into a pipelike structure called the tubule. The pores of the capillaries are of such a size that small molecules in the blood, such as glucose and urea, can pass through with the water to form urine. In a normal kidney, large molecules, such as proteins, cannot readily get through the pores. Since most blood proteins carry negative electrical charges, even the smaller proteins in the blood cannot easily get through the pores, because they are repelled by the negative charge on each pore.

The glomerular filtration rate (GFR) is a measure of how much filtering the kidneys perform in a given period of time. Anyone with a high blood sugar and normal kidneys will have an excessively high GFR. This is in part because blood glucose draws water into the bloodstream from the surrounding tissues, thus increasing blood volume, blood pressure, and blood flow through the kidneys. A GFR that is one-and-a-half to two times normal is commonplace in diabetics with high blood sugars prior to the onset of permanent injury to their kidneys. These people may typically have as much glucose in a 24-hour urine collection as the weight of 5 to 50 packets of sugar. According to an Italian study, an increase in blood sugar from 80 mg/dl to 272 mg/dl resulted in an average GFR increase of 40 percent even in diabetics with severe kidney disease. Before we knew about glycosylation of proteins and the other toxic effects of glucose upon blood vessels, it was speculated that the cause of diabetic kidney disease (nephropathy) was this excessive filtration (hyperfiltration).

The metabolism of dietary protein produces waste products such as urea and ammonia, which contain nitrogen. It therefore had been speculated that in order to clear these wastes from the blood, people eating large amounts of protein would have elevated GFRs. As a result, diabetics have been urged to reduce their protein intake to low levels. Studies by an Israeli group, however, of people on high-protein (meat-eating) and very low protein (vegetarian) diets, disclosed no difference in GFR. Furthermore, over many years on these diets, kidney function was unchanged between the two groups. A report from Denmark described a study in which Type I diabetics without discernible kidney disease were put on protein-restricted diets, and experienced a very small change in GFR and no change in other measures of kidney function. These would suggest that the currently prevailing admonition to all diabetics to reduce protein intake is unjustified.

Recent studies on diabetic rats have shown the following: Rats with blood sugars maintained at 250 mg/dl rapidly develop diabetic nephropathy. If their dietary protein is increased, kidney destruction accelerates. Diabetic rats at the same laboratory, with blood sugars maintained at 100 mg/dl, live full lives and never develop nephropathy, no matter how much protein they consume. Diabetic rats with high blood sugars and significant nephropathy have shown total reversal of their kidney disease after blood sugars were normalized for several months.

Other studies have enabled researchers to piece together a scenario for the causes of diabetic nephropathy, where glycosylation of proteins, abnormal clotting factors, abnormal platelets, antibodies to glycosylated proteins, and so on, join together to injure glomerular capillaries. Early injury may only cause reduction of electrical charge on the pores. As a result, negatively charged proteins such as albumin leak through the pores and appear in the urine. Glycosylated proteins leak through pores much earlier than normal proteins. High blood pressure, and especially high serum insulin levels, can increase GFR and force even more protein to leak through the pores. If some of these proteins are glycosylated, they will stick to the mesangium, the tissue between the capillaries. Examination of diabetic glomeruli indeed discloses large deposits of glycosylated proteins and antibodies to glycosylated proteins in capillary walls and mesangium. As these deposits increase, the mesangium compresses the capillaries, causing pressure in the capillaries to increase and larger proteins to leak from the pores. This leads to more thickening of the mesangium, more compression of the capillaries, and acceleration of destruction. Eventually the mesangium and capillaries become a mass of scar tissue. Independently of this, both high blood sugars and glycosylated proteins cause mesangial cells to produce type IV collagen, a fibrous material that further increases their bulk.

Many studies performed on humans show that when blood sugars improve, GFR improves and less protein leaks into the urine. When blood sugars remain high, however, there is further deterioration. There is a point of no return, where a glomerulus has been so injured that no amount of blood sugar improvement can revive it.

Nowadays many diabetics who have lost all kidney function are treated by artificial kidneys (dialysis machines) that remove nitrogenous wastes from the blood. In order to reduce the weekly number of dialysis treatments, which are costly and unpleasant, patients are severely restricted in their consumption of dietary protein. Instead of using large amounts of carbohydrate to replace the lost calories, many dialysis centers now recommend olive oil to their diabetics. Olive oil is high in monounsaturated fats, which are believed to lower the risk of heart disease.

In summary: Diabetic nephropathy does not appear if blood sugar is kept normal. Dietary protein does not cause diabetic nephropathy, but can possibly (still uncertain) accelerate the process once there has been a considerable amount of kidney damage. Dietary protein has no substantial effect upon the GFR of healthy kidneys, certainly not in comparison to the GFR increase caused by elevated blood sugar levels.*

RESTRICTIONS ON SALT INTAKE: ARE THEY REASONABLE FOR ALL DIABETICS?

Many diabetics have hypertension, or high blood pressure. About half of all people with hypertension will experience blood pressure elevations when they eat substantial amounts of salt. Hypertension accelerates glomerulopathy (destruction of the glomerulus) in people with chronically elevated blood sugars, but in Type I diabetes, hypertension usually appears after, not before, the appearance of significant amounts of albumin in the urine. Is it therefore appropriate to ask all diabetics to lower their salt intake?[†] Let us look at a few of the mechanisms involved in the hypertension that some diabetics experience.

People with advanced glomerulopathy will inevitably develop hypertension in part because GFR is severely diminished. These people can-

---

* Your physician might find informative the following articles on this subject: "Molecular and Physiological Aspects of Nephropathy in Type I Diabetes Mellitus," by Raskin and Tamborlane, *Jnl Diabetes and Its Complications,* 1996, 10:31–37; "The Effects of Dietary Protein Restriction and Blood Pressure Control on the Progression of Chronic Renal Disease," by S. Klahr et al., *New England Jnl Med,* 1994, 330:877–884; also, in the same issue of *New England Jnl Med,* the editorial "The Role of Dietary Protein Restriction in Progressive Azotemia" (pp. 929–930).

† A study of older individuals who were rotated between low-, moderate-, and high-salt diets demonstrated that those on low-salt diets experienced significantly more sleep disturbances, and had more rapid heart rates and higher serum norepinephrine (adrenaline) levels. An international study called Intersalt, covering 10,079 people in 32 countries, reported in 1988 that "salt has only small importance in hypertension." More recently, another study showed that salt restriction increases insulin resistance and thus can indirectly increase blood pressure.

not make enough urine, and therefore retain water. Excessive water in the blood causes elevated blood pressure. There are many other ways hypertension can be caused by high blood sugars.

The mere presence of high blood sugar will cause water to leave tissues and enter the bloodstream, even experimentally in nondiabetics. It is not unusual to observe reduction in blood pressure concomitant with control of blood sugar. Studies have shown that many, and possibly most, hypertensive nondiabetics are insulin-resistant, and therefore have high serum insulin levels. In addition to causing elevation of serum triglycerides and reduction in serum HDL in nondiabetics, high serum insulin levels have long been known to foster salt and water retention by the kidneys. Furthermore, excessive insulin stimulates the sympathetic nervous system, which in turn speeds up the heart and constricts blood vessels, causing further increase in blood pressure. Thus Type II diabetics who eat lots of carbohydrate, and therefore will tend to make excessive insulin, can readily develop hypertension. Type I diabetics treated with the usual industrial doses of insulin to cover high-carbohydrate diets are likewise more susceptible to hypertension. One dramatic study showed that in hypertensive individuals, blood pressure is directly proportional to serum insulin level. A report from Nottingham, England, showed that a brief infusion of insulin and glucose would increase blood pressure in normal men without changing their blood sugars.

Why don't all diabetics on high-carbohydrate diets or all poorly controlled diabetics have hypertension?

One reason is that the body has several very efficient systems for unloading sodium (a component of salt) and water. One of the more important of these systems is controlled by a hormone manufactured in the heart called atrial naturietic factor (ANF). When the heart is expanded by even a slight fluid overload, it produces ANF. The ANF then signals the kidneys to unload sodium and water. Hypertensive individuals, and the children of two hypertensive parents, tend to produce much lower amounts of ANF than do normal people. Nonhypertensive diabetics apparently are able to produce enough ANF to control the blood pressure effects of high blood sugars and high serum insulin levels, provided they do not have moderately advanced kidney disease. Indeed, a study, in which some of my patients participated, showed that diabetics with high blood sugars produce significantly more ANF than those with lower blood sugars.

How does all this apply to you? First, you and your physician should know if you have glomerulopathy. This is readily determined if the tests suggested in Chapter 2 are performed. If these tests are abnormal, your physician may advise you to reduce your salt intake.

Whether your renal risk profile is normal or abnormal, your resting blood pressure should also be measured. A proper measurement requires that you first be seated in a *quiet* room, without conversation, for 15–30 minutes. Blood pressure should be measured every 5 minutes, until it drops to a low value and then starts to increase. The lowest reading is the significant one. If you get nervous in the doctor's office, then you should measure your own blood pressure at home in a similar fashion. Repeated measurements, with low values just exceeding 135/85, suggest that your blood pressure is "borderline." (The American Diabetes Association suggests that 120/80 be considered borderline for younger diabetics.) You may benefit from dietary salt reduction. The only way to find out is to check your blood pressure while on your current salt intake, and again after following a low-salt (sodium) diet for at least three weeks. Your physician can give you guidelines for such a diet, and you can consult nutritional tables such as those in the books listed in Chapter 3. I would suggest that resting blood pressures be measured several times a day, and at the same hours each day, throughout the study. Blood pressures can then be averaged, and the averages compared. If your blood pressure drops significantly on the low-salt diet, your physician may urge you to keep the salt intake down. Alternately, he may want you to take small amounts of supplemental potassium, which tends to offset the effects of dietary salt on blood pressure. Recent studies suggest that as many as 40 percent of hypertensive patients (the so-called low-renin hypertensives) may show lower blood pressures when they take calcium supplements.

WHAT ABOUT DIETARY FIBER?

"Fiber" is a general term that has come to refer to the undigestible portion of many vegetables and fruits. Some vegetable fibers, such as guar and pectin, are soluble in water. Another type of fiber, which some of us call roughage, is not water-soluble. Both types appear to affect the movement of food through the gut (soluble fiber slows processing in the upper digestive tract, while insoluble fiber speeds digestion farther down). Certain insoluble fiber products, such as psyllium, have long been used as laxatives. Consumption of large amounts of dietary fiber is usually unpleasant, because both types can cause abdominal discomfort, diarrhea, and flatulence. Sources of insoluble fiber include most salad vegetables. Soluble fiber is found in many beans, such as garbanzos, and in certain fruits, such as apples.

I first learned of attempts at using fiber as an adjunct to the treatment of diabetes about twenty years ago. At that time, Dr. David Jenkins, in England, reported that guar gum, when added to bread, could reduce the maximum postprandial blood sugar rise from an entire meal by 36 percent in diabetic subjects. This was interesting for several reasons. First of all, the discovery occurred at a time when few new approaches to controlling blood sugar had appeared in the medical literature. Second, I missed the high-carbohydrate foods I had given up, and hoped I might possibly reinstate some. I managed to track down a supplier of powdered guar gum, and placed a considerable amount into a folded slice of bread. I knew how much a slice of bread would affect my blood sugar, and so as an experiment, I used the same amount of guar gum that Dr. Jenkins had used, and then ate the concoction on an empty stomach. The chore was difficult, because once moistened by my saliva, the guar gum stuck to my palate and was difficult to swallow. I did not find any change in the subsequent blood sugar increase. Despite the unpleasantness of choking down powdered guar gum (which is often used in commercial products such as ice cream as a thickener), I repeated this experiment on two more occasions, with the same result. Subsequently, some investigators have announced results similar to those of Dr. Jenkins, yet other researchers have found no effect on postprandial blood sugar. In any event, a reduction of postprandial blood sugar by only 36 percent really isn't adequate for our purpose, since we're shooting for the same blood sugars as nondiabetics. This means virtually no rise after eating.

Dr. Jenkins also discovered, however, that the chronic use of guar gum resulted in a reduction of serum cholesterol levels. This is probably related to the considerable recirculation of cholesterol through the gut. The liver secretes some cholesterol into bile, which is released into the upper intestine. This cholesterol is later absorbed lower in the intestines, and eventually reappears in the blood. Guar binds the cholesterol in the gut, so that rather than being absorbed, it appears in the stool.

In the light of these very interesting results, other researchers studied the effect of foods (usually beans) containing other soluble forms of fiber. When beans were substituted for faster-acting forms of carbohydrate, postprandial blood sugars in diabetics increased more slowly, and the peaks were even slightly reduced. Serum cholesterol levels were also reduced by about 15 percent. But subsequent studies, reported in 1990, have uncovered flaws in the original reports, casting serious doubt upon any direct effect of these foods upon serum lipids. In any event, postprandial blood sugars were rarely normalized by such diets.

Many popular articles and books have appeared advocating "high-fiber" diets for everyone — not just diabetics. Somehow, "fiber" came to mean all fiber, not just soluble fiber, even though the only viable studies had utilized such products as guar gum and beans.

In my experience, reduction of dietary carbohydrate is far more effective in preventing blood sugar increases after meals. The lower blood sugars, in turn, bring about improved lipid profiles.

A recent food to join the high-fiber trend is oat bran. This has gotten a lot of play in the popular press. Recently, a patient of mine started substituting oat bran muffins for protein in her diet. Before she started, her $HgbA_{1C}$ (see Chapter 2) was within the normal range and her ratio of total cholesterol to HDL was very low (meaning her cholesterol risk ratio was low). After three months on oat bran, her $HgbA_{1C}$ became elevated and her cholesterol-to-HDL ratio nearly doubled. I tried one of her tiny oat bran muffins after first injecting 3 units of fast-acting insulin (nearly as much as I use for an entire meal). After 3 hours, my blood sugar went up by about 100 mg/dl, to 190 mg/dl. This illustrates the adverse effect that most oat bran preparations can have upon blood sugar. The reason for this is that most such preparations contain flour. On the other hand, I find that certain bran products, such as the bran crackers listed in Chapter 10, raise blood sugar very little. This is because, unlike most packaged bran products, they contain mostly bran and little flour. They therefore have very little carbohydrate. You can perform similar experiments yourself — just use your blood glucose meter. Beware of commercial "high-fiber" products that promise cholesterol reduction. If they contain carbohydrate, they must at least be counted in your meal plan and will probably render little or no improvement in your lipid profile.

Fiber, like carbohydrate, is not essential for a healthy life. Just look at the Eskimos and other hunting populations that survive almost exclusively on protein and fat, and don't develop cardiac or circulatory diseases.*

WHAT DIET WILL WORK FOR YOU?

Actual results are the yardstick for an appropriate diet. We have the tools for self-monitoring of blood sugar and blood pressure. We have tests for measuring kidney function, HgbA$_{1C}$, thrombotic risk profiles, and lipid profiles (see Chapter 2). Under your doctor's supervision, try our diet recommendations for at least two months. Then try any other diet plan for two months and see what happens. The differences may not be in the direction that the popular literature would predict.

---

* As this book was going to press, a report appeared entitled "Dietary Fiber, Glycemic Load, and Risk of Non-Insulin-Dependent Diabetes in Women" (*Jnl Amer Med Assoc* 1997; 277: 472–477). This study of 65,173 nurses and former nurses found a strong association between diets high in starch, flour, and sweet foods and the development of Type II diabetes. Furthermore, consumption of minimally refined grain (such as bran without flour) lowered this risk. The combination of high glycemic foods and low intake of unrefined insoluble fiber was associated with a 2.5-fold higher incidence of diabetes. If you remember our discussion of beta cell burnout (pages 38–40), this should come as no surprise.

Don't Permit Hospitalization to Impair Your Blood Sugar Control

I f ever it is necessary for you to become a hospital patient in the United States, the chances are overwhelming that no reasonable thought will be given to controlling your blood sugar. Most of the medical orthodoxy doesn't do it anywhere else, so why should they do it in the hospital?

The reasons, of course, are many: lack of blood sugar control skills on the part of most hospital medical staff; unawareness of the importance of normal or near-normal blood sugars in the face of illness or surgery; and an almost pathological fear of hypoglycemia (and the potential for lawsuits if it occurs). Many if not most hospital dietitians have been indoctrinated by the ADA, with the result that diabetic inpatients are forced to eat "normal" high-carbohydrate foods and are deprived of protein and fat. Some of my patients tell stories of having to sneak in their own insulin, throw out hospital food, and fight tooth and nail with well-meaning but uninformed hospital personnel.

Many studies of hospitalized patients have demonstrated that elevated blood sugar delays surgical healing, delays recovery from infections, and leaves patients open to new infection. It also has been shown to increase death rate of patients who have been hospitalized from heart attack or stroke, and increases the likelihood of a new stroke or heart attack.

What can you do to help keep your blood sugars under control while in the hospital?

Most of my patients live great distances from my office, so that I am not the admitting physician or surgeon when they are hospitalized, and as such I am not in a position to write their orders, help control their diets, and directly oversee their medical care.

After sharing the frustration of my patients over the years, I've come up with a letter that has worked repeatedly for elective hospitalization, such as for surgeries planned in advance. As you will see, it relies on the prevailing fear of litigation that appropriately permeates the medical care system in this country. This letter should be sent by you or your diabetologist to the admitting physician, with a copy to the hospital administrator. I've composed the letter as if you were writing it, since the odds are that you are not under the care of a diabetologist. It can, of course, be modified to suit your circumstances.

Dear Dr. _____:

*I am scheduled for admission to your hospital on _____, _____.
I have Type [I or II] diabetes and am naturally concerned about control of my blood sugars while hospitalized.*

It is now generally accepted that elevated blood sugar levels impede recovery, prolong hospitalization, and increase the incidence of hospital death. Major health problems brought about by inappropriate blood sugar elevations during hospitalization have justifiably led to litigation.

Since I have been successful at keeping my blood sugars essentially normal around the clock, I naturally expect equivalent care while I'm in the hands of medical professionals.

I currently take the following medications for controlling my blood sugars:

[List here doses, times, and purposes of medications: "basal insulin (or OHA) to cover the fasting state — must receive even if not eating," "prelunch (breakfast, supper) insulin (or OHA), to be skipped if meal is skipped." Detail also any use of insulin or glucose tablets for correcting off-target blood sugars, etc. Also indicate your target blood sugar. You may also include a sample GLUCOGRAF sheet and request that all medications used by the hospital be listed on it if you are not capable of listing them yourself.]

My hospital orders should call for a "normal diet" and not a "diabetic diet," so that I can select my own meals.

Routine intravenous fluids should not contain caloric substances such as glucose, fructose, lactose, or lactated Ringer's solution (except for treatment of blood sugars that are below my target). All of these substances will raise my blood sugar to unacceptable levels. Normal or half-normal saline solutions are perfectly adequate for routine hydration.

If I am conscious and without cognitive impairment, I should have full responsibility for treatment of my diabetes — without outside interference.

My blood sugar meter and blood sugar control medications, including insulin syringes, should not be confiscated by hospital personnel. This is a barbaric practice that is rapidly being abandoned in modern hospitals. *

If I am unable to care for my own blood sugars, I expect that the hospital staff will exercise every effort to maintain my blood sugars within the range of [00–00].

Sincerely,

cc: [Hospital administrator]
*   [Close relative or friend]*

---

* Many hospital pharmacies do not stock the products that we commonly utilize in this book, such as 25–30-unit insulin syringes, ultralente insulin, and Humalog (lispro).

APPENDIX C

Drugs That May Affect Blood Glucose Levels

By
MICHAEL D. JOHNSON, Pharm. D.
Clinical Instructor of Pharmacy Practice
Washington State University
   and
STEPHEN M. SETTER, Pharm. D.
Fellow in Geriatrics
Washington State University
   and
JOHN R. WHITE, JR., Pharm. D.
Associate Professor of Pharmacy Practice
Washington State University

The drugs included in this appendix are ones that have been documented to alter blood glucose levels. Patient response to a specific drug is highly variable, and can be affected by other treatments such as diet, exercise, route of administration or dosage of insulin or oral hypoglycemic agents, and so on. In the following tables, the level of expected response and the probability of such a response occurring is quantified by observing the following three significance levels:

+   Low probability of occurrence and/or low level of glucose alteration expected in most patients.

++   Probability of occurrence in most patients is high, but degree of glucose alteration may or may not be clinically significant.

+++   High probability of occurrence, clinically significant in many cases.

Drugs That May Increase Blood Glucose Levels

Drug	Mechanism of Action	Clinical Significance
acetazolamide (Diamox)	Unknown, but may enhance insulin elimination. Also may increase elimination of sulfonylureas.	+
alcohol (ethanol)	Chronic heavy ingestion may worsen glucose tolerance and may also increase the metabolism of tolbutamide (Orinase). Small quantities may result in chlorpropamide-alcohol flush reaction or hypoglycemia.	+
asparaginase (Elspar)	May be related to inhibition of insulin synthesis (diabetic ketoacidosis has been reported).	++
beta-adrenergic antagonists	Inhibit insulin secretion. May take weeks for reversal after discontinuation. Cardioselective beta blockers are less likely to produce this effect.	++
caffeine	Stimulation of gluconeogenesis (noted only with high doses).	+
calcium channel antagonists	Inhibit insulin secretion.	+
clonidine	May be related to release of growth hormone. The effect is transient, and is usually associated with a high dose of clonidine.	+
diazoxide (Hyperstat IV)	Inhibits insulin secretion. Decreases utilization of glucose.	+++
diuretics	May be related to hypokalemia leading to a decrease in insulin secretion. Thiazides show a greater increasing effect than loop diuretics, which show	+++

Drug	Mechanism of Action	Clinical Significance
	a greater effect than potassium-sparing diuretics.	
epinephrine-like agents (sympathomimetics, decongestants, anorexiants)	Increase glycogenolysis and gluconeogenesis.	++
glucagon	Increases glycogenolysis.	+++
glucocorticosteroids	Increase gluconeogenesis; depress insulin action.	+++
glycerol	Unknown, probably related to volume depletion (hyperglycemic hyperosmolar nonketotic coma has been reported).	++
Immunosuppressives (cyclosporin/tacrolimus [Prograf])	May induce insulin resistance.	++
interferon (alpha and beta)	Unknown (interferon-beta may worsen DKA).	+
lithium salts (Eskalith, Lithane, Lithobid)	May decrease insulin secretion.	+
niacin	Unknown.	++
nicotine	Vasoconstriction leading to a decreased absorption of injected insulin.	++
oral contraceptives	Unknown. High-dose combination products can cause impaired glucose tolerance due to decreased insulin receptor binding, which is very minimal with newer low-dose combination products.	++
pentamidine (Pentam 300, NebuPent)	Promotes pancreatic toxicity (toxic to beta cells).	+++
phenytoin (Dilantin)	Inhibits insulin secretion.	++

Drug	Mechanism of Action	Clinical Significance
rifampin (Rifadin, Rimactane)	Enhances metabolism of tolbutamide (Orinase).	+
ritonavir (Norvir)	Unknown, possibly due to pancreatic toxicity.	+
sugar-containing syrups	Increased sugar load.	++
thyroid hormones	Thyroid replacement in previously hypothyroid patients increases the metabolic clearance of insulin and oral hypoglycemic agents.	++

Drugs That May Cause Hypoglycemia

Drug	Mechanism of Action	Clinical Significance
alcohol (ethanol)	Impairs gluconeogenesis and increases insulin secretion.	+++
anabolic steroids	Decrease glucose tolerance.	+
angiotensin-converting enzyme inhibitors (ACEIs)	Possibly improve insulin sensitivity, particularly in skeletal muscle.	+
beta-adrenergic antagonists	Inhibit glycogenolysis; attenuate signs and symptoms of hypoglycemia.	++
chloramphenicol (Chloromycetin)	May inhibit metabolism of sulfonylureas.	++
chloroquine (Aralen)	Unknown. (Hypoglycemia leading to death has been reported in overdose situations.)	++
clofibrate (Atromid-S)	Unknown. Concomitant use with a sulfonylurea may cause displacement of sulfonylurea from protein binding sites, decreased insulin resistance, or competition for renal tubular secretion.	+

Drug	Mechanism of Action	Clinical Significance
coumarins/dicumarol (warfarin [Coumadin])	Inhibit hepatic clearance of tolbutamide (Orinase) and chlorpropamide (Diabinese).	++
disopyramide (Norpace)	Unknown. Appears to result from endogenous insulin secretion.	++
growth hormone	Unknown. Noted in cases of growth hormone replacement with somatotropin where fasting insulin levels increased. Three weekly doses were divided into daily doses and the problem resolved.	++
MAO inhibitors	May increase insulin release and decrease sympathetic response to hypoglycemia.	+
pentamidine (Pentam 300, NebuPent)	Causes cytolytic response in pancreas accompanied by release of insulin.	+++
phenylbutazone (Azolid, Butazolidin)	Reduces clearance of sulfonylureas.	++
salicylates	Increases insulin secretion and sensitivity; may alter pharmacokinetic disposition of sulfonylureas.	++
saquinavir (Invirase)	Unknown.	+
serotonin anorexiants (fenfluramine [Pondimin] and dexfenfluramine [Redux])	Increase insulin sensitivity and also enhances the effects of sulfonylureas.	++
sulfonamides	Alter clearance of sulfonylureas.	+
triazole antifungals (fluconazole [Diflucan] and itraconazole [Sporanox])	Enhance the effect of sulfonylureas.	+++

Recipes for Low-Carbohydrate Meals

Recipes by
TIMOTHY J. AUBERT, C.W.C.

Throughout these recipes the abbreviation CHO is used for carbohydrate (CHO stands for carbon, hydrogen, and oxygen, the elements that make up carbohydrates) and PRO for protein. Each recipe shows the number of servings provided and the approximate grams of carbohydrates and ounces of protein in each serving. (If you are adapting these recipes or creating your own and consulting nutrition books, remember that to convert *grams* of protein to *ounces* of a protein food, you divide by 6.)

The recipes are meant to be examples of what can be done within a low-carbohydrate meal plan. They certainly can be modified. If a recipe calls for less carbohydrate than required by your meal plan, add some vegetables, salad, bran crackers, et cetera, to the meal to make up the difference. Refer to Chapter 10 for some typical suggestions.

Using these recipes without understanding how to follow a meal plan is inappropriate. Reread Chapters 9–11 to refresh your memory, if necessary. Look especially at the box entitled "No-No's in a Nutshell," on pages 130–131. It is likely that any vegetable *not* listed in that section is suitably low in fast-acting carbohydrate. Remember that ⅔ cup of cooked low-carbohydrate vegetables is equivalent to 6 grams carbohydrate, as is 1 cup of mixed green salad.

PREPARING POWDERED ARTIFICIAL SWEETENERS

As you know, the paper packets containing granulated, so-called sugar-free sweeteners usually contain about 96 percent glucose, making them inappropriate for diabetics. You can prepare your own granulated sweetener for use in some of the following recipes by crushing or grinding Equal (aspartame) tablets (not packets) or saccharin tablets in one of the following ways:

- between two spoons
- in a pepper mill
- in a small electric coffee grinder

Aspartame (but not saccharin) will lose its taste if added to food before cooking, so it must be used only after cooking. You may prefer to use stevia (page 64), since it is sold as powder or liquid and is not degraded by heat.

SUBSTITUTIONS

A number of these recipes include bran crackers. Some have been written for Bran-a-Crisp crackers (3 grams carbohydrate each) and others for G/G Scandinavian Bran Crispbread (2 grams carbohydrate each). Feel free to substitute one brand for the other (1 Bran-a-Crisp cracker equals 1½ G/G crispbreads).

If a recipe calls for oil, the selection is up to your taste. I sometimes use oil in place of butter if quantities are very small. For example, I cook omelets in peanut oil because I like its taste.

All standard vinegars are acceptable for these recipes except for balsamic vinegar, which is inevitably sweetened.

SAUCES

Here is a selection of sauces that are called for in the later recipes. They can be stored in the refrigerator for up to 3 days without impairment of flavor. They should not be frozen.

Dijon Mustard Butter

12 servings, 2 Tbsp each	*Per serving: 0.7 gm CHO, 0.04 oz PRO*	
	CHO (gm)	PRO (gm)
2 Tbsp minced shallots	3.4	0.6
1¼ cups (2½ sticks) butter, softened	—	2.5

	CHO	PRO
3 Tbsp Dijon mustard	3.0	—
1 tsp lemon juice	0.43	0.03
1 Tbsp Worcestershire sauce	1.0	—
Tabasco sauce to taste	0.5	—

Sauté shallots in 1 teaspoon of the butter. In a food processor, combine shallots with all other ingredients until smooth. Place on parchment paper or on plastic wrap. Roll butter in the paper or wrap until you have a 1-inch-diameter cylinder. Refrigerate until butter is needed. Slice into ¼-inch pieces to use (3 slices = 1 tablespoon).

Lemon Butter

4 servings, 2 Tbsp each	*Per serving: 0.7 gm CHO, 0.05 oz PRO*	
	CHO (gm)	PRO (gm)
½ cup (1 stick) unsalted butter, softened	—	1.0
2 Tbsp lemon juice	2.6	0.2
Salt and white pepper to taste	—	—

In a food processor, combine all ingredients until smooth. Roll butter into a 1-inch-diameter cylinder as directed for Dijon Mustard Butter, above, and refrigerate until needed. Slice into ¼-inch pieces to use (3 slices = 1 tablespoon).

Lemon Pepper Butter

4 servings, 2 Tbsp each	*Per serving: 0.7 gm CHO, 0.05 oz PRO*	
	CHO (gm)	PRO (gm)
½ cup (1 stick) butter, softened	—	1.0
2 Tbsp lemon juice	2.6	0.2
⅛ tsp salt	—	—
⅛ tsp white pepper	—	—
Lemon pepper seasoning, to taste	—	—

In a food processor, combine all ingredients until smooth. Roll butter into a 1-inch-diameter cylinder as directed for Dijon Mustard Butter, above, and refrigerate until needed. Slice into ¼-inch pieces to use (3 slices = 1 tablespoon).

Ginger Scallion Butter

12 servings, 2 Tbsp each	*Per serving: 0.5 gm CHO, 0.07 oz PRO*	
	CHO (gm)	PRO (gm)
1¼ cups (2½ sticks) butter, softened	—	2.5
4 minced scallions	1.85	0.45
¼ tsp minced garlic	0.5	0.08
½ tsp minced fresh ginger	0.65	0.1
1 Tbsp minced parsley	0.6	0.3
1 Tbsp soy sauce	1.2	1.2
1 Tbsp lemon juice	1.3	0.1

In a food processor, combine all ingredients until smooth. Roll butter into a 1-inch-diameter cylinder as directed for Dijon Mustard Butter, above, and refrigerate until needed. Slice into ¼-inch pieces to use (3 slices = 1 tablespoon).

Tarragon Butter

12 servings, 2 Tbsp each	*Per serving: 1.7 gm CHO, 0.11 oz PRO*	
	CHO (gm)	PRO (gm)
¾ cup white wine	7.2	0.6
1 bay leaf	0.3	0.1
7 black peppercorns, crushed	0.7	0.1
3 Tbsp tarragon vinegar	—	—
2 Tbsp minced shallots	4.8	0.7
1 cup heavy cream	6.6	4.9
¾ cup (1½ sticks) butter, softened	—	1.5
½ tsp chopped fresh tarragon	0.8	0.4
Pinch salt and white pepper	—	—

Combine wine, bay leaf, crushed peppercorns, vinegar, and shallots in a nonreactive pan. Bring to a boil and reduce to about 2 tablespoons. Strain, removing bay leaf and crushed peppercorns. Reduce cream by half in a separate pan and add to the wine reduction. Gradually whisk in the butter over low heat. When all the butter is dissolved, add the chopped fresh tarragon and season to taste.

Spicy Mustard Sauce

16 servings, 2 Tbsp each	*Per serving: 2.3 gm CHO, 0.11 oz PRO*	
	CHO (gm)	PRO (gm)
½ cup minced shallots	19.2	2.8
¼ cup cider vinegar	—	—
1 tsp black peppercorns, cracked	1.4	0.2
1 bay leaf	—	—
1 cup dry white wine	9.6	—
1 cup heavy cream	6.6	4.9
1½ cups (3 sticks) unsalted butter, softened	—	3.0
Dijon style mustard, to taste	—	—
Creole mustard (or any other spicy mustard) to taste	—	—

Combine the first 5 ingredients in a small nonreactive saucepan and reduce to ⅓ cup. Add heavy cream and reduce mixture by half. Strain and
return to the stove. Cut softened butter into small pieces and slowly add
to the sauce while whisking. After all the butter is incorporated, add the
mustard to taste.

Court Bouillon

8 servings, 1 cup each	*Per serving: 2.4 gm CHO, 0.05 oz PRO*	
	CHO (gm)	PRO (gm)
2½ quarts water	—	—
½ cup vinegar	—	—
2 Tbsp salt	—	—
½ pound onions, peeled and sliced	19.2	2.4
Pinch dried thyme leaves	—	—
1½ bay leaves	—	—
½ bunch parsley stems	—	—
¼ tsp black peppercorns	0.35	0.05

Combine all ingredients except peppercorns in a large saucepan. Simmer for 50 minutes. Add peppercorns and simmer for an additional 10
minutes. Strain, cool, and store in airtight container in refrigerator.

BREAKFAST

Breakfast is the meal where you may find you miss carbohydrate the most. No more home fries or hash browns, toast, pancakes, French toast, waffles, cereals, and the like. The recipe suggestions that follow can put some zip back into breakfast while keeping carbohydrates way down.

Mushroom Omelet with Bacon

1 serving   *Per serving: 3.1 gm CHO, 2.8 oz PRO*

	CHO (gm)	PRO (gm)
2 slices bacon	—	4.0
1 fresh mushroom, sliced	1.5	0.35
Butter to taste	—	—
2 eggs	1.2	12.0
1 Tbsp cream	0.4	0.3
Salt and pepper to taste	—	—

Pan-fry bacon and remove to paper towel to drain. Sauté sliced mushroom in butter for 2–3 minutes. In a small bowl, mix eggs with cream, then add to mushrooms. Cook eggs without stirring for 2 minutes, or until desired firmness. Season with salt and pepper to taste. Roll or fold omelet and turn out on a plate. Serve with the bacon.

Scrambled Eggs with Onions, Peppers, and Stripples

1 serving   *Per serving: 5.3 gm CHO, 2.4 oz PRO*

	CHO (gm)	PRO (gm)
2 slices Stripples	2.0	2.0
2 eggs	1.2	12.0
1 Tbsp cream	0.4	0.3
Butter to taste	—	—
1 Tbsp minced onion	0.9	0.3
1 Tbsp minced green pepper	0.8	—
Salt and pepper to taste	—	—

Microwave Stripples and set aside. Combine eggs and cream thoroughly in a small bowl. Heat butter in sauté pan, add eggs, and cook for 1 minute. Add minced onion and pepper. Season with salt and pepper to taste and cook to desired consistency.

Ham and Cheese Omelet

1 serving   *Per serving: 3.6 gm CHO, 6 oz PRO*

	CHO (gm)	PRO (gm)
2 eggs	1.2	12.0
1 Tbsp cream	0.4	0.3
Butter to taste	—	—
1 slice (2 oz) ham, diced or julienned	—	12.0
2 oz cheese, grated or sliced thin	2.0	12.0
Salt and pepper to taste	—	—

Mix together eggs and cream in a small bowl. Heat butter in sauté pan and cook egg mixture 1–2 minutes without stirring. Place ham and cheese on top and season to taste with salt and pepper. Either roll or fold the eggs and cook to desired consistency.

Sausage and Egg or Ham and Egg Open Sandwich

This recipe was developed by Amy Z. Kornfeld and Hank Kornfeld

1 serving   *Per serving: 6 gm CHO, 4.7 oz PRO*

	CHO (gm)	PRO (gm)
2 sausage patties, 1 oz each, or 2 slices ham, turkey, or salami	—	12.0
1 Tbsp butter or 1 tsp vegetable oil	—	—
2 eggs	1.2	12.0
2 G/G crispbreads	4.0	—
2 slices cheese (about ¾ ounce total)	0.8	4.0

Brown sausage, ham, turkey, or salami and drain off fat. Keep warm in 250°F oven. Heat butter or oil in a nonstick skillet until water drops sprinkled on surface skitter across. Break eggs into pan. Fry eggs for 2–3 minutes over medium heat. If desired, flip them over and fry for another minute or so. Put crispbreads on an ovenproof plate and place eggs on top. Cover with sausage, ham, turkey, or salami, and top off with cheese. Warm briefly in oven to melt cheese.

French Bran Toast

This is another recipe from Amy Z. Kornfeld and Hank Kornfeld

1 serving   *Per serving: 7 gm* CHO, *1 oz* PRO

	CHO (gm)	PRO (gm)
2 Bran-a-Crisp crackers	6.0	—
2 tsp water	—	—
1 egg or egg substitute	0.6	6.0
¼ tsp cinnamon	—	—
⅛ tsp nutmeg	—	—
⅛ tsp vanilla extract	—	—
Artificial maple or fruit-flavored baking extract, to taste	—	—
1 Tbsp cream	0.4	0.3
1 tsp vegetable oil	—	—
Melted butter to taste	—	—
1 or more ground or crushed Equal tablets, or a pinch of stevia powder	—	—

Soak crackers in 2 teaspoons water for 5 minutes, or just long enough to soften. Meanwhile, in a broad shallow bowl beat egg or egg substitute with cinnamon, nutmeg, vanilla, and other flavor extract. Add 1 Tbsp cream and beat gently. Place softened wafers in egg mixture for 1–2 minutes. Heat nonstick skillet until water droplets sprinkled on surface skitter across. Add oil to skillet and spread it around with a folded paper towel. Place egg-soaked wafers in pan and cook over medium heat for about 3 minutes per side. When done remove from pan and pour on melted butter, or sprinkle to taste with the ground Equal tablets or stevia powder.

Pancakes

Amy Z. Kornfeld and Hank Kornfeld also suggested this substitute
for traditional pancakes

1 serving   *Per serving: 5 gm* CHO, *1.1 oz* PRO

	CHO (gm)	PRO (gm)
2 G/G crispbreads	4.0	—
1 egg, beaten	0.6	6.0
⅛ tsp nutmeg	—	—
¼ tsp cinnamon	—	—
⅛ tsp vanilla extract	—	—
Artificial vanilla, orange, or almond baking extract, to taste	—	—
1 Tbsp cream	0.4	0.3
1 tsp vegetable oil	—	—
Melted butter to taste	—	—
1 or more Equal tablets, ground, or pinch stevia powder	—	—

Grind crispbreads in blender, food processor, or electric coffee grinder
to a flourlike consistency. Combine egg, nutmeg, cinnamon, vanilla,
baking extract, and cream in bowl. Add ground crispbreads and mix.
Heat nonstick skillet. When hot, add oil to skillet and spread it around
with a paper towel. Add ¼ of batter to skillet. Cook for 2 minutes. Turn
carefully and cook other side for another 2 minutes, to produce first
pancake. Repeat 3 times to produce 3 more pancakes. Cover with melted
butter. Sprinkle pancakes with ground Equal or stevia powder.

SOUPS

Cucumber Soup

4 servings, about ¾ cup each   *Per serving: 3.9 gm* CHO, *0.16 oz* PRO

	CHO (gm)	PRO (gm)
1 whole cucumber, peeled and sliced	8.3	2.1
½ cup chopped fennel	6.3	1.1
1 Tbsp Erivan whole-milk yogurt	0.75	0.75
½ cup cold water	—	—

| ½ tsp fresh dill | — | — |
| Lemon pepper seasoning to taste | — | — |

In a blender combine sliced cucumber, fennel, yogurt, water, and dill. Purée until smooth, season with lemon pepper seasoning, and serve.

Leek Soup

2 servings, about 1½ cups each	*Per serving: 9.8 gm CHO, 0.25 oz PRO*	
	CHO (gm)	PRO (gm)
1 medium leek, cleaned and chopped into ½-inch pieces	17.6	1.9
1 Tbsp butter	—	0.1
2 cups water	—	—
1 cube Knorr's chicken bouillon	2.0	0.8
Salt and pepper to taste	—	—

In a 2-quart pan sauté leek with butter until wilted. Add water and bouillon cube. Bring to a boil. Reduce heat and simmer for 6 minutes. Season with salt and pepper and serve.

Zucchini Soup

3 servings, about 1½ cups each	*Per serving: 3.2 gm CHO, 0.35 oz PRO*	
	CHO (gm)	PRO (gm)
4 medium zucchini, cleaned and sliced	4.0	3.5
1½ Tbsp chopped onion	1.35	0.15
1 Tbsp butter	—	0.1
3 Tbsp hot water	—	—
1 cube Knorr's chicken bouillon, crushed	2.0	0.8
Salt, pepper, garlic powder to taste	—	—
⅓ cup heavy cream	2.2	1.63

In a 2-quart pan, sauté zucchini and onion in butter until tender. Transfer vegetables to a blender and purée. Add hot water with crushed bouillon cube; blend for 1–2 minutes. Season with salt, pepper, and garlic powder to taste. Serve hot or cold. Add cream to individual portions, about 2 tablespoons per serving.

SALAD

Asparagus and Artichoke Salad

	CHO (gm)	PRO (gm)
2 servings *Per serving: 4 gm CHO, 0.3 oz PRO*		
4 spears asparagus	2.6	1.3
Lightly salted boiling water	—	—
½ cup canned artichoke hearts, drained	4.0	2.0
2 Tbsp oil	—	—
1 Tbsp cider vinegar	—	—
1 tsp prepared mustard	—	—
½ clove garlic, minced	0.5	0.1
1 tsp minced onion	0.9	0.3
Basil, thyme, oregano, salt, and pepper to taste	—	—

Cook asparagus in a small amount of lightly salted boiling water for about 4 minutes, or until tender. Drain and refresh in ice water or cold water. Once cool, cut into inch-long pieces and place in a bowl. Cut drained artichoke hearts in half. Add to asparagus. Combine oil, vinegar, mustard, garlic, and onion and mix well. Add basil, thyme, oregano, and salt and pepper to taste. Pour this dressing over asparagus and artichokes, toss gently but thoroughly, and serve.

POULTRY

Turkey Melt

	CHO (gm)	PRO (gm)
2 servings *Per serving: 3.5 gm CHO, 1.8 oz PRO*		
2 G/G crispbreads	4.0	2.0
2 slices turkey, 1 oz each	—	12.0
2 cooked Stripples	2.0	2.0
2 slices cheese, ½ oz each	1.0	6.0

Place G/G crispbreads in a small broiler pan and lay turkey and cooked Stripples on top. Cover with cheese. Place in a 325°F oven or toaster oven until cheese is thoroughly melted. Serve hot.

Grilled Chicken with Tarragon Butter

1 serving *Per serving: 3.8 gm CHO, 6.2 oz PRO*

	CHO (gm)	PRO (gm)
1 Tbsp oil	—	—
1 Tbsp lemon juice	1.3	0.1
1 tsp chopped fresh tarragon	1.6	0.8
Salt and pepper to taste	—	—
½ chicken breast (6 oz)	—	36.0
1 Tbsp Tarragon Butter (page 335)	0.9	0.34

Combine oil, lemon juice, chopped tarragon, salt, and pepper. Pour mixture over chicken breast and let marinate for at least 15 minutes. Grill chicken to desired doneness. Top with pats of Tarragon Butter.

Chicken Shish Kebab with Vegetables

1 serving *Per serving: 12 gm CHO, 4.3 oz PRO*

	CHO (gm)	PRO (gm)
4 oz chicken, cut into 1-inch cubes	—	24.0
1 oz yellow onion, cut into 1-inch squares	2.4	0.3
1 oz red bell pepper, cut into 1-inch squares	4.8	0.7
1 oz green bell pepper, cut into 1-inch squares	4.8	0.7
Salt and pepper to taste	—	—

Thread chicken, onion, and pepper pieces alternately on skewer. Season with salt and pepper and grill until chicken is fully cooked.

Chicken Dijon

1 serving *Per serving: 0.35 gm CHO, 4 oz PRO*

	CHO (gm)	PRO (gm)
4 oz chicken breast	—	24.0
Salt and pepper to taste	—	—
1 Tbsp Dijon Mustard Butter (page 333)	0.35	0.13

Season chicken breast with salt and pepper. Grill, bake, or broil to desired doneness. Place chicken on plate, put pats of Dijon Mustard Butter on top, let melt, and serve hot.

Lemon Chicken

1 serving	Per serving: 0.35 gm CHO, 4 oz PRO	CHO (gm)	PRO (gm)
4 oz chicken breast		—	24.0
Salt and pepper to taste		—	—
1 Tbsp Lemon Butter (page 334)		0.35	0.025

Season chicken breast with salt and pepper. Grill, bake, or broil to desired doneness. Place chicken on a plate, put pats of Lemon Butter on
top and let melt. Serve hot.

Broiled Chicken Salad

1 serving	Per serving: 1.9 gm CHO, 4 oz PRO	CHO (gm)	PRO (gm)
4 oz chicken breast		—	24.0
2 Tbsp salad oil		—	—
1 Tbsp vinegar		—	—
1 Tbsp chopped onion		0.9	0.3
1 clove garlic, minced		1.0	0.2
Basil, parsley, chives, and salt and pepper to taste		—	—

Grill or broil chicken. Cool and cut into ¼-inch strips. Combine oil,
vinegar, onion, garlic, basil, parsley, chives, and salt and pepper to taste.
Serve cold over chicken strips.

Additional vegetables (up to ⅔ cup) or salad greens (up to 1 cup)
may be chopped and added to taste. Be sure they are not on the No-No's
list on pages 130–131, and make sure you add their CHO content to your
computation.

Grilled Marinated Duck Breast

4 servings	Per serving: 0.85 gm CHO, 4.1 oz PRO	CHO (gm)	PRO (gm)
4 duck breasts, 4 oz each		—	96.0
2 Tbsp soy sauce		1.6	1.5
3 Tbsp water		—	—

	CHO	PRO
¼ Tbsp chopped fresh ginger	0.8	0.15
1 clove garlic, chopped	1.0	0.2
Salt and pepper to taste	—	—

Trim duck breasts of visible fat, if necessary, and place in a large bowl. Combine all the remaining ingredients in a small bowl and pour over duck. Turn duck breast over to evenly coat. Let duck marinate for several hours or overnight, turning occasionally. Remove duck from marinade and grill or sauté, skin side down, until golden brown. Turn breasts over and cook 1–2 minutes more. Remove duck from grill or sauté pan. Duck should be medium rare to medium. Slice on the diagonal to serve hot with vegetables or salad.

BEEF, LAMB, AND VEAL

Note that serving size for most recipes in this section is 4 ounces protein. This does not imply any preference for this particular amount. In fact, many people will want more protein. If this is the case for you, simply eat a larger serving or increase recipe ingredients proportionately.

Grilled Cheeseburger with Canadian Bacon

1 serving   Per serving: 2 gm CHO, 4 oz PRO

	CHO (gm)	PRO (gm)
2½ oz hamburger patty	—	15.0
Salt and pepper to taste	—	—
1 slice cooked Canadian bacon (1 oz)	0.5	6.0
1 slice cheese (½ oz)	0.5	3.0
1 slice pickle	1.0	—

Season hamburger to taste and grill or fry until almost cooked to desired doneness. Place Canadian bacon and cheese on top and let the cheese melt. Serve with slice of pickle.

Grilled Steak with Mushroom Sauce

4 servings   *Per serving: 2.3 gm* CHO*, 4 oz* PRO

	CHO (gm)	PRO (gm)
4 small steaks, 4 oz each	—	96.0
Salt and pepper to taste	—	—
Oil	—	—
4 oz mushrooms, caps sliced, stems chopped	1.6	0.7
3 Tbsp butter	—	0.4
1 oz minced shallots	4.8	0.7
1 sprig thyme	0.45	0.05
½ bay leaf, crumbled	0.1	0.05
¼ cup dry red wine	2.4	—
¼ cup water	—	—

Preheat grill. Season steaks with salt and pepper, coat lightly with oil, and set aside.

On medium to high heat, in a small saucepan, sauté sliced mushroom caps in butter until soft. Remove mushrooms and keep warm. In the same saucepan, sauté shallots until shallots become translucent. Add the chopped mushroom stems and cook until moisture is released. Add thyme, bay leaf, red wine, water, and salt and pepper to taste. Simmer to reduce sauce by ¼.

While sauce is simmering, grill steaks to desired doneness. Strain sauce, add the precooked mushroom caps, heat, and serve over steaks.

Broiled Steak with Red Wine Sauce

4 servings   *Per serving: 1.8 gm* CHO*, 4 oz* PRO

	CHO (gm)	PRO (gm)
4 small steaks, 4 oz each	—	96.0
Salt and pepper to taste	—	—
¾ cup dry red wine	6.0	—
1 clove garlic, minced	1.0	—
1 tablespoon butter	—	0.1

Preheat broiler. Season steaks with salt and pepper. Broil until done. Remove steaks from broiler pan and keep warm.

Drain fat from pan. On top of stove, add wine to the pan juices and bring to boil, scraping bottom of pan. Add garlic and seasoning to taste. Simmer sauce to reduce by ¼, and swirl in butter just before serving. Spoon some of the sauce over each steak.

Marinated Flank Steak

5 servings	Per serving: 0.4 gm CHO, 8 oz PRO	
	CHO (gm)	PRO (gm)
2½ lb flank steak	—	240.0
2 cloves garlic, minced	2.0	0.4
½ cup olive oil	—	—
¼ cup red wine vinegar	—	—
¾ cup white wine vinegar	—	—
Salt and pepper to taste	—	—

Place flank steak in a shallow glass baking dish. Combine remaining ingredients in a small bowl and mix well. Pour over steak and cover dish with plastic wrap. Marinate meat 12–24 hours, refrigerated, turning occasionally.

Remove steak from refrigerator about 1 hour before you are ready to cook it. When grill is hot, remove steak from marinade and grill approximately 8 minutes per side for medium rare. To serve, carve in thin slices, cutting diagonally across the grain.

Filet Mignon with Green and
Black Peppercorn Sauce

2 servings	Per serving: 2.2 gm CHO, 4 oz PRO	
	CHO (gm)	PRO (gm)
8 oz filet mignon	—	48.0
1 Tbsp oil	—	—
Salt and pepper to taste	—	—
¼ cup dry red wine	2.4	—
6 whole green peppercorns	1.0	—
6 whole black peppercorns	1.0	—
1 tablespoon butter	—	0.1

Preheat oven to 350°F. Lightly coat filet with oil and season with salt and pepper. Set aside.

Heat an oven pan on top of the stove. When very hot, place filet in it and sear on all sides. Place pan with filet in oven, and bake (8 minutes for rare, 10–12 minutes for medium, or 15–18 minutes for well done). Remove pan from oven, place filet on a plate, and keep it warm.

Deglaze pan with wine on stovetop, scraping all drippings from bottom of pan. Add peppercorns. Simmer until liquid is reduced by ¼ of original amount, then swirl in butter. Divide filet mignon into two equal portions, pour sauce over, and serve.

Broiled Steak Salad

1 serving *Per serving: 2.1 gm CHO, 4 oz PRO*

	CHO (gm)	PRO (gm)
4 oz lean steak	—	24.0
2 Tbsp oil	—	—
1 Tbsp vinegar	—	—
1 Tbsp chopped onion	0.9	0.3
1 clove garlic, minced	1.0	0.2
Basil, parsley, and salt and pepper to taste	—	—

Grill or broil steak to desired doneness. Cool and cut into ¼-inch strips. Combine remaining ingredients thoroughly in a bowl, then add steak and mix. Correct the seasoning.

Additional vegetables (up to ⅔ cup) or salad greens (up to 1 cup) may be chopped and added to taste. Be sure they are not on the No-No's list on pages 130–131, and make sure you add their CHO content to your computations.

Lamb Shish Kebab

4 servings *Per serving: 8 gm CHO, 4.2 oz PRO*

	CHO (gm)	PRO (gm)
1 lb lamb, cut into 1-inch cubes	—	96.0
Salt and pepper to taste	—	—
4 oz yellow onion, cut into 1-inch squares	9.6	1.2
4 oz green bell pepper, cut into 1-inch squares	19.2	2.8

	CHO	PRO
8 whole mushrooms	3.2	1.4
Oil, to coat	—	—

Preheat broiler or grill. Season lamb cubes with salt and pepper. On skewers alternate pieces of lamb, onion, green pepper, and whole mushrooms. Lightly brush with oil and broil or grill to desired doneness.

Veal Scallopini

1 serving   *Per serving: 7 gm* CHO, *6.8 oz* PRO

	CHO (gm)	PRO (gm)
6 oz veal cutlets for scallopini	—	36.0
Salt and pepper to taste	—	—
2 Tbsp full-fat soy flour, to lightly coat veal	3.8	3.6
2 Tbsp butter	—	0.3
1 tsp minced shallots	0.85	0.15
3 Tbsp white wine	1.8	—
3 Tbsp water	—	—
1 Tbsp chopped parsley	0.6	0.03

Season veal with salt and pepper and lightly coat with soy flour. Heat sauté pan and add 1 tablespoon butter. Sauté veal until golden brown on both sides. Remove from pan and keep warm. Add shallots to pan drippings and sauté briefly. Remove pan from heat and add white wine. Scrape bottom of pan to get all the drippings, add water, and simmer to reduce sauce slightly. Add the parsley and 1 tablespoon butter to finish the sauce. Season to taste. Place finished veal on a platter, pour sauce over veal, and serve.

PORK

Pork Chops with Horseradish Sauce

2 servings   *Per serving: 3 gm* CHO, *3.7 oz* PRO

	CHO (gm)	PRO (gm)
4 Tbsp grated fresh horseradish	1.6	1.8
¼ cup cider vinegar	—	—

¼ cup water	—	—
½ cup sour cream	4.0	3.2
1 egg yolk	0.3	2.8
½–1 Equal tablet, crushed, or stevia to taste (optional)	—	—
Salt and pepper to taste	—	—
2 small pork chops, each about 4 oz with bone	—	36.0

Soak horseradish in vinegar and water to cover for 15 minutes or more. In the top of a double boiler, combine sour cream, egg yolk, crushed Equal tablet or stevia, and salt and pepper to taste. Stir over, not in, hot water until thick and smooth. Drain horseradish in a strainer, pressing to remove excess liquid, and add to the sauce. Adjust seasoning, cover sauce, and keep warm.

Season pork chops with salt and pepper. Grill, bake, or broil to desired doneness and serve with warm horseradish sauce.

Stir-Fried Pork with Sweet and Sour Cabbage

1 serving   *Per serving: 5.8 gm CHO, 4.3 oz PRO*

	CHO (gm)	PRO (gm)
½ cup shredded red cabbage	2.1	0.5
½ cup shredded white cabbage	1.9	0.5
½ cup bean sprouts	0.6	0.7
Pinch cumin seeds	—	—
1 Tbsp cider vinegar	—	—
½–1 Equal tablet, crushed, or stevia to taste	—	—
Salt and pepper to taste	—	—
1 Tbsp oil	—	—
4 oz pork tenderloin, cut into strips ¼ inch thick	—	24.0
2 Tbsp dry white wine	1.2	—

In a large sauté pan or medium pot, combine red cabbage, white cabbage, and 2 tablespoons water. Cook over medium heat until the cabbage wilts. Add bean sprouts, cumin seeds, vinegar, and crushed Equal tablet or stevia to taste. Season with salt and pepper. Cook over low heat for 3–5 minutes, or until vegetables are tender. Cover and keep warm. In a medium sauté pan or wok, heat 1 tablespoon oil. Season pork strips with salt and pepper. Add to hot oil, and stir constantly to prevent scorching. When the pork is almost cooked through (this will take just 2–3 minutes), add white wine and cook another minute or so to let the alcohol boil away. Serve with the cabbage.

SEAFOOD

Grilled Salmon with Lemon Pepper Butter

1 serving   *Per serving: 1.3 gm CHO, 8 oz PRO*

	CHO (gm)	PRO (gm)
8 oz salmon steak	—	48.0
Oil, to coat	—	—
Salt and pepper to taste	—	—
½ Tbsp lemon juice	0.65	0.05
2 Tbsp Lemon Pepper Butter (page 334)	0.65	0.3

Preheat grill or broiler. Coat salmon with oil and season with salt and pepper. Place salmon on heated grill or broiler pan and grill about 4 minutes per side. When the salmon is ready to be turned over, be careful not to break the meat apart. After the salmon is turned, pour ½ tablespoon of lemon juice over it and finish cooking. Remove fish from grill and place on a heated plate. Cover with Lemon Pepper Butter and serve.

Pan-Fried Swordfish with Ginger Scallion Butter

1 serving   *Per serving: 7.3 gm CHO, 4.5 oz PRO*

	CHO (gm)	PRO (gm)
¼ cup soy sauce	2.4	2.4
2 Tbsp dry white wine	1.2	0.1
¼ tsp minced garlic	0.5	0.08
1 tsp minced fresh ginger	1.3	0.2
2 scallions, minced	0.93	0.23
½ Tbsp lemon juice	0.65	0.05
4 oz swordfish steak	—	24.0

	CHO	PRO
Salt and pepper to taste	—	—
2 Tbsp butter	—	0.3
1 Tbsp Ginger Scallion Butter (page 335)	0.25	0.2

Combine first 6 ingredients (soy sauce through lemon juice) in a shallow glass bowl and place swordfish steak in it, turning to coat both sides. Allow the fish to marinate for 30 minutes. Remove swordfish and blot dry. Season with salt and pepper. Heat butter in a sauté pan over medium-high heat. When butter starts to foam, add fish and cook to desired doneness. Remove fish from pan and place on a heated plate. Serve with pats of Ginger Scallion Butter on top.

Trout Amandine

1 serving	*Per serving: 3.4 gm CHO, 5.2 oz PRO*	
	CHO (gm)	PRO (gm)
5 oz trout fillet	—	30.0
Salt and pepper to taste	—	—
2 Tbsp butter	—	0.3
2 Tbsp slivered almonds	1.72	1.68
1 Tbsp lemon juice	1.3	0.1
2 tsp chopped parsley	0.4	0.2

Season trout on both sides with salt and pepper. Sauté the trout in 1 tablespoon butter until almost cooked. Remove to a warm plate and keep warm (fish will continue cooking). Pour excess butter from sauté pan. Add remaining tablespoon butter and let brown slightly. Add the almonds and brown them. Just before serving, stir in lemon juice and parsley, and pour sauce over trout.

Bluefish with Spicy Mustard Sauce

1 serving	*Per serving: 2.3 gm CHO, 4.1 oz PRO*	
	CHO (gm)	PRO (gm)
2 Tbsp Spicy Mustard Sauce (page 336)	2.3	0.68
4 oz bluefish steak	—	24.0
Oil to coat bluefish	—	—
Salt and pepper to taste	—	—

Preheat grill or broiler. Make Spicy Mustard Sauce and keep warm. Lightly coat bluefish with oil and season with salt and pepper. Cook to desired doneness and serve napped with mustard sauce.

Tuna Melt

1 serving	Per serving: 6 gm CHO, 8.2 oz PRO	
	CHO (gm)	PRO (gm)
1 can (6 oz) tuna fish	—	36.0
2 Tbsp mayonnaise	—	—
Pepper to taste	—	—
2 G/G crispbreads	4.0	1.0
2 oz cheese slices	2.0	12.0

Drain tuna and mix with mayonnaise and pepper. Mound tuna mix on G/G crispbreads and top with cheese slices. Place in oven or toaster oven at 350°F until cheese is fully melted.

Poached Salmon with Lemon Pepper Butter

2 servings	Per serving: 2.7 gm CHO, 4.1 oz PRO	
	CHO (gm)	PRO (gm)
2 cups Court Bouillon (page 336)	4.8	0.48
8 oz salmon fillet, skin on	—	48.0
2 Tbsp Lemon Pepper Butter (page 334)	0.65	0.35

Make Court Bouillon and Lemon Pepper Butter and keep warm. In a covered sauté pan large enough to hold the fish in one layer, heat Court Bouillon to about 165°F. Place salmon in it, cover, and simmer gently for 10–12 minutes, or until fully cooked. Remove fish from poaching liquid and drain. Divide fish, place on 2 warm plates, and cover with Lemon Pepper Butter.

Salmon Salad

	3 servings	Per serving: 1.8 gm CHO, 4.4 oz PRO	
		CHO (gm)	PRO (gm)
1 can (13 oz) salmon		—	78.0
1 rib celery, chopped		1.5	0.3
¼ cup chopped onion		1.8	0.25
1 tsp chopped parsley		—	—
¼ spear pickle, chopped		1.0	—
Lemon pepper seasoning, to taste		—	—
2–3 Tbsp mayonnaise		—	—
1 Tbsp prepared mustard		—	—
½ tsp minced chives		—	—
Salt and pepper to taste		—	—

Place salmon in a large bowl with next 8 ingredients (celery through chives) and mix well. Season to taste with salt and pepper and chill. Serve cold.

QUICHES AND SOUFFLÉS

Quiche Lorraine

	4 servings	Per serving: 9.7 gm CHO, 3.6 oz PRO	
		CHO (gm)	PRO (gm)
10 G/G crispbreads, crushed		20.0	10.0
5 Tbsp butter, softened		—	0.7
5 slices bacon		0.16	9.8
1½ cups (6 oz) shredded Swiss cheese		6.0	36.0
½ cup chopped scallions		3.7	0.9
1 cup heavy cream		6.6	4.9
4 eggs, separated		2.4	24.0
¼ tsp nutmeg		—	—
¼ tsp salt		—	—
Pepper to taste		—	—

Preheat oven to 350°F. To make crust, combine crushed crispbreads with softened butter. Press mixture into an 8-inch pie pan, making sure that it is of even thickness all over.

Cook bacon until crisp. Let cool, then crumble. In a bowl, combine all other ingredients except the egg whites. Whip whites to soft peaks and then fold into mixture. Stir in the crumbled bacon. Pour into the cracker crust and bake for 30–40 minutes, or until top is light to golden brown.

Cheese Quiche

3 servings   *Per serving: 10.7 gm CHO, 4.3 oz PRO*

	CHO (gm)	PRO (gm)
10 G/G crispbreads, crushed	20.0	10.0
5 Tbsp butter, softened	—	0.7
¼ cup grated Parmesan cheese	1.5	10.0
½ tsp dry mustard	—	—
¼ tsp salt	—	—
¼ tsp pepper	—	—
¾ cup (3 oz) shredded Swiss cheese	3.0	18.0
¾ cup (3 oz) shredded cheddar cheese	3.0	18.0
3 eggs, separated	1.8	18.0
½ cup heavy cream	3.3	2.45

Preheat oven to 350°F. To make crust, combine crushed crispbreads with softened butter. Press mixture into an 8-inch pie pan, making sure that it is of even thickness all over. In a bowl, combine remaining ingredients except egg whites. Whip whites to soft peaks, then fold into the cheese mixture and pour into the pie crust. Bake for 30–40 minutes, or until top is light to golden brown.

Spinach Soufflé

6 servings   *Per serving: 6.9 gm CHO, 2.9 oz PRO*

	CHO (gm)	PRO (gm)
2 Tbsp butter	—	0.3
¼ cup full-fat soy flour	7.5	7.3
10 oz frozen chopped spinach, thawed, squeezed to remove excess moisture	10.0	8.0
¼ cup grated Parmesan cheese	1.5	10.0
1 clove garlic, minced	1.0	0.2
½ tsp salt	—	—
¼ tsp pepper	—	—

1 tsp prepared mustard	—	—
1 cup milk	11.4	8.0
1½ cups (6 oz) cheddar cheese, shredded	6.0	36.0
6 eggs, separated	3.6	36.0
½ tsp cream of tartar	0.6	—

Preheat oven to 350°F. Use a bit of the butter and soy flour to lightly grease and flour an 8-inch soufflé dish. In a large bowl, combine all ingredients, including the spinach, except egg whites. Whip whites to soft peaks and then fold into the other ingredients. Pour the mixture into the greased and floured dish. Bake for 30–40 minutes, or until top is light to golden brown.

Zucchini Soufflé

6 servings	Per serving: 7.1 gm CHO, 1.7 oz PRO	
	CHO (gm)	PRO (gm)
2 Tbsp butter	—	0.5
¼ cup full-fat soy flour	7.5	7.3
¼ cup grated Parmesan cheese	1.5	10.0
1 lb zucchini, sliced	15.2	6.4
1 medium onion, chopped	6.9	0.9
1 garlic clove, minced	1.0	0.2
¼ cup dry white wine	2.4	0.8
2 Tbsp minced parsley	0.4	0.2
1 Tbsp lemon juice	1.3	0.1
2 Tbsp diced pimiento	2.0	—
½ tsp cream of tartar	0.6	—
Nutmeg, pinch, or to taste	—	—
Salt and pepper to taste	—	—
6 eggs, separated	3.6	36.0

Preheat oven to 350°F. Use a bit of the butter and soy flour to lightly grease and flour an 8-inch soufflé dish. Heat remaining butter in a sauté pan and sauté zucchini slices, onion, and garlic until zucchini becomes translucent. Put sautéed mixture into food processor and pulse to mince. Pour into a large bowl and add the rest of the soy flour and all remaining ingredients except the eggs. In a separate bowl, beat egg *yolks* until frothy. Blend into the mixture. In a separate bowl, beat egg *whites* into soft peaks. Carefully fold into the zucchini mixture and pour mixture into prepared soufflé dish. Bake for 30–40 minutes, until top is light to golden brown.

DESSERTS

Chocolate Vanilla Cheesecake

8 servings   *Per serving: 4.9 gm CHO, 1.8 oz PRO*

	CHO (gm)	PRO (gm)
1 tsp butter	—	0.04
2 Tbsp full-fat soy flour	3.8	3.6
6 eggs, separated	3.6	36.0
6 Equal tablets, crushed, or powdered stevia to taste	—	—
1 lb cream cheese	11.2	36.8
1 cup sour cream	8.0	6.4
6 drops vanilla extract	0.6	—
¼ cup cocoa powder	12.0	4.0

Preheat oven to 350°F. Butter an 8- or 9-inch springform pan and dust with soy flour. In a large bowl, beat egg yolks with Equal or stevia until foamy. Add cream cheese, sour cream, and vanilla extract, and beat until fluffy. In a separate bowl, beat egg whites until stiff. Fold into cream cheese mixture. Pour half the mixture into the springform pan. Mix cocoa powder into remaining half, then spoon it over vanilla mixture already in pan. Bake until golden (about 25–30 minutes).

Individual Chocolate Soufflés

4 servings   *Per serving: 2.9 gm CHO, 1.8 oz PRO*

	CHO (gm)	PRO (gm)
4 eggs, separated	2.4	24.0
4 Equal tablets, crushed, or stevia to taste	—	—
8 oz cream cheese, cut into small pieces	5.6	18.4
1 Tbsp sour cream	0.5	0.4
1 Tbsp cocoa powder	3.0	1.0

Beat egg yolks with crushed Equal tablets or stevia until foamy. Add cream cheese, sour cream, and cocoa powder. Beat until very smooth. In a separate bowl, beat the egg whites until they form stiff peaks, then fold into the cream cheese mixture. Pour into individual soufflé cups and bake at 350°F for 15–20 minutes, or until golden brown.

Rhubarb Pie

6 servings   Per serving: 8.8 gm CHO, 0.6 oz PRO

	CHO (gm)	PRO (gm)
10 G/G crispbreads, crushed	20.0	5.0
5 Tbsp butter, softened	—	0.7
2 packets Jell-O unsweetened lemon pudding mix	13.0	—
1 cup sour cream	8.0	6.4
1 egg, separated	0.6	6.0
Equal tablets, crushed, or stevia to taste	—	—
2 cups rhubarb cut into 1-inch pieces	11.2	2.4

Preheat oven to 350°F. To make crust, combine crushed crispbreads with softened butter. Press mixture evenly into an 8-inch pie pan. Combine lemon pudding mix, sour cream, egg yolk, and Equal tablets or stevia. Beat until smooth. In separate bowl, beat egg white until stiff peaks form. Fold the egg white into pudding mixture. Put cut rhubarb into pie shell and cover with lemon pudding mixture. Bake at 350°F for 25–30 minutes, or until golden brown.

Beignet

This recipe was created by my patient Elise Bahar,
a nineteen-year-old fine arts student.

1 serving   Per serving: 2.9 gm CHO, 1.4 oz PRO

	CHO (gm)	PRO (gm)
1 cup vegetable oil	—	—
1 egg	0.6	6.0
1 Tbsp full-fat soy flour	1.9	1.8
1 Tbsp heavy cream	0.4	0.3
Stevia to taste	—	—
Cinnamon to taste	—	—

Heat vegetable oil for about 5 minutes in a 2-quart saucepan while you mix the batter. Beat egg, soy flour, cream, and stevia in a bowl until fully mixed. Drop a small amount of batter into hot oil. If the drop rises to the top, pour rest of batter into hot oil. Wait until edges of beignet are golden, then flip to other side. When edges are golden, remove beignet from oil and place on paper towel to drain. Sprinkle with powdered cinnamon.

Foot Care for Diabetics

lthough it is not directly related to the normalization of blood sugars, I have included this short but important section on foot care because of the constant danger diabetes poses.

The incidence of limb-threatening ulcerations in diabetics is very high, affecting about one in seven patients. Nonhealing "diabetic" ulcerations are the major cause of leg, foot, and toe amputations in this country, after traumatic injuries such as motor vehicle accidents. These ulcerations do not occur spontaneously; they are always preceded by gradual or sudden injury to the skin by some external factor. Preventing such injuries can prevent their sad consequences.

Virtually all diabetics who have experienced ongoing higher-than-normal blood sugars for more than five years suffer some loss of sensitivity to pain, pressure, and temperature in their feet. This is because elevated blood sugars injure and can eventually destroy all sensory nerves in the feet. Furthermore, the nerves that control the shape of the foot are likewise injured, with a resultant deformity that includes "claw" or "hammer" toes, high arch, and prominent bones at the bases of the toes on the underside of the foot. The nerves that stimulate perspiration in the feet are also affected. This results in the classic dry, often cracked skin that we see on diabetic feet. Dry skin is both more easily damaged and slower to heal than is normal moist skin, and cracks permit entry of infectious bacteria.

Elevated blood sugar also causes impairment of circulation in the arteries of the legs, as well as in the arteries and small capillary blood vessels that supply the skin of the feet. In order to heal, injured skin can require fifty times the blood flow of normal skin. If this increase in flow is unavailable, the injury will deteriorate, becoming gangrenous, and facilitate an infection that spreads up the leg. This infection may not respond to antibiotics.

Blood circulation to the normal foot can readily increase one hundredfold, if necessary, in order to conduct the heat of warm objects away from the skin. Impaired circulation may make this impossible, and the resultant burn may not even cause pain.

A deformed foot with bony prominences (knuckles of toes, tips of toes, heels, and bases of toes at soles) may be continually rubbed or pressed by shoes. This foot is frequently unable to perceive the extent of such pressure and may not heal readily if injured. It can be burned at relatively low temperatures.

The following guidelines are therefore essential for all diabetics, to prevent foot injury and the potentially grave consequences that may ensue:

- Never walk barefoot, either indoors or out.
- Purchase shoes or sneakers late in the day, when foot size is the greatest. Shoes must be comfortable at the first wearing and should not require breaking in. Request shoes with deep toe boxes. Pointed-toe shoes should not be worn, even if the tips are blunted (as in many men's styles). Suitable, very comfortable shoes are manufactured by Rockport. A variety of appropriate, dressy styles can be purchased at Eneslo in New York City. A number of currently available brands of athletic shoes and walking shoes are especially accommodating and even have removable insoles so that orthotics (see below) will fit, without making the shoe too tight. If necessary, I prescribe orthopedic or custom oxfords for certain of my patients.
- Inspect the insides of your shoes daily for foreign objects, torn lining, protruding nails, or bumps. Have them repaired if you find any of these.
- Don't wear sandals with thongs.
- Try to change to a different pair of shoes each day of the week.
- Ideally, your feet should be examined daily for possible injury or signs of excessive pressure from shoes — blisters, cracks or other openings in the skin, pink spots, or calluses. Be sure to check be-

tween your toes. Use a mirror or have another person inspect your soles, if necessary. Contact your physician immediately if any of these signs are found.

- If the skin of your feet is dry, lubricate the entire foot. Suitable lubricants include mink oil, olive oil, any vegetable oil, vitamin E oil, and emulsified lanolin. Do not use petroleum jelly (Vaseline), mineral oil, or baby oil, as they are not absorbed by the skin.
- Do not smoke cigarettes. Nicotine causes closure of the valves that permit blood to enter the small vessels that nourish the skin.
- Keep feet away from heat. Therefore no heating pads, hot water bottles, or electric blankets. Do not place feet near sources of warmth such as radiators or fireplaces. Baths and showers should feel cool — not even lukewarm. Temperature should be estimated with your hand or a bath thermometer, not with your feet. Water temperature should be less than 92°F, as even this temperature can cause burns when circulation is impaired. A bath thermometer is suggested.
- Do not soak your feet in water, even if so instructed by a physician. This causes macerated skin, which breaks down more easily and doesn't heal well. When bathing or showering, get in, get washed, and get out. Don't soak. Beware of rain, swimming pools, and any environment that may wet your feet or your shoes.
- Do not put adhesive tape or other adhesive products like corn plasters in contact with your feet. Fragile skin might be peeled off when the tape is removed.
- Do not put any medications in contact with your skin that are not prescribed by your physician. Many over-the-counter medications, such as iodine, salicylic acid, and corn-removal agents, are dangerous.
- If the skin of your feet is dry, your cardiologist should try to avoid medicines called beta blockers for hypertension or heart disease, as these can inhibit perspiration that moistens the feet.
- Do not attempt to file down, remove, or shave calluses or corns. This is dangerous. Do not permit podiatrists, pedicurists, or anyone else to do so. If calluses are present, show them to your physician. Ask him or her to arrange for your shoes to be stretched, prescribe new shoes, or supply you with appropriate orthotic inserts. Your physician may instruct you in the use of a shoe stretcher or "ball and ring" to modify ill-fitting footwear.

- Do not trim your toenails if you cannot see them clearly. Ask a friend or relative, podiatrist, or your physician to do this for you. If the corners of your nails are pointed, you can file them with an emery board or have someone else trim them.
- If you have thickened toenails, ask your physician to have clippings tested for fungus infection. If infection is present, he should prescribe tincture of fungoid. This solution must be applied *twice* daily to the nails to be effective. It must be used for about twelve months to effect a cure.
- Don't wear stockings or socks with tight elastic bands. Don't use garters. Don't wear socks with holes or that have been darned.
- Phone your physician immediately if you experience any injury to your foot. I consider even a minor injury to be an emergency. Procrastination can be disastrous.

GLOSSARY

Adrenaline: See **Epinephrine.**

Aerobic exercise: Activity that is mild enough to permit muscles to function for extended periods without developing an oxygen deficit. Examples include jogging, casual biking, slow swimming, walking, dancing. See also **anaerobic exercise.**

Alpha cells: The cells of the pancreas that produce **glucagon.**

Amino acids: The "building blocks" of proteins. Protein molecules are strings of amino acids bound together in various sequences and patterns. Amino acids can be partially converted to glucose by the liver, very slowly.

Anaerobic exercise: Strenuous activity that causes a temporary oxygen deficit in the muscles being exercised. Such exercise can be performed only briefly before you run out of breath or the muscle fatigues. Anaerobic exercise utilizes eighteen times as much glucose as aerobic exercise for a given amount of work. It tends to build muscle bulk and thereby reduce insulin resistance. Examples include sprinting, uphill biking, pushups, speed-swimming, repetitive lifting of heavy weights. See also **aerobic exercise.**

Atherosclerosis: Injury to the lining of any large artery. This can eventually lead to total blockage of the artery and loss of the tissues or organs to which it supplies blood. Also called arteriosclerosis or macrovascular disease.

Autonomic neuropathy: Damage to autonomic nerves by chronically elevated blood sugars. Autonomic nerves control bodily functions that are not consciously controlled — such as heart rate, digestion, sweating, erections of the penis, blood pressure, bladder tone, and dilation and constriction of the pupils of the eyes.

Basal: In discussions of blood sugar control, refers to the fasting state. Basal insulin refers to long-acting insulins administered in just the right doses to prevent blood sugar rise while fasting. Basal doses of oral hypoglycemic agents are just the right doses of long-acting pills to prevent blood sugar rise while fasting.

Beta blockers: Medications used for the treatment of high blood pressure or angina (heart pain) that tend to relax the muscular walls of arteries and slow the rate and contractility of the heart.

Beta cell burnout: Destruction of pancreatic **beta cells** caused by over-stimulation of insulin production or by toxic effects of high blood sugars.

Beta cells: Cells located in the pancreas that produce and store insulin and release it into the bloodstream.

Blood glucose: Blood sugar.

Blood glucose profile: A record of blood sugars (glucose) measured a number of times daily for a period of several days or weeks. Often accompanied by related data on meals, medications, exercise, infection or illness, and any other matters that may affect blood sugar levels.

Blood glucose self-monitoring: The act of measuring and recording your own blood sugars, usually utilizing a single drop of finger-stick blood and a blood glucose meter.

Carbohydrate: One of the three basic sources (protein, fat, carbohydrate) of calories or energy in foods. Carbohydrate molecules are usually chains of sugars strung together like beads on a necklace. Of the three basic caloric foods, carbohydrate raises blood sugar the most.

cc: Cubic centimeter. A measure of volume; 1/1000 of a liter or quart.

Complex carbohydrate: Made from longer, more complex chains of sugars, some are digested more slowly and raise blood sugar less rapidly than **simple carbohydrate.**

Counterregulatory hormones: Hormones produced by the body, often in times of stress or illness, that bring about an increase in blood sugar. These include **glucagon, epinephrine,** cortisol, and growth hormone.

Coverage: The practice of injecting fast-acting insulin to lower an elevated blood sugar. Coverage may also refer to the use of a fast-acting insulin or oral hypoglycemic agent to cover a meal, thereby preventing a postprandial blood sugar rise.

C-peptide: A byproduct of insulin production by the pancreas, which when measured in the blood indicates how much insulin was recently made. People who make no insulin make no C-peptide.

Creatinine clearance: A kidney function test that estimates the **glomerular filtration rate.** It requires a 24-hour urine collection and a small sample of blood.

Crystalline insulin: See **regular insulin.**

Dawn phenomenon: An apparent reduction in the effectiveness of insulin in lowering or maintaining blood sugar due to rapid clearance of insulin from the bloodstream by the liver. It may begin about an hour before arising in the morning and continue for 2–3 hours after awakening.

Delayed stomach-emptying: See **gastroparesis.**

DKA: Diabetic Ketoacidosis. See **Ketoacidosis.**

Epinephrine: A hormone produced by the adrenal glands in response to stresses such as pain, fright, anger, and hypoglycemia. Elevated blood levels of epinephrine can cause tremors and increases of heart rate and blood sugar. Also called adrenaline.

Fasting blood glucose, fasting blood sugar: Blood sugar value when measured before the first meal of the day, usually at least 12 hours after any prior consumption of food.

Fat: One of the three basic sources (protein, fat, carbohydrate) of calories or energy in foods. High in calories, it can be found in milk, cheese, egg yolk, meat, fish, fowl, nuts, oils, and some vegetables. Consumption of fat does not directly affect blood sugar.

Fibrinogen: A precursor of fibrin, which is the structural element of blood clots. Elevated levels of fibrinogen in the blood can be caused by high blood sugars and are associated with increased risk for heart attacks, strokes, retinopathy, kidney damage, and other complications of diabetes.

Fructose: A sugar occurring especially in fruits, fruit juices, and honey.

Gastroparesis: A neuropathy caused by prolonged blood sugar elevation, which can severely impair the muscular and secretory activities of the stomach. Gastrointestinal discomfort may be present after meals. Blood sugars after meals may be unpredictable because of a random effect upon the rate of stomach-emptying. Also called delayed stomach-emptying and gastroparesis diabeticorum.

Glomerular filtration rate (GFR): The kidneys filter blood by means of about 6 million microscopic glomeruli. The GFR is a measure of how much filtering the kidneys perform in a given time period. See also **glomerulus.**

Glomerulopathy: The condition of damaged glomeruli.

Glomerulus: The microscopic filtering unit of the kidneys that removes water and other substances from blood, thereby creating urine.

Glucagon: A hormone produced by the alpha cells of the pancreas that causes blood sugar to increase.

Glucograf II data sheet: A preprinted form used by diabetics for recording blood sugar measurements, medications, exercise, and meals. Illustrated on page 75.

Gluconeogenesis: The conversion of amino acids (the building blocks of proteins) to glucose by the liver.

Glucophage: See **metformin.**

Glucose: A naturally occurring sugar, which when measured in the blood is called blood sugar. Glucose is the building block of most carbohydrates.

Glucose challenge: An event, such as a high-carbohydrate meal, that can raise blood sugar significantly.

Glucose transporters: Specialized protein molecules that migrate from inside a cell to the surface. They protrude from the surface and bind blood glucose in order to bring it into the cell.

Glycation: The binding of glucose to proteins of blood or body tissues. Glycation, or glycosylation, of proteins can adversely affect their structure and function, leading to many of the complications of diabetes.

Glycogen: A starchy substance formed from glucose that is stored in the liver and muscles. It can be rapidly converted back to glucose by the action of certain counterregulatory hormones.

Glycosylation: See **glycation.**

Glycosylated hemoglobin: By measuring the glycation, or glycosylation, of hemoglobin, the principal protein of red blood cells, we can estimate one's average blood sugar over the prior four months. See also **glycation.**

H: The abbreviation for lispro insulin used in this book. See **Humalog.**

HDL: Abbreviation for high-density lipoprotein. A submicroscopic particle found in the blood that transports **cholesterol** and **triglycerides**

from arterial walls to the liver. Also known as "the good cholesterol." High blood levels of HDL are believed to offer protection from coronary artery disease, peripheral vascular disease, and stroke. See also **LDL.**

Hemoglobin A$_{1C}$ (HgbA$_{1C}$): The most commonly measured indicator of **glycosylated hemoglobin.**

High-density lipoprotein: See **HDL.**

Humalog (H): Brand name for a new, clear, "ultra fast-acting" insulin. Also known generically as lispro.

Hyperglycemia: Abnormally high blood sugar.

Hyperinsulinemia: Elevated blood insulin level.

Hyperlipidemia: A vague term that commonly refers to any of a number of abnormalities of fatty substances in the blood. These may include elevated triglycerides, elevated LDL (the "bad cholesterol"), or low levels of HDL (the "good cholesterol"). Also called dyslipidemia.

Hypertension: High blood pressure.

Hypoglycemia: Abnormally low blood sugar.

Hypoglycemia unawareness: Inability to experience or perceive the physical symptoms of low blood sugar.

Hypotension: Abnormally low blood pressure.

IDDM: Abbreviation for insulin-dependent diabetes mellitus; see **Type II diabetes.**

Impaired glucose tolerance (IGT): A mild or early form of diabetes that can slowly cause many of the long-term complications of "full-blown" diabetes. Frequently precedes the onset of diabetes. A treatable disorder.

Insulin: A hormone produced by the beta cells of the pancreas gland that facilitates the entry of glucose into most cells of the body. Insulin is also the fat-building hormone.

Insulin receptors: Molecules on the surface of most cells of the body that bind circulating insulin. It is the binding of insulin by a cell that facilitates the entry of glucose into the cell.

Insulin resistance: Reduced sensitivity of the body to insulin's effects on blood sugar.

Intramuscular (IM): Used to describe an injection (as of lispro insulin) into muscle in order to speed up its action.

Islets: Also called islets of Langerhans. Clusters of cells in the pancreas that include the beta cells, which make insulin.

Ketoacidosis: An acute, life-threatening condition caused by the combination of very high blood sugars and dehydration. It involves high blood levels of ketones, including acetone, and an acidification of the blood.

L: See **Lente insulin.**

Lactose: A sugar found in milk and cottage cheese that is converted to glucose by the liver.

LDL: Abbreviation for low-density lipoprotein, a particle in the blood that deposits **cholesterol** and **triglycerides** in arterial walls. Elevated LDL is a risk factor for coronary artery disease and peripheral vascular disease. More important as a measure of disease risk than the LDL value itself is the ratio of LDL to HDL. For accurate measurement, a "direct LDL" test must be ordered. See also **HDL.**

Lente insulin (L): An intermediate-acting insulin that lowers or maintains blood sugar for a period of about 10 hours after injection.

Lipid profile: A battery of measurements of fatty substances in the blood. It may include **LDL,** total cholesterol, **triglycerides, HDL.**

Lipoprotein(a): A lipoprotein that increases risk of heart attack by interfering with the body's mechanism for dissolving blood clots. Abbreviated Lp(a).

Lipoproteins: Submicroscopic particles that carry fatty substances such as cholesterol and triglycerides through the bloodstream. Examples of lipoproteins include HDL, LDL, apolipoproteins, and lipoprotein(a).

Lispro: See **Humalog.**

Low-density lipoprotein: See **LDL.**

Lower esophageal sphincter (LES): A muscular band near the lower end of the esophagus, a tube connecting the throat to the stomach. Normal contraction of this band after swallowing prevents regurgitation of stomach contents.

Macrovascular: Relating to large blood vessels.

Maturity-onset diabetes: See **Type II diabetes**.

Metformin: Sold under the brand name Glucophage, this OHA is one of the most effective that we have. Rather than increasing insulin production and "burning out" pancreatic beta cells, it increases the body's sensitivity to its own or injected insulin. See also **Troglitazone.**

mg/dl: Milligrams per deciliter. The unit of blood sugar measurement in the United States. See also **mmol/l.**

Microaneurysms: Ballooning of microscopic blood vessels, caused by destruction of cells that line the outer walls of these vessels. Microaneurysms are often found in the retinas of the eyes of diabetics who have had elevated blood sugars for prolonged periods.

Microangiopathy: Injury to small blood vessels, commonly found in long-standing poorly controlled diabetes. A major cause of blindness and kidney disease in diabetics.

Microvascular: Relating to small blood vessels.

mmol/l: Millimoles per liter. The international unit of blood sugar measurement. See also **mg/dl** (1 mmol/l = 18 mg/dl).

Monounsaturated fats: Fats whose molecules contain fatty acids that are missing one pair of hydrogen atoms. These fats are believed to offer protection from vascular disease because their consumption lowers serum **LDL** and raises **HDL** in some high-risk individuals.

Nephropathy: Damage to kidneys. In this book, the term is limited to damage caused by diabetes.

Neuroglycopenia: A blood sugar so low that inadequate glucose is getting into the brain. As a result, cognition, coordination, and level of consciousness may become severely impaired. A severe form of **hypoglycemia.**

Neuropathy: Damage to nerves. In this book, the term is limited to damage caused by diabetes.

Neurotransmitters: The chemical "messengers" of the central and peripheral nervous systems.

NIDDM: Abbreviation for non-insulin-dependent diabetes mellitus. Not entirely accurately used interchangeably with the term Type II diabetes, or maturity-onset diabetes. See **Type II diabetes.**

Oral hypoglycemic agent (OHA): Pill used to lower blood sugar in Type II diabetes.

Pancreas: A large abdominal organ that manufactures insulin, glucagon, and other hormones, secreting them into the bloodstream. The pancreas also produces digestive enzymes and bicarbonate, which are secreted into the upper gastrointestinal tract, beyond the stomach.

Phase I insulin response: A sudden release of insulin by the pancreas in response to a **glucose challenge,** such as a meal. This may represent the release of stored insulin granules. Usually impaired in early diabetes.

Phase II insulin response: The continued slower release of (probably newly manufactured) insulin from the pancreas that occurs after the phase I insulin response.

Platelets: Small particles in the blood that play a major role in causing blood to clot.

Polyunsaturated fats: Fats made from fatty acids that are missing two or more pairs of hydrogen atoms. Dietary consumption appears to offer reduction of elevated serum **LDL** levels for some individuals.

Postprandial: After a meal.

Postural hypotension: A sudden drop in blood pressure upon standing.

Preprandial: Before a meal.

Progressive exercise: A planned exercise program wherein the work required per session becomes greater and greater over a period of weeks, months, or years.

Protein: One of the three basic sources (protein, fat, carbohydrate) of calories or energy in foods. The principal nutritional component of fish, poultry, lean meat, and egg white, it is also present in other foods in lesser amounts. The major component of most human tissues other than fat and water.

Pyloric valve: A muscular band at the exit of the stomach that relaxes to permit stomach-emptying in normal individuals. In people with diabetic gastroparesis, the pyloric valve may be randomly in spasm and delay stomach-emptying.

R: See **regular insulin.**

Regular insulin, or **regular (R)**: A commonly used clear, rapid-acting insulin. Also called crystalline insulin.

Renal: Relating to the kidney.

Renal risk profile: A series of tests that can reflect damage suffered by the kidney.

Retinopathy: Injury to the retina, or light-sensing surface, in the rear of the eye. Usually caused by chronically high blood sugars in diabetics.

R-R interval study: A quantitative, objective test for **autonomic neuropathy**. The test is similar to an electrocardiogram, but the patient breathes deeply while the test is under way.

Simple carbohydrate: A carbohydrate that can be rapidly converted to glucose by the digestive process. Also called simple sugar.

Stevia: A sugarless, herbal sweetener, sold as liquid or powder in health food stores.

Subcutaneous: Below the skin but above muscle, as in a subcutaneous injection.

Sucrose: Table sugar. The sucrose molecule consists of one glucose molecule bound to one fructose molecule.

Sugars: A group of chemical compounds consisting of six carbon atoms bound to hydrogen and oxygen atoms. Most sugars taste sweet and can be converted to glucose (blood sugar) by the body. Some sugars are formed by the joining together of two other sugars. Sugars are the simplest **carbohydrates**.

Sulfonylureas: A class of oral hypoglycemic agents that are chemically related to sulfa. They lower blood sugar by stimulating pancreatic beta cells to make more insulin, and carry with them a danger of "burning out" those cells.

Thrombotic risk profile: A group of blood tests that can reflect the tendency of blood to clot prematurely, thereby increasing the risk for heart attacks, poor circulation, and certain types of stroke. These tests include fibrinogen and lipoprotein(a).

Total cholesterol: The sum of serum **HDL** plus serum **LDL** plus approximately one-fifth of serum **triglycerides**.

Triglycerides: Substances found in blood and fatty tissues comprising the storage form of fat. Each triglyceride molecule consists of three fatty acid molecules bound to a glycerol molecule. Serum triglyceride is frequently elevated when blood sugar is high. Elevated levels can be a risk factor for vascular disease.

Troglitazone: Sold under the brand name Rezulin. This is another oral hypoglycemic agent that like **metformin** lowers insulin resistance and thereby lowers the likelihood of **beta cell burnout.** It is much less likely than metformin to cause gastrointestinal side effects.

Truncal obesity: A form of obesity, also called central or visceral obesity, in which the circumference of the waist is greater than the circumference of the hips (in males) or greater than 80 percent of the hip circumference in females.

Type I diabetes: A type of diabetes, usually appearing before the age of forty-five, that involves total or near total loss of the capacity to produce insulin. Also called insulin-dependent diabetes mellitus (IDDM), autoimmune diabetes, or juvenile-onset diabetes.

Type II diabetes: The type of diabetes that usually appears after the age of forty-five and is commonly associated with obesity. It usually involves partial loss of insulin-producing capability, diminished non-insulin-mediated glucose transport, and resistance to the glucose transport effects of insulin. Also called non-insulin-dependent diabetes mellitus (NIDDM), insulin-resistant diabetes, or maturity-onset diabetes.

UL: See **ultralente insulin.**

Ultralente insulin (UL): A very long-acting, cloudy insulin.

Unit: A measure of the biological effectiveness of insulin at reducing blood sugar. The lines on the scale of an insulin syringe usually measure increments of 1 unit. The lines on some newer syringes represent increments of ½ unit.

Vagus nerve: The single largest nerve in the body, and the main neural component of the part of the nervous system that regulates the autonomic (involuntary) functions of the body, including heart rate, blood pressure, breathing, and digestion.

Vascular: Relating to the vasculature, or blood vessels.

Visceral obesity: See **truncal obesity.**

INDEX